W0043493

CLINICS IN ANDROLOGY

E.S.E. HAFEZ, *series editor*

VOLUME 3

1. J.C. Emperaire, A. Audebert, E.S.E. Hafez, eds., Homologous artificial insemination. 1980, ISBN 90-247-2269-1.

2. L.I. Lipshultz, J.N. Corriere Jr., E.S.E. Hafez, eds., Surgery of the male reproductive tract. 1980, ISBN 90-247-2315-9.

4. J. Bain, E.S.E. Hafez, eds., Diagnosis in andrology. 1980, ISBN 90-247-2365-5.

5. G.R. Cunningham, W.-B. Schill, E.S.E. Hafez., eds., Regulation of male fertility. 1980, ISBN 90-247-2373-6.

6. E.S.E. Hafez, E. Spring-Mills, eds., Prostatic carcinoma. 1980, ISBN 90-247-2379-5.

series ISBN 90-247-2333-7

DESCENDED AND CRYPTORCHID TESTIS

edited by

E.S.E. HAFEZ

Reproductive Physiology Laboratory Andrology Research Unit
C.S. Mott Center for Human Growth and Development
Wayne State University School of Medicine, Detroit, Michigan, USA

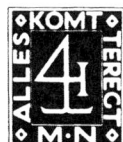

1980

MARTINUS NIJHOFF PUBLISHERS
THE HAGUE/BOSTON/LONDON

Distributors:

for the United States and Canada

Kluwer Boston, Inc.
160 Old Derby Street
Hingham, MA 02043
USA

for all other countries

Kluwer Academic Publishers Group
Distribution Center
P.O. Box 322
3300 AH Dordrecht
The Netherlands

Library of Congress Cataloging in Publication Data   CIP

Main entry under title:

Descended and cryptorchid testis.

  (Clinics in andrology; v. 3)
  Includes index.
  1. Testis. 2. Cryptorchism. I. Hafez, E.S.E. II. Series.
QP255.D47   617'.463   80-10303

ISBN-13: 978-94-009-8842-2   e-ISBN-13: 978-94-009-8840-8
DOI: 10.1007/978-94-009-8840-8

TABLE OF CONTENTS

Contributors   VII

Preface   IX

I. DESCENDED TESTIS

1. Development of normal testis   5
    J.C. CZYBA, C. GIROD

2. Functional histology of descended testis   14
    E.S.E. HAFEZ

3. Germ cells   21
    LUCIA CASTELLANI-CERESA

4. Ultrastructure of spermiogenesis in normal and pathological testis   32
    MARINA CAMATINI

5. Acrosomal formation and malformation   44
    SHIRLEY SIEW, PHILIP TROEN, HOWARD R. NANKIN

6. Peritubular tissue   62
    E. BUSTOS-OBREGÓN

7. The blood-testis barrier   73
    S. FURUYA, Y. KUMAMOTO, M. MORI, S. SUGIYAMA

8. Neuro-endocrine control of spermatogenesis   94
    C. GIROD, J.C. CZYBA

9. Biogenesis of androgens and estrogens by the normal testis   109
    B.K. TSANG, G.A. KINSON

II. CRYPTORCHID TESTIS

10. Normal and abnormal testicular descent in some mammals   125
    C.J.G. WENSING, B. COLENBRANDER, H.M.W. VAN STRAATEN

11. Etiology of testicular descent   138
    F. HADŽISELIMOVIĆ, B. HERZOG

12. Germ cell lines in the normal and cryptorchid testis   148
    FRANCO COTELLI, MARCO ERRAGUTI, MARCELLO GAMBACORTA, CARLA LORA LAMIA DONIN

13. Functional morphology of cryptorchid Leydig and Sertoli cells   158
    F. HADŽISELIMOVIĆ, B. HERZOG

14. Estrogen-induced cryptorchidism in animals   166
     F. Hadžiselimović, B. Herzog, E. Krušlin

III. TESTICULAR PATHOLOGY   177

15. Varicocele: mechanisms of action and deleterious effects on the human testis   179
     A.H. El-Beheiry, E.S.E. Hafez

16. Testicular tumours in cryptorchid testis   185
     S. Omar, S. El-Badawi

     Subject index   188

CONTRIBUTORS

BUSTOS-OBREGÓN, E.: Department of Cellular Biology and Genetics, University of Chile, Casilla 6556, Santiago-7, Chile

CAMATINI, MARINA: Laboratory of Comparative Anatomy, Department of Zoology, State University of Milan, Via Celoria 10, 20133 Milan, Italy

CASTELLANI-CERESA, LUCIA: Laboratory of Cytology, Department of Zoology, State University of Milan, Via Celoria 10, 20133 Milan, Italy.

COLENBRANDER, B.: Department of Anatomy, School of Veterinary Medicine, State University of Utrecht, Bekkerstraat 141, 3572 SG Utrecht, The Netherlands

COTELLI, FRANCO: Laboratorio di Microscopia Elettronica, Istituto di Zoologia, State University of Milan, Via Celoria 10, 20133 Milan, Italy

CZYBA, J.C.: Department of Histology, Embryology and Cytogenetics, Faculté de Médecine Grange-Blanche, 8 avenue Rockefeller, 69008 Lyons, France

EL-BADAWI, S.: Departments of Surgery and Radiotherapy, Cancer Institute, University of Cairo, Egypt (23 Amin El-Rafi Street, Dokky, Giza, Egypt)

EL-BEHEIRY, A.H.: Department of Dermatology, Venereology and Andrology, Alexandria University School of Medicine, Alexandria, Egypt

ERRAGUTI, MARCO: Laboratorio di Microscopia Elettronica, Istituto di Zoologia, State University of Milan, Via Celoria 10, 20133 Milan, Italy

FURUYA, S.: Department of Urology, Sapporo Medical College, Sapporo 060, Japan

GAMBACORTA, MARCELLO: Istituto di Anatomia Patologica, E.O., 'Ca Granda', Niguarda, Milan, Italy

GIROD, C.: Department of Histology-Embryology and Cytogenetics, Faculté de Médecine Alexis-Carrel, rue Guillaume Paradin, 69008 Lyons, France

HADŽISELIMOVIĆ, F.: Pediatric Department, University Children's Hospital, Romergasse 8, 4005 Basel, Switzerland

HAFEZ, E.S.E.: Reproductive Physiology Laboratory, Andrology Research Unit, C.S. Mott Center for Human Growth and Development, Wayne State University School of Medicine, Detroit, Michigan 48201, USA

HERZOG, B.: University Clinic for Pediatric Surgery, University Children's Hospital, Romergasse 8, 4005 Basel, Switzerland

KINSON, G.A.: Department of Physiology, School of Medicine, Faculty of Health Sciences, University of Ottawa, Ottawa, Ontario K1N 9A9, Canada

KRUŠLIN, E., Sandoz AG, Rothausstrasse 61, 4133 Schweizerhalle, Switzerland

KUMAMOTO, Y.: Department of Urology, Sapporo Medical College, Sapporo 060, Japan

LORA LAMIA DONIN, CARLA: Laboratorio di Microscopia Elettronica, Istituto di Zoologia, State University of Milan, Via Celoria 10, 20133 Milan, Italy

MORI, M.: Department of Pathology, Sapporo Medical College, Sapporo 060, Japan

NANKIN, HOWARD R.: Division of Endocrinology and Metabolism, University of South Carolina School of Medicine, Columbia, South Carolina 29201, USA

OMAR, S.: Departments of Surgery and Oncology, Cancer Institute, University of Cairo, Egypt (11 Bollus Hanna Street, Dokky, Cairo, Egypt)

SIEW, SHIRLEY: Department of Pathology, Michigan State University, Fee Hall, East Lansing, Michigan 48824, USA

STRAATEN, H.W.M. VAN: Department of Anatomy, School of Veterinary Medicine, State University of Utrecht, Bekkerstraat 141, 3572 SG Utrecht, The Netherlands

SUGIYAMA, S.: Department of Dermatology, Sapporo Medical College, Sapporo 060, Japan

TROEN, PHILIP: Department of Medicine, School of Medicine, University of Pittsburgh and Montefiore Hospital, 3459 Fifth Avenue, Pittsburgh, Pennsylvania 15213, USA

TSANG, B.K.: Animal and Cell Physiology Group, National Research Council of Canada Division of Biological Sciences, Ottawa, Ontario, Canada

WENSING, C.J.G.: Department of Anatomy, Vakgroep Funktionele Morphologie, State University of Utrecht, Bekkerstraat 141, 3572 SG Utrecht, The Netherlands

PREFACE

During the past decade extensive investigations have been done on the testis. Since the observations have been published in many different journals, it seemed appropriate to bring together and summarize some of the pertinent findings in a single volume.

Twenty-eight scientists and clinicians from nine countries have contributed to this book. They have reviewed the literature and presented their own, new observations on the developmental, anatomical, physiological, biochemical and pathological aspects of the descended and cryptorchid testis. In addition, several contributors have evaluated the usefulness of certain animals as models for systematically studying specific aspects of cryptorchidism. It is hoped that this volume will serve as a useful summary and reference for those working in this area and that it will encourage further research in testicular physiopathology.

The editor thanks the contributors for their enthusiasm, cooperation and meticulous writing of the chapters. The support of the Departments of Gynecology/Obstetrics and the Department of Physiology of Wayne State University School of Medicine, Detroit and the assistance from the staff of Martinus Nijhoff are gratefully acknowledged. The cheerful cooperation of Miss Lori Rust and Miss Penny Stoops who helped to type and assemble the volume is most deeply appreciated.

E.S.E. HAFEZ
Detroit, Michigan
USA

DESCENDED AND CRYPTORCHID TESTIS

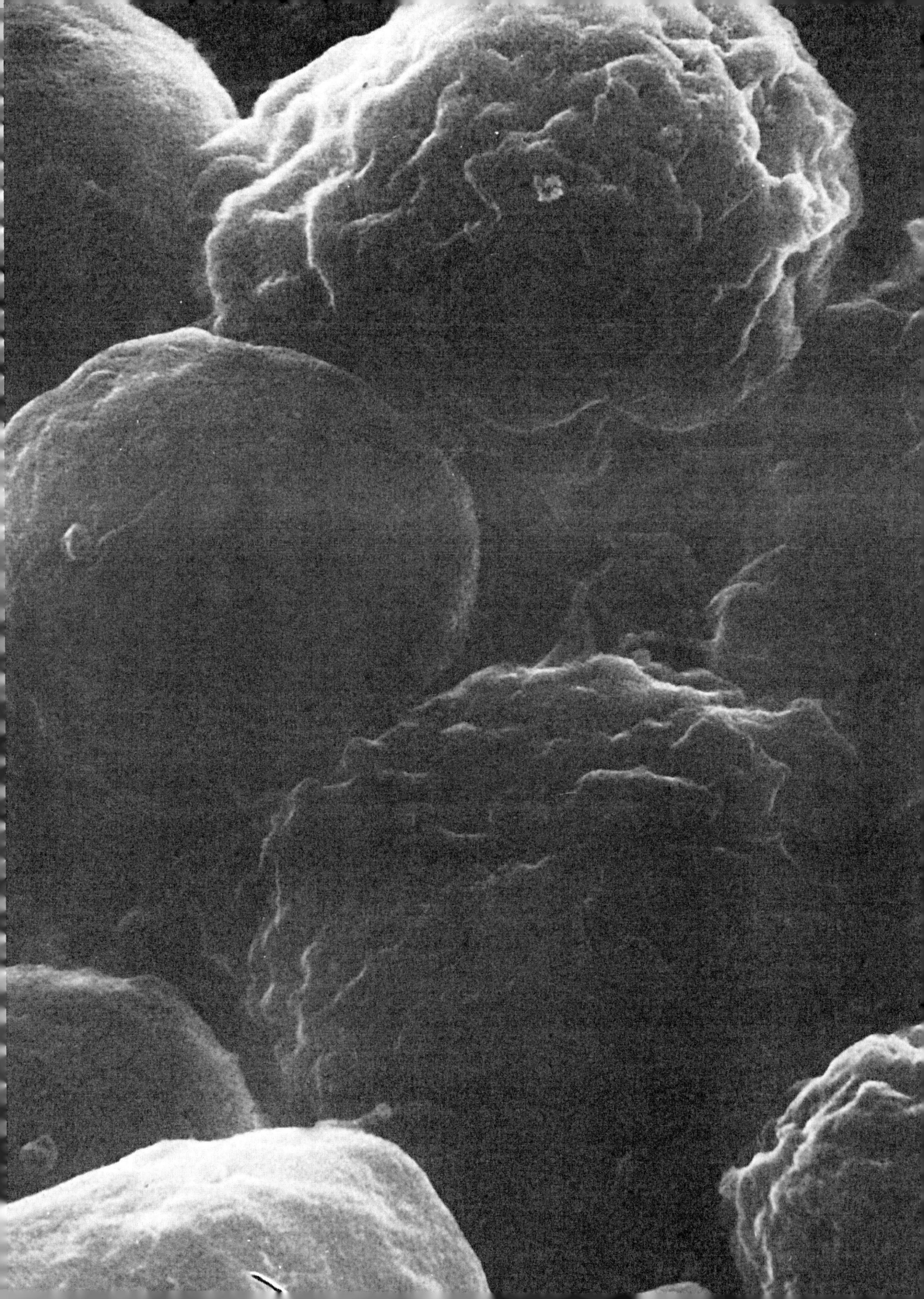

I. DESCENDED TESTIS

1. DEVELOPMENT OF NORMAL TESTIS

J.C. CZYBA and C. GIROD

The embryological development of the male genital apparatus comprises two major stages. The first lasts from the middle of the third week to the end of the sixth week of embryonic life, and is the period of construction of the primordia of the genital apparatus. This is called the *indifferent stage* because the nature of the development is common to both the male and the female sex. At the end of this period, when both the gonads and the systems of canals (Wolffian ducts and Müllerian ducts) which connect them with the urogenital sinus are present, there is still no morphological feature which indicates the eventual destiny of the embryo as male or female; this is only revealed by the chromosome complement which is, of course, determined at fertilization. The second stage begins at the seventh week and consists initially of *testicular differentiation* by the transformation of the undifferentiated gonad in genetically male embryos. This testicular differentiation is controlled by the Y heterochromosome and passes through several phases before its completion at puberty. The testicular hormone secretions are responsible, from a very early stage, for the differentiation of the male reproductive tract from the Wolffian ducts, the urogenital sinus and the primordia of the external genitalia.

1. INDIFFERENT STAGE

The undifferentiated gonad develops between the middle of the third week and the end of the sixth week of embryonic life, and results from the formation and organization of two separate elements:

- *primordial germ cells*, stem cells which will give rise to the germinal line; and
- *the gonadal blastema*, or *common somatic blastema*, a tissue into which the germ cells migrate

and which will later serve as their support and will assist in the microscopic organization of the eventual male or female gonads.

The undifferentiated gonad develops in contact with the *mesonephros* and very quickly establishes connections with some of the mesonephrotic tubules.

1.1. Primordial germ cells

1.1.1. Appearance and detection. Primordial germ cells appear during the third week in the connecting stalk very close to the entoblastic cells of the allantoic diverticulum, or even among these entoblastic cells. Several authors have reported this origin in man, without, however, being able to establish that these cells are directly derived from the entoblast (see Falin 1969). These cells are larger (14-18 μm) than the entoblastic cells, and they can be identified by their easily recognizable alkaline phosphatase activity in the cytoplasm. During their fourth week their abundant ribonucleoprotein and glycogen, which can easily be demonstrated by histochemical reactions, indicates their intense metabolic activity. The germ cells are morphologically identical in either male or female embryos.

1.1.2. Migration into the genital ridge. During the fourth week the longitudinal delimitation of the embryo causes the posterior extermity to roll up, carrying the allantoic diverticulum including the germ cells into the interior of the embryo. Simultaneously with this *passive migration*, caused by the differential growth of the neighbouring tissues, the germ cells undertake an *active migration* by amoeboid movements. At the 25th day some germ cells migrate into the ventral border of the primitive hindgut, at the 27th day they pass around the lateral borders, and, at the 28th day, they reach the root of the dorsal mesentery from whence they move from each side to the median region of the metanephros where they enter into a localized thickening of the coelomic epithelium covering the metanephros which is called the *genital ridge*. The name *germinal epithelium* for the epithelium of the genital ridge was proposed by Waldeyer in 1890, but the term should be abandoned as this epithelium gives rise to no germ cells.

It is not easy to determine the number of germ cells formed in the connecting stalk or the number which reach the genital ridge, especially as these cells multiply during their migration. It is also probable that some cells may be lost en route. Finally, although most of the germ cells migrate by displacement through the dorsal mesentery, it cannot be ruled out that some of them might reach the genital ridge through the bloodstream; this type of migration has been observed in mammals and birds.

This gathering of the primitive germ cells in a precise region of the embryo implies a phenomenon of tissue recognition. By analogy with findings in several classes of vertebrates it may be supposed that the genital ridge exerts an attractive effect on the germ cells by a chemotactic mechanism. The diffusible substance which is recognized by the germ cells has, however, not yet been isolated. This substance, which is probably of a simple chemical composition, appears to have no zoological specificity since, both in-vivo and in-vitro 'attracting substance' from mammals is capable of stimulating and orienting the displacement of primitive germ cells from birds.

1.2. Common somatic blastema

1.2.1. Organization and evolution of the blastema. The region of the mesonephros opposite to the genital ridge undergoes considerable transformations which are common to both male and female embryos.

During the fourth week (while the migration of the primitive germ cells is in progress) the mesenchyma subjacent to the genital ridge forms an aggregation of cells called the gonadal blastema, the common somatic blastema or the paramesonephric blastema (Gropp and Ohno 1966). This aggregation continues and increases during the fifth week. By the sixth week the blastema is clearly separated from the coelomic epithelium by a looser mesenchymatous zone in which germ cells may be seen.

The elements of the common blastema are characterized by progressively denser cords of mesenchymatous cells with alkaline phosphatase activity in relation, anteriorly, with the gathering primitive germ cells and, posteriorly, with the mesonephric tubules.

The common blastema is constituted in several stages. Initially, some of the cells of the genital ridge (multilayered epithelium) are involved in the formation of the blastema – in fact, during the fifth week of development, the basal membrane of the coelomic epithelium can no longer be seen. The blastema cells, which are essentially formed at the expense of the mesenchymatous cells, then become separated from the coelomic epithelium. The primitive germ cells are sandwiched between the common blastema and the coelomic epithelium (which is now unilayered, and again limited by a basal membrane). The deeper region of the blastema differentiates into a system of canals which form a network of anastomoses in relation with mesonephric tubes; this is the beginning of the formation of the first urogenital connections.

Two properties of the common somatic blastema should be emphasized. The formation of the blastema is independent of the presence of primitive germ cells, in fact, it occurs even in the absence of germinal elements. The blastema cells exert an influence on the maintenance and development of the germ cells, and germ cells which stray out of the neighbourhood of the blastema degenerate.

1.2.2. Primary sex cords. The old-fashioned concept of the 'primary sex cords', epithelial cords derived from the coelomic epithelium of the genital ridge and inserted into the subjacent mesenchyma, can no longer be considered valid. Similarly the notion of a cortical zone of the undifferentiated gonad derived from the coelomic epithelium, and a medullary zone formed by a localized differentiation of cells of the mesenchyme of the mesonephros should be abandoned.

Well-characterized primitive germ cells are recognizable in the common somatic blastema and in the superficial coelomic epithelium; therefore, the 'primary sex cords' are simply the cells of the common somatic blastema. However, as mentioned above, although this differentiation is mainly of mesenchymatous origin, some of the cells are derived from proliferation of the coelomic epithelium.

2. DIFFERENTIATION OF THE TESTIS

Testicular differentiation starts at the beginning of the seventh week. The common blastema cells differentiate and become organized into, on the one hand, the *testicular cords* into which the primary germ cells migrate and, on the other, the *interstitial Leydig cells*. The morphological basis for gametogenesis and hormone activity is thereby assured (see Figure 1).

Shortly before birth, the testicles descend into the scrotum. During childhood, the genital apparatus changes very little; its growth is slow. The final stage in its ontogenesis occurs at adolescence during the process of puberty which is, itself, initiated by the activation of the hypothalamo-hypophyseal apparatus.

During puberty the testicles begin to produce viable gametes capable of fertilization.

2.1. Prenatal stages

2.1.1. Morphogenesis of the testis. The mesenchyma situated beneath the coelomic epithelium thickens to form a peripheral connective sheet composed initially of cells which take on a fusiform shape, and of fibers of reticulin – the *tunica albuginea*. At the eighth week septa, or septal connective tissues, develop from the interior surface of the tunica albuginea and demarcate the testicular lobes.

Two types of cells develop within the common blastema: *Sertoli cells*, which form solid cellular blocks constituting the *testicular cords (or seminiferous cords)*, and *Leydig cells*, which are situated in the interstitial spaces between the cords. In each lobe, the testicular cord branches out to give rise to two or three definitive testicular cords. Each testicular cord is covered by a basal lamina which will eventually be replaced by the lamina propria around the seminiferous tubules.

2.1.1.1. Germ cells. The germ cells migrate towards the interior from their initial peripheral localization and penetrate into the interior of the testicular cords where they continue to multiply actively. They are then called *gonocytes*, and are characterized by their regular round or oval shape. Ultrastructurally, they have a large, spherical central nucleus with dispersed chromatin and a voluminous reticulated nucleolus; their cytoplasm contains dispersed ribosomes, a small endoplasmic reticulum, a variable Golgi apparatus, and a few lysosomes (Gondos and Hobel 1971; Wartenberg et al. 1971).

The gonocytes move progressively towards the periphery of the cords where they are to be found in pairs near the basal membrane. At this stage in their evolution these germ cells have been called *type II gonocytes, prospermatogonia, primitive type A spermatogonia,* or *fetal spermatogonia* (see Gondos 1977). At the twelfth week, these cells often have connecting bridges (Wartenberg et al. 1971). This phenomenon, which also occurs in the adult testicle, therefore appears early; it has been interpreted as the ultrastructural reflection of an incomplete cytokinesis, and, more precisely, as a means of synchronization of spermatogenic maturation.

The number of germ cells in the cords increases up to the seventeenth week and many mitoses can be seen up to that time. Thereafter the number of mitoses diminishes, to cease entirely around the twentieth week, whereas the number of degenerating germ cells increases.

Three successive stages in the evolution of germ cells in the fetal testicle can thus be described: primitive germ cells, gonocytes, and fetal spermatogonia (or prospermatogonia). Prospermatogonia have been divided into three different types (Wartenberg 1978): multiplying (M), transitional-1 (T1) and transitional-2 (T2).

2.1.1.2. Sertoli cells. In the testicular cords, at the seventh week, the mesenchymatous cells from the common blastema develop into Sertoli cells; they enlarge and progressively envelop the gonocytes, entering into very close contact with them (Jost et al. 1974). The germ cells can easily be distinguished by their elongated shape, their irregular invaginated nucleus, and the abundance of their cytoplasmic organelles; within their cytoplasm can be found numerous free ribosomes, polyribosomes, glycogen, a moderately-developed rough endoplasmic reticulum, elongated mitochondria, lysosomes, and a well-developed Golgi apparatus. The degeneration of the gonocytes is accompanied by the appearance of phagosomes in the Sertoli cells. The earliest Sertoli cells have a pale cytoplasm, but two weeks after their appearance another population of darker cells develops. These two populations each exercise a distinctive physiological control over the primitive

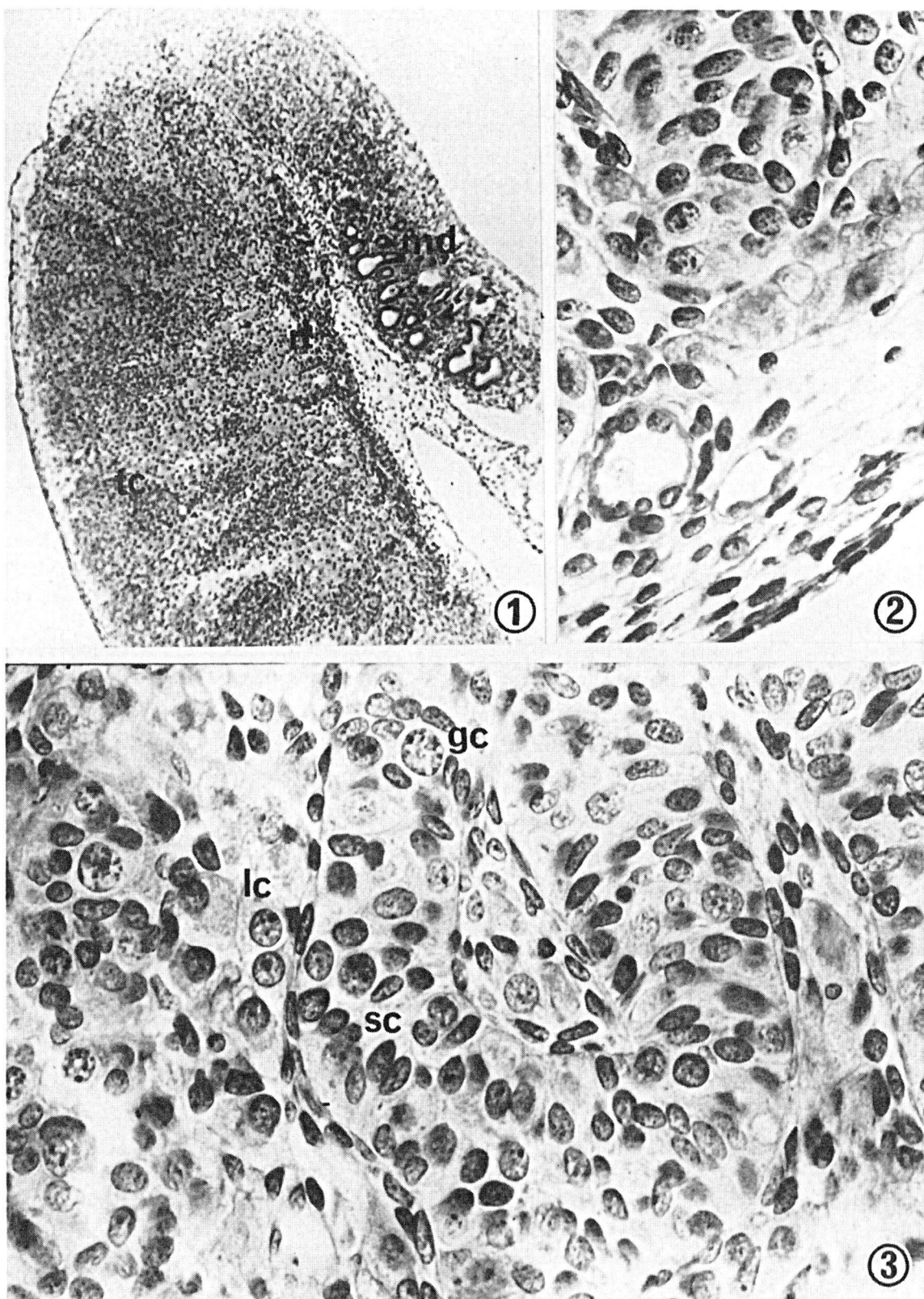

Figure 1. Embryonic human testis at the eighth week: (1) general appearance: short, straight testicular cords (tc) connect with the rete testis (rt); mesonephric ducts (md) are visible in the mesorchium; (2) peripheral region of the gonad: the cords are separated from the surface epithelium by small cells which will later form the tunica albuginea by fiber formation; (3) testicular cords are separated by developing connective tissue containing the earlier Leydig cells (lc) - germ cells (gc) are incorporated in the cords among Sertoli cells (sc).

germ cells and they are given the names 'meiosis-preventing (MP) Sertoli cells', and 'meiosis-inducing (MI) Sertoli cells' (Wartenberg 1978).

Several authors believe that the Sertoli cells are directly derived from the coelomic epithelium of the genital ridge (Gier and Marion 1970; Gondos 1974).

2.1.1.3. Leydig cells. Situated between the testicular cords, the Leydig cells may be recognized from the eighth week onwards by their increasingly oval shape. Electron microscopy shows a rapid augmentation of their smooth endoplasmic reticulum and mitochondria, whereas the proportion of free ribosomes and rough endoplasmic reticulum diminishes (Pelliniemi and Niemi 1969; Holstein et al. 1971; Gondos 1975). Histochemical reactions reveal the enzymatic equipment for steroidogenesis (Jirasek 1971).

Ultrastructural observations permit the description of four phases in the evolution of the fetal Leydig cells: (1) a pre-differentiation shape (up to the eighth week) corresponding to the presence of mesenchymatous cells; (2) a differentiation phase (eighth to fourteenth week) characterized by the infiltration of the cells between the testicular cords; (3) a maturation phase (fourteenth to eighteenth week) when the interstitial gland of the fetal testicle occupies approximately half the organ; and (4) an involution phase (eighteenth to fourteenth week) characterized by the degeneration and disappearance of the Leydig cells. It should be noted that the evolutionary cycle of the ultrastructure of the fetal Leydig cells correlates with a cycle of secretion of chorionic gonadotropin (Hooker 1970).

The time at which differentiation occurs and the duration of the differentiated appearance depend upon the species considered; in species other than humans the regression is most frequently postnatal.

2.1.1.4. Peritubular cells. The membrana propria develops progressively from the mesenchymatous cells of the intertubular spaces which differentiate into fibroblasts, some of which become myoid cells with contractile ability. The organization of the membrana propria is dependent upon the production of androgens by the Leydig cells (De Kretser et al. 1975).

2.1.2. Associated structures. At the time when the somite number is complete, the genital ridge,

covered by mesoblastic epithelium, expands from the sixteenth to the twenty-fourth somite. Between the eighth and eleventh weeks, the testis shortens and broadens, and is suspended from the adjacent mesonephros by a mesorchium. Degeneration of the mesonephros leaves a cranial diaphragmatic fold anchoring the testis to the primordium of the diaphragm, and a caudal inguinal fold which reaches the wall of the body in the future inguinal area. Immediately posterior to the mesonephros and continuous with it, an undifferentiated nephrogenic mesenchyma (nephric blastema) is penetrated by a Wolffian diverticulum (urethral bud). The urethral bud and the nephric blastema join to form the future kidney – the metanephros, which begins an antero-dorsal ascent and rotation. The residual nephrogenic cord becomes the gubernaculum testis visible in the free edge of the inguinal fold.

The blood vessels connect with the gonad through the mesorchium. In the fetal testis the major vascular trunks under the tunica albuginea are parallel to the surface. Capillaries form around the seminiferous and rete cords.

At the beginning of the third month, the caudal end of the abdominal cavity forms the vaginal processes (processus vaginalis) which herniate through the abdominal wall into the already-formed scrotal swellings to produce the inguinal canal.

2.1.3. Descent of the testis. Until the seventh month, the testis remains in its place of origin, ventral to somites 16 to 24 at the level of the anterior iliac spine. The migration of the testis into the scrotum, usually called 'descent', begins during the eighth month and may be complete two weeks later, or still incomplete at birth (Scorer 1964). Three stages can be distinguished in this descent: nephric displacement, transabdominal movement, and inguinal passage (Gier and Marion 1970).

The stage of gonadal movement resulting from nephric changes is complete in the sixty-day human fetus; the cephalic ligament tends to hold the testis anteriorly, but the gubernaculum, together with the mesonephric and Müllerian ducts, progressively move the gonad posteriorly as the metanephros presses anteriorly into the space recently vacated by the mesonephros.

The enlarging metanephros, the liver, and the gut all apply pressure on the testis, while the gubernaculum, anchored deeply within the groin, keeps it under continuous tension. Elongation of the lumbar region keeps the cord taut, and this results in movement of the gonad to a position immediately posteroventral to the tip of the kidney. Simultaneously, the evagination of the processus vaginalis extends around the gubernaculum and forms a hernia into the inguinal canal, which becomes a channel reaching the scrotum at 112 days. This elongation of the processus vaginalis is accompanied by movement of the testis which is pulled against the inguinal ring, where it remains for some time. This last stage is reached at about 150 days.

Inguinal passage, the last stage of descent, consists of movement of the testis from the peritoneal cavity into the lumen of the channel, and occurs after the seventh month.

Pressure from the expanding visceral organs certainly plays the most important role in moving the gonad. Contraction of the inguinal ring and pressure from the oblique muscles move the testis beyond the external inguinal ring. The processus vaginalis progresses into the scrotum together with the gubernaculum which shortens and thickens, leading the tail epididymis into the scrotal folds.

2.2. Evolution during childhood, and pubertal maturation of the testis

At birth, the seminiferous tubules have a diameter approximately equal to those of the fetus (60-70 microns). They have the appearance of solid cords. At the centre of some of them, cellular debris corresponding to degenerated spermatogonia can be observed. Virtually no Leydig cells can be seen in the intertubular spaces; these are occupied by cells with pycnotic nuclei and a vacuolated cytoplasm, and some fibroblast-like cells (Figure 2).

During childhood, up to the age of 10–11 years, the seminiferous tubules do not increase in diameter, but become long and sinuous. The spermatogonia have a characteristic appearance: they are large cells situated near to the lamina propria of the tubule, with large nucleolated nuclei, sometimes in mitosis, and with a chromophobic cytoplasm (thus apparently different from the fetal spermatogonia).

In children older than eight years, binucleated and hypertrophied spermatogonia may be observed. Leydig cells appear to be absent until the age of nine or ten years, and do not appear in any number until an average age of twelve years. One can observe the progressive transformation of fibroblast-like cells into rounded or elongated cells with a highly chromophilic cytoplasm. In fact, the acquisition of enzyme equipment specific for steroidogenesis precedes the morphological differentiation, and continues until the process of spermatogenesis is active in the tubules.

At puberty the testicles increase in total volume. The seminiferous tubules attain a considerable diameter; the following mean diameters have been reported: 72 microns at ten years, 85 microns at twelve years, 100–150 microns at fifteen years, and over 150 microns in the adult. The tubes develop a lumen. The spermatogonia show an intense mitotic activity and signs of cellular differentiation can be observed. These spermatogonia quickly give rise to spermatocytes, but spermiogenesis is much slower to develop. The MI Sertoli cells differentiate to become mature Sertoli cells, the fundamental difference being the appearance of junctional specializations of the plasma membrane which contribute to the blood-testis barrier.

3. FUNCTIONS OF THE DEVELOPING TESTIS

3.1. Androgenic secretion

3.1.1. Male differentiation of the reproductive tract. The studies of Jost (1972) have shown that the masculinization of the genital tract occurs only in the presence of the fetal testicles; if the fetus is castrated, the genital tract develops as female. Also, the morphological and functional development of the fetal Leydig cells is dependent on the fetal hypophysis. More recent studies using testosterone antagonists, hormone-binding techniques, and organ culture methods have confirmed and extended these initial observations.

There is a close relationship between steroid production by the fetal testicle and the masculine-type differentiation of structures derived from the Wolffian ducts. The active substance is testosterone, and the capacity for masculinization is present for only a specific time period.

The formation, in the testicles, of testosterone from pregnenolone can be detected from the eighth week with a maximum activity near the thirteenth week, followed by a diminution to a very low level after the twenty-first week (Siiteri and Wilson 1974).

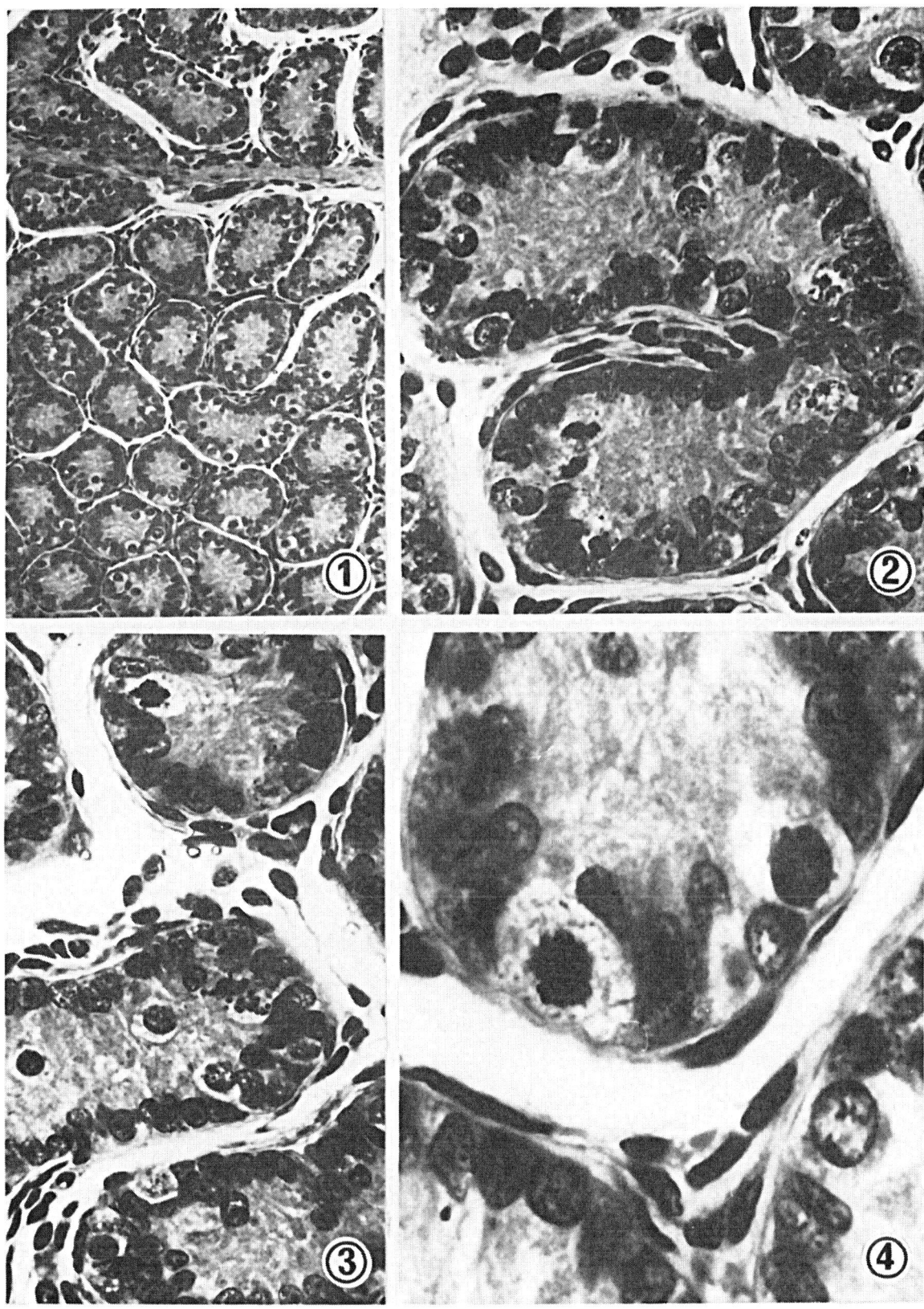

Figure 2. Seminiferous tubules of the child: (1, 2) general appearance at two different magnifications. The tubules contain only Sertoli cells and spermatogonia. No Leydig cells can be seen in the interstitial spaces; (3, 4) spermatogonia in mitosis.

3.1.2. Sexual differentiation of the central nervous system. Harris's studies have shown that, for several animal species, an essential role in the development of the brain is played by the testosterone secreted by the fetal testicle. This action is possible only during a very brief critical period covering a few days before and after birth. The animal which has experienced this action in the neonatal period will, after puberty, have a male-type libido, and its hypothalamic control of gonadotropins will be tonic and not cyclic.

It has not been possible to verify these observations in man. However, during the first three months after birth one can observe a progressive increase in the plasmatic concentration of testosterone in baby boys to about half that in adult men. The concentration then diminishes over a period of three to seven months to normal childhood values (Forest et al. 1974).

3.1.3. Puberty. Although the childhood levels of plasmatic testosterone are very low, the gonads can be stimulated by gonadotropins as in the adult. It is as though the feedback control system of the gonads was regulated at a low level. Puberty is set off by a rapid rise in the plasmatic concentration of gonadotropins which stimulate an important secretion of the testicular steroids which are responsible for the appearance of secondary sexual characteristics.

3.2. Müllerian-inhibiting activity

The regression of the Müllerian ducts during the differentiation of the reproductive tract is not due to testicular steroids, but rather to a substance secreted by the Sertoli cells, and not yet isolated (Josso 1974).

3.3. Causes of differentiation of the testis

3.3.1. Genetic control. Mammalian testicular differentiation occurs only when all, or part, of the Y chromosome is present in at least some of the embryonic cells. The unique role of the Y is to divert the spontaneous tendency of the undifferentiated embryonic gonad to form an ovary, and to force it to form a testis.

The regulating gene on the Y which determines testicular function is directly responsible also for a protein of the plasma membrane called HY antigen. This HY antigen constitutes the recognition signal which allows the direct interactions between the migratory germ cells and the elements of the genital ridge, which result in the differentiation of Sertoli cells and of testosterone-producing interstitial cells.

The Y chromosome has no influence on the ability of somatic cells to respond to testosterone. If female (XX) fetuses are treated with exogenous testosterone, they develop a purely male-type reproductive tract instead of ovaries. The response of somatic cells to testosterone depends upon the presence of nuclear and cytoplasmic proteins which are normally present in the cytoplasm of both male and female cells. These proteins are synthesized under the control of a gene in the locus *Tfm* on the X chromosome.

It would appear, then, that male development is induced by two principal regulatory genes: one gene on the Y chromosome which controls testicular formation, and one on the X chromosome which determines the sensitivity to androgens. If the Y gene controlling testicular formation is suppressed by mutation, the XY cells form ovaries instead of testicles. If the *Tfm* locus on the X chromosome has undergone mutation preventing the synthesis of the androgen receptor proteins, the Y chromosome still causes the differentiation of testosterone-secreting testicles, but the rest of the reproductive tract will spontaneously develop as female (see Ohno et al. 1978a). The cases of testicular differentiation in 46 XX individuals have been interpreted as the action of the Y regulator gene which has been fixed, by translocation, onto an X chromosome.

3.4. Causes of testicular descent

Many hypotheses have been advanced to explain the causes of testicular descent, but none are entirely satisfactory.

3.4.1. Mechanical causes. Two elements appear to influence the migration of the testicles: the gubernaculum testis or scrotal ligament, and the peritoneal canal which surrounds the testis forming the vaginalis. The gubernaculum does not appear to be firmly anchored to the scrotum, and so the scrotal ligament would not seem to be able to exert a traction on the testicle. The gubernaculum might play a part in dilating, by its volume, the inguinal canal in preparation for the descent of the testicle. Another part is probably played by abdominal pressure on the cylinder comprising the gubernaculum and the testis, each increase in pressure due to prenatal uterine contractions or to postnatal cries and strainings causing an advance of the testicles.

3.4.2. Hormonal causes. The descent of the gonad might depend on the secretion of chorionic gonado-

tropins. Childhood cryptorchidism has been successfully treated by injections of HCG. The gonadotropins would act by the stimulation of androgen production in the fetal adrenal cortex. These androgens would then induce a dilatation of the inguinal canal.

REFERENCES

Bressler RS: Hormonal control of postnatal maturation of the seminiferous cord. Ann Biol Anim Bioch Biophys 18(2B): 535, 1978.

Byskov AG: The meiosis-inducing interaction between germ cells and rete cells in the fetal mouse gonad. Ann Biol Anim Bioch Biophys 18(2B): 327, 1978.

Carlon N, Stahl A: Les premiers stades du développement des gonades chez l'homme et les vertébrés supérieurs. Path Biol 21(8): 903, 1973.

Charney CW, Conston AS, Meranze DR: Testicular developmental histology. Ann NY Acad Sci 55: 597, 1952.

Czyba JC, Cosnier J, Girod C, Laurent JL: Ontogenesis de la sexualidad humana: desarrollo de los aparatos genitales y del comportamento sexual. Barcelona, Eunibar, 1978.

De Kretser DM, Kerr JB, Paulsen CA: The peritubular tissue in the normal and pathological human testis: an ultrastructural study. Biol Reprod 12: 317, 1975.

Falin LI: The development of genital gland and the origin of germ cells in human embryogenesis. Acta Anat 72(2): 195, 1969.

Forest MG, Sizonenko-Cathiard AM, Bertrand J: Hypophyso-gonadal function in human during the first year of life I: evidence for testicular activity in early infancy. J Clin Invest 32: 65, 1974.

Furuya S, Kumamoto Y, Sugiyama S: Fine structure and development of Sertoli junctions in human testis. Arch Androl 1(3): 211, 1978.

Gier HT, Marion GB: Development of the mammalian testis. In: The testis. Johnson AD, Gomes WR, Vandemark NL (eds). New York, Academic Press, 1970, vols 1, 2.

Gillman J: The development of the gonad in man. Contrib Embryol 210: 811, 1948.

Gondos B: Intercellular bridges and mammalian germ cell differentiation. Differentiation 1: 177, 1973.

Gondos B: Testicular changes associated with the initiation of spermatogenesis. Ann Clin Lab Sci 5: 4, 1975.

Gondos B: Testicular development. In: The testis. Johnson AD, Gomes WR (eds). New York, Academic Press, 1977, vol 4, p 1.

Gondos B, Connel CJ: Cellular interrelationships in the fetal rabbit testis. Arch Androl 1(1): 19, 1978.

Gondos B, Hobel CJ: Ultrastructure of germ cell development in the human fetal testis. Z Zellforsch 119: 1, 1971.

Gould SF, Bernstein MM: Fine structure of fetal human testis and epididymis. Arch Androl 2(2): 93, 1979.

Gropp A, Ohno S: The presence of a common embryonic blastema for ovarian and testicular parenchymal (follicular, interstitial and tubular) cells in cattle. Bos Taurus Z Zellforsch 74(4): 505, 1966.

Hochereau de Reviers M-T, Courot M: Sertoli cells and development of seminiferous epithelium. Ann Biol Anim Bioch Biophys 18(2B): 573, 1978.

Holstein AF, Wartenberg H, Vossmeyer J: Zur Cytologie der pränatalen Gonadentwicklung beim Menschen III: die Entwicklung der Leydigzellen im Hoden von Embryonen und Feten. Z Anat Entwicklungsgesch 135: 43, 1971.

Hooker CW: The intertubular tissue of the testis. In: The testis. Johnson AD, Gomes WR, Vandemark NL (eds). New York, Academic Press, 1970, vol 1, p 483.

Jirasek JE: Development of the genital system and male pseudohermaphroditism. Baltimore, Johns Hopkins Press, 1971.

Josso N: Müllerian-inhibiting activity of human fetal testicular tissue deprived of germ cells by in-vitro irradiation. Pediatr Res 8: 755, 1974.

Jost A: A new look on the mechanisms controlling sex differentiation in mammals. Johns Hopkins Med J 130: 38, 1972.

Jost A, Magre S, Cressent M: Sertoli cells and early testicular differentiation. In: Male fertility and sterility. Mancini RE, Martini L (eds). New York, Academic Press, 1974.

Lemen CN: A study of the development and structural relationships of the testis and gubernaculum. Surg Gynec Obstet 110: 164, 1960.

Ohno S, Ciccarese S, Nagai Y, Wachtel S: H-Y antigen in testes of XX (BALB) XY (C3H) chimaeric male mouse. Arch Androl 1(1): 103, 1978a.

Ohno S, Nagai Y, Ciccarese S: Testicular cells lysostripped of H-Y antigen organize ovarian follicles-like aggregates. Cytogenet Cell Genet 20: 351, 1978b.

Pelliniemi LJ, Niemi M: Fine structure of the human foetal testis I: the interstitial tissue. Z Zellforsch 99: 507, 1969.

Prasad MRN: Gonadotropic control of the development of testis and accessory organs. In: Gonadotropins and gonadal function. Mondgal NR (ed). New York, Academic Press, 1974, p 199.

Saenger P, Levine LS, Watchel SS, Korth-Schutz S, Doberne Y, Koo GC, Lavengood RW, German JL, New MI: Presence of H-Y antigen and testis in 46 XX true hermaphrodism: evidence for Y chromosomal function. J Clin Endocr 43(6): 1234, 1976.

Scorer CG: The descent of the testis. Arch Dis Child 39: 605, 1964.

Siiteri PK, Wilson JD: Testosterone formation and metabolism during male sexual differentiation in the human embryo. J Clin Endocr Metab 38: 113, 1974.

Van Wagenen G, Simpson ME: Embryology of the ovary and testis in *Homo sapiens* and *Macaca mulatta*. New Haven, Yale University Press, 1965.

Wartenberg H: Human testicular development and the role of the mesonephros in the origin of a dual Sertoli cell system. Andrologia 10: 1, 1978.

Wartenberg H, Holstein AF, Vossmeyer J: Zur Cytologie der pränatalen Gonadentwicklung beim Menschen II: Elektronmikroskopische Untersuchungen über die Cytogenese und fetalen Spermatogonien im Hoden. Anat Embryol 134: 165, 1971.

Watchel SS, Koo GC, Ohno S: H-Y antigen and male development. In: The testis in normal and infertile men. Troen P, Nankin HR (eds). New York, Raven, 1977, p 35.

2. FUNCTIONAL HISTOLOGY OF DESCENDED TESTIS

E.S.E. HAFEZ

1. DEVELOPMENTAL CHANGES IN DESCENDED TESTIS

From birth until shortly before puberty the testis is rather static, showing tubules of small diameter, with no basement membrane, and is populated by two types of cells: (1) cells with deeply-staining elongated basophilic nuclei and no definite cellular membrane which are the progenitors of Sertoli cells, and (2) primary spermatogenic cells which have a definite cellular membrane, rounded nuclei and light-staining eosinophylic cytoplasm (Table 1, Table 2). In the immature testes the sex cords (future seminiferous tubules) do not have a lumen and have no spermatogenic activity. The gonocytes (stem spermatogonia) divide by mitosis, but do not differentiate into primary spermatocytes. In the pubertal testis the germ cells undergo spermatogenic differentiation, whereas the supporting cells differentiate into Sertoli cells. Leydig cells are present at birth due to the effect of circulating maternal gonadotropins, and disappear a few weeks after birth. Thus, in a prepubertal testis, the interstitium contains no Leydig cells (Girgis and Hafez 1977).

At puberty the histology of the testis is dramatically changed. The adult testis is characterized by large diameter of the tubules; a thin but definite basement membrane; a thin tubular wall two or three layers thick, and full and regular spermatogenic activity from basal spermatogonium, primary

Table 1. Structural differentiation of the descended testis (Bartsch et al. 1978).

Stage	Seminiferous tubules	Peritubular connective tissue	Interstitial tissue
Neonate (one year)	Made of two types of gonocytes (primitive germ cells); located in centre of tubule with tendency to migrate toward basement membrane; oval-shaped spermatogonia and Sertoli cells contact basement membrane.	Composed of the basement membrane of one layer, a collagen fiber zone, and fibroblasts; fibroblasts form concentric rings around tubule.	Fetal Leydig cells are well developed.
Prepuberty	Gonocytes are absent; spermatogonia A and B and spermatocytes and Sertoli cells complete the transformation to S_a and S_b types. S_a type is most common.	Certain widening without quantitative changes: basement membrane still consists of one layer without knob formation; collagen fiber layer is wider; and cellular layer is composed of fibroblasts; fibroblasts differentiate into myofibroblasts.	Precursors of Leydig cells grouped around vessels at 4-8 years of age.
Puberty	Tubules acquire a lumen development of all stages until spermatozoa with a few degenerating cells; Sertoli cells increase 4-5 times in size and increase in number; sperm appear with full development of Sertoli cells; tubules acquire certain contractility.	Under the influence of FSH and LH ultrastructural changes occur; basement membrane becomes multilayered with knob formation, collagen fibers run in an orderly fashion.	Leydig cells well differentiated with remarkable increase in smooth endoplasmic reticulum; Reinecke's crystalloids are absent.

Table 2. Structural differences of seminiferous tubules and Sertoli cells in prepubertal or pubertal testis.

	Prepubertal	Pubertal
Seminiferous tubule		
diameter	60-105	100-200
spermatogonia count	8-18	105-244
spermatocyte-sperm	absent	absent
		present
lumen	absent	absent
		present
Sertoli cell		
shape	cuboidal or columnar	radially elongated
nucleus	oval	irregularly infolded
endoplasmic reticulum	moderate	abundant
lipid droplet	seldom	regularly present
cytoplasmic filament and microtubule	moderate	abundant

spermatocyte, secondary spermatocyte and spermatid to terminal spermatozoa. The typical adult A-pale or A-dark spermatogonia only appear during puberty. Lodged between spermatogenic cells are the Sertoli cells with their prominent nuclei and wavy cytoplasm in which spermatids are embedded. A narrow compact interstitium contains well-formed Leydig cells closely applied to the outer walls of seminiferous tubules. The lumen is often present, especially if the tubular section is exactly transverse, commonly containing sloughed spermatogenic cells. Only a few spermatozoa can be noted, as once formed they are dislodged into the lumen (Girgis and Hafez 1977).

Thus, differentiation between prepubertal and postpubertal testis is easy and definite and, since the difference is due to the effect of pituitary gonadotropins, the biopsy serves as a parameter of pituitary gonadotropic function and for the diagnosis of cases of prepubertal hypogonadotropic hypogonadism. Since the testis exerts a feedback influence on FSH secretion, severely damaged seminiferous tubules are usually associated with high FSH (De Kretser et al. 1972).

2. KINETICS OF SPERMATOGENESIS

Spermatogenesis involves remarkable structural and ultrastructural differentiation including spermatogonial stem cell renewal, the two meiotic reduction divisions and the process of spermiogenesis, where the young round spermatids differentiate into mature spermatids.

A major portion of the cytoplasm of the sperm is eliminated prior to its release into the tubular lumen. The excess cytoplasm (residual cytoplasm) is separated from the neck and proximal flagellar regions at the time of sperm release. Once freed this residual cytoplasm is transported to the base of the seminiferous tubule where it is degraded by the Sertoli cell. The excess of cytoplasm is also eliminated at the head of the spermatid. Several methods have been used to evaluate spermatogenic activity (Table 3).

Table 3. Score count to evaluate testicular function as judged by histological characteristics.

Score	Histological criteria*
10	Full spermatogenesis
9	Many late spermatids, disorganized epithelium
8	Few late spermatids
7	No late spermatids; many early spermatids
6	No late spermatids; few early spermatids
5	No spermatids, many spermatocytes
4	No spermatids, few spermatocytes
3	Spermatogonia only
2	No germinal cells, Sertoli cells only
1	No seminiferous epithelium

* Each tubule is scored according to histological data (adapted from De Kretser and Holstein 1976: Johnsen 1970).

Long tubular projections of the spermatid with bulbous endings, the tubulobulbar complexes, form by invaginating into the Sertoli cell. The bulbous and tubular portions are devoid of organelles and are in direct continuity with the cytoplasm surrounding the head of the spermatid. Tubulobulbar complexes formed during spermiation undergo phagocytosis by the Sertoli cell. Upon the regression of tubulobulbar processes the perinuclear space around the head shrinks to allow a close relationship of the spermatid plasma membrane and acrosome around the nucleus.

The time required for spermatogenesis varies among mammalian species: in man spermatogenesis requires 74 ± 4 days (Heller and Clermont 1964). It would appear that once spermatogonia have begun the spermatogenic process, they progress through the developmental changes or degenerate. This fact is of importance in assessing the response of the testis to agents which supposedly stimulate spermatogenesis as they should be used for at least 70-80 days before conclusions can be drawn (De Kretser 1974). Six cell associations have been identified in the seminiferous tubule cycle (Clermont 1963; Heller and Clermont 1964). Not all spermatogenic stages are seen in the same section, because of the nature of the spermatogenic cycle, so that study of serial sections is essential for proper reading of the biopsy. Four stages of progressive changes in the morphology of the spermatid are noted: Golgi phase, cap phase, acrosome phase and maturation phase (Table 4).

Testicular changes are the result of damage, deficiencies or an underlying genetic error. Such changes are necessarily limited by structural elements of the testes and their potentialities as well as the nature and intensity of the inducing agent and the point or points at which it is maximally felt. Thus

Table 4. Cytological characteristics of spermatogenic cells in descended testis.

Spermatogenic stage type	*Cytological characteristics*
Spermatogonium	ovoid nucleus with deeply-stained dust-like chromatin
Ad (dark)	a pale-staining nuclear vacuole in centre of nucleus
	one or two nucleoli closely applied to nuclear membrane
A (pale)	disoid or ovoid nucleus with pale-stained very fine granulated chromatin
	one or two nucleoli attached to nuclear envelope
	spherical nucleus with clumps or granules of heavily-stained chromatin distributed along nuclear membrane, centrally-located nucleolus
B	spherical nucleus with clumps or granules of heavily-stained chromatin distributed along nuclear membrane, centrally-located nucleolus
Primary spermatocytes general characteristics	earliest modification of primary spermatocyte; what characterizes it from spermatogonia is the appearance of very fine single leptotene threads
	three of four nucleoli, one main nucleolus and two or three secondary nucleoli; secondary and main nucleoli are similar and all of them are related to acrocentric chromosomes
(preleptotene)	spherical nucleus with deeply-stained granulated chromatin accumulating on nuclear membrane nucleolus
prophase (first division)	nucleus undergoes progressive swelling
	chromatin assumes characteristics of leptotene, zygotene and pachytene
Secondary spermatocytes	spherical homogeneous nucleus with finely-granulated chromatin and some larger deeply-stained globular masses
	nucleolus is very inconspicuous and is absent much of the time
	not frequently observed because of their short life span
Spermatid Golgi phase	newly-formed spermatids have a spherical nucleus with Golgi zone, mitochondria, centrioles, and chromatoid body, well-demarcated nucleus, elaborate small granules which stain vividly with PAS
cap phase	proacrosomic granules coalesce to form a single-layer acrosome granule closely attached to surface of nucleus
	head cap expands around acrosomic granule and grows over surface of nucleus
	acrosomic granule and head cap stained well by PAS
acrosome phase	acrosome's nucleus and flagellum undergo remarkable modifications
	nucleus migrates to periphery of cell; nuclear chromatin condenses into coarse dense granules
maturation phase	spermatid rotates and acrosome becomes directed toward wall of seminiferous tubule
Basement membrane	a homogeneous moderately electron-dense layer, 0.3-0.4 μm thick, in direct contact with the bases of the spermatogonia and Sertoli cells; membrane may protrude into tubule indenting these cells

Source: Burgos et al. (1970); Clermont (1970); Courot et al. (1970); Hooker (1970); Solari and Tres (1970); Vilar et al. (1970); Girgis and Hafez (1977); Fabbrini and Hafez (1980).

the same type of lesion may be produced by more than one agent and the same agent may produce more than one characteristic feature.

Disturbance of spermatogenic cells may occur with or without associated peritubular changes. Selective damage may be produced by toxic agents such as cytostatic drugs (Vilar 1974), nitrofurantoins (Nelson and Bunge 1957), sulfa drugs, excessive smoking, heavy metal poisoning, fever and high temperature, and hormonal dysfunction associated with varicocele and cryptorchidism (Table 5).

Table 5. Structural differences between descended and cryptorchid testis.

Morphometrical parameters	Descended	Cryptorchid
No. of Sertoli cell nuclei/cm³	1461×10^6	1617×10^6
Single cell volume (μm^3)	491	429
Volume density of spermatogonia/cm³	.0056	.0021
Volume density of degenerating cells	.0012	.0018

Source: Adapted from Bartsch et al. (1978).

3. SERTOLI CELLS

The nucleus is irregularly shaped and its membrane presents numerous pores. The inner aspect of the nuclear membrane is electron-dense due to the presence of a fibrous lamina (Table 6). The outer aspect presents a concentric arrangement of 50 Å cytoplasmic filaments. The chromatin is dispersed with some perichromatin granules (Bustos-Obregón and Esponda 1977). Microtubules are abundant in Sertoli cells at certain stages of the spermatogenic cycle. With the elongation of the spermatids, their long axis becomes perpendicular to the basement membrane; their nucleus is located in a deep recess in the Sertoli cell, and most of the cytoplasm is displaced caudally around the base of the flagellum, extending toward the lumen of the seminiferous tubule. Owing to the syncytial nature of the developing germ cells, the residual lobules of spermatid cytoplasm are connected to one another by intercellular bridges which result from incomplete cytokinesis in the germ cell divisions of spermatogenesis (Fawcett 1975).

The mitochondria are numerous, generally very long and have lamellar crystae generally oriented transversely. In the basal cytoplasm they are randomly oriented, 'cup-shaped', and contain vesicular crystae. The Golgi complex consists of a few short parallel cisternal and small vesicles, numerous lysosomes, autophagic and heterophagic vacuoles and lipid droplets. Lipid droplets vary according to a true 'lipid cycle' which corresponds to the cycle of seminiferous epithelium. Sertoli cells contain two types of crystals: (1) Charcot-Böttcher crystalloids, 10-25 μm long and 2-3 μm thick, and (2) smaller crystals 1-5 μm long and about 1 μm thick.

In the depths of the apical invaginations of Sertoli cells there are parallel bundles of filaments which appear to course circumferentially in the thin layer of cytoplasm between the inner surface of the cell membrane and a fenestrated cisterna of endoplasmic reticulum. In this zone the filaments develop during condensation of spermatid nucleus and thus seem to represent a peculiar device for maintaining attachment of the Sertoli cell; each cell has subsurface cisternae and bundles of filaments connected with its apposed membranes. These arrangements represent extensive and unique junctional complexes involving two adjacent Sertoli cells. The outer leaflets of the membranes are 150-200 Å apart, but in some areas they approach to within 20 Å of one another in accord with the gap junctions of other cellular types.

Junctional specializations between the Sertoli cells have both gap and tight junctions, as adjudged by uranyl acetate staining, electron-opaque tracer and freeze fracture techniques (Dym 1973; Dym and Fawcett 1970; Nagano and Suzuki 1976a, 1976b). These gap junctions gradually disappear in the course of postnatal development of the testis, while the tight junctions appear to increase in size and number. In the mature testis, special tight junctions are characterized by three components: (1) multiple punctata pentalaminar membrane fusions; (2) subsurface cisternae of endoplasmic reticulum oriented in parallel with the Sertoli cell plasma membrane; and (3) bundles of microfilaments between the Sertoli cell plasma membrane and the associated subsurface cisternae (Fawcett 1975; Fawcett et al. 1976).

Sertoli cells actively participate in the spermatogenic process; they undergo clinical changes of the endoplasmic reticulum, mitochondria, the 'cycle of glycogen' and 'cycle of lipids'. There is a close relationship between quantity and location of the glycogen and the stage of the spermatogenic cycle

Table 6. Major structural characteristics of Sertoli cells and Leydig cells.

	Sertoli cell	*Leydig cell*
General characteristics	Closely associated with germinal cells; outlines of germinal cells occupy deep recesses of conforming shape on base of Sertoli cells; tall columnar extending from base of epithelium to lumen of seminiferous tubule; laterally directed cytoplasmic processes cause intimate wrapping around spermatogonia with elaborate infolding of cytoplasmic membranes and ingested spermatozoa, especially spermatids; three types of vacuoles: (a) small clear vacuoles, (b) small, faintly osiohilic vacuoles, (c) large lucent vacuoles with a dark rim.	Polygonal epithelioid cells scattered or more often irregularly grouped in angular spaces or in stands along the intertubular spaces; finely granular cytoplasm contains vacuoles representing lipid globules which dissolve during specimen preparation; cytoplasm stains by many acid dyes with little affinity for basic dyes; cell contains glycogen, hydrolytic enzymes (lipases, estrases and phosphatases) and oxidative enzymes; aggregate in clusters in close proximity to blood vessels but separated from them by perivascular fibrosis, cell is polygonal in form and 15-20μm in diameter, surrounded by a typical plasmalemma with fold or microvilli; abundant smooth endoplasmic reticulum consists of interconnected membrane tubules 800-1200 Å in diameter.
Organelles in cytoplasm	Numerous, long and slender mitochondria; mitochondria in basal cytoplasm are randomly oriented, whereas those in the supranuclear columnar portion of cell are parallel to cell axis; multiple separate Golgi elements scattered through basal cytoplasm in supranuclear region.	Scattered patches of rough endoplasmic reticulum interconnect with smooth endoplasmic reticulum; mitochondria are elongated or rounded and contain cristae of lamellar or less frequently tubular formation; Golgi complex made up of 4-6 flat-ended sacs closely pressed together, with small vesicles at their periphery; cytoplasm contains lipid droplets, Reinke crystals, microtubules, and microfilaments; lysosomes, digestive vacuoles and residual bodies containing pigment.
Nucleus	Infolded; karysomes and peripheral clumps of heterochromatin that characterize nuclei or most somatic cell types are lacking; nucleoplasm homogeneous with large proportion of euchromatin with fine fibrogranular texture.	Large, oval, or round with a thin peripheral rim of heterochromatin, broken only at the sites of pores through the nuclear envelope; one or two prominent nucleoli.

Source: De Kretser (1967, 1968); Fawcett (1975); Christensen (1975); Bustos-Obregón and Esponda (1977).

(Fabbrini et al. 1969). Glycogen accumulates during the first stage, whereas there is a sharp decrease in the amount of Sertolian glycogen in the sixth, second and third stages. For example glycogen accumulates in the dark spermatogonia only before the transformation of spermatogonium A into spermatogonium B (Fabbrini et al. 1969). There is an increase of lipid content immediately after spermiation due to phagocytosis of residual bodies.

4. TUBULAR WALL

The tubular wall is a complex structure made of five layers: a typical basement membrane next to the basal surface of the Sertoli cell; an internal acellular layer, containing collagen fibers, glycoproteins and hyaluronic acid; an internal cellular layer made of spindle-shaped cells (myoid cells or 'peritubular smooth muscle cells' – p.s.m. cells); and an external cellular layer consisting of fibroblast. The acellular layers probably act as a cushion against microtrauma and variations in hydrostatic or osmotic pressure whereas the basement membrane probably constitutes a sort of selective filter for some proteins (Fabbrini and Hafez 1980). The fibroblasts probably participate in the barrier mechanism. The peritubular connective tissue is made of regularly alternating 2-6 (variable) layers of collagen fibers and (contractile) myoid cells beneath the basement membrane. The external surface is covered by a basement membrane and it may be in close association with some microfibrillar material.

Peritubular changes are always associated with disturbed spermatogenesis of varying degrees according to the extent of peritubular thickening leading in advanced cases to complete tubular 'hyalinization' with or without residual Sertoli cells. Hyalinization is the accumulation of apparently amorphous material between seminiferous epithelium and myoid cells. Tubular hyalinization may be generalized or localized. The generalized type is mostly progressive and its course is unaffected by treatment.

Another common anomaly is 'peritubular fibrosis', which is excessive proliferation in the lamina propria of seminiferous tubules.

5. INTERSTITIAL TISSUE

The space between the seminiferous tubules which is filled with irregular meshwork of loose connective tissue containing Leydig cells, fibroblasts, macrophages, mast cells and nonmyelinated nerve cells occupies one third of the testicular volume (Table 6). Interstitium is usually narrow and compact. Rarely it shares in fibrosis with the walls of the seminiferous tubules as in postinflammatory fibrosis.

Leydig cells are normally present in small clusters wedged or thinly spread out in relation to the outer walls of seminiferous tubules. Leydig cells are absent in prepubertal testes, show hyperplasia in cases of primary testicular dysfunctions, which may be diffuse in character as in progressive tubular hyalinization or localized to areas of focal necrosis or in masses and sheets as in Klinefelter's syndrome.

Several methods have been developed to evaluate frequency distribution and volume of interstitial cells, e.g. point counting or the Leydig-Sertoli cell ratio (Ahmad et al. 1969; Heller et al. 1971). For example, Leydig cell numbers do not increase in normal men treated with HCG, but the cells become consistently larger, an indication of hypertrophy rather than hyperplasia (Heller and Leach 1971).

6. UNDESCENDED TESTIS

Cryptorchidism represents the common anomaly of

sexual differentiation in man. Many concepts have been advanced, but the mechanisms which cause descent of the testis are not clearly understood. In the rat, the gubernaculum as a receptor or responder organ for testicular descent appears to be a structure worthy of scrutiny, since it is conspicuous during descent of the testis, but virtually disappears after descent is completed. Cryptorchidism is associated with severe damage of Sertoli cells, spermatogonia and the tubular membrane of the seminiferous tubules. Dramatic changes occur in the germinal epithelium of the cryptorchid testis, some of which are irreversible and more pronounced with increasing age.

It appears that testicular descent is an androgen-mediated event requiring an intact hypothalamic-pituitary-testicular axis. Any anomaly or disturbance affecting this pathway or any defect either in the synthesis or action of androgen may lead to abnormal testicular descent. Wensing and his associates used a pig as experimental animal. A swelling reaction of the extraabdominal part of the gubernaculum brings about the migration of the testis into the inguinal canal; subsequent regression of this swollen gubernaculum enables the testis to move to its final position. It would appear that testosterone, estradiol and gonadotropins are not important regulatory hormones in the migration of the male gonad.

Cryptorchidism is an endocrine disorder which affects about one percent of men. Bilateral and unilateral cryptorchidism is frequently associated with infertility, impaired LH response to LH-RH and cytological changes in Leydig cells. Experimentally-induced cryptorchidism in experimental animals causes a decreased testicular testosterone content. Prepubertal cryptorchidism does not represent a definite cause of immune lesions for the cryptorchid and/or scrotal testis as judged by antigens and antibodies.

REFERENCES

Ahmad KN, Lennox B, Mac WC: Estimation of the volume of Leydig cells in man. Lancet 2: 461, 1969.
Bartsch G, Oberholzer M, Holliger O, Wever J, Weber A, Rohr HP: Stereology: a new quantitative morphological method to study epididymal function. Andrologia 10: 31-42, 1978.
Burgos MH, Vitale-Calpe R, Aoki A: Fine structure of the testis and its functional significance. In: The testis, Johnson AD, Gomes WR, Vandemark NL (eds), New York, Academic Press, 1970, vol 1, p 551-649.
Bustos-Obregón E, Esponda P: Ultrastructure of the nucleus of human Sertoli cells in normal and pathological testis. Andrology 119, 1977.
Christensen AK: Leydig cells. In: Handbook of physiology, sec 7: Endocrinology; vol 5: Male reproductive system, Greep RO, Astwood EB (eds), Baltimore, Williams and Wilkins, 1975.
Clermont Y: The cycle of the seminiferous epithelium in men. Am J Anat 112: 35, 1963.

Clermont Y: Dynamics of human spermatogenesis. In: The human testis, Rosemberg E, Paulsen CA (eds), New York, Plenum, 1970, p 47-61.

Courot M, Hochereau de Reviers M-T, Ortavant R: Spermatogenesis. In: The testis, Johnson AD, Gomes WR, Vandemark NL (eds), New York, Academic Press, 1970, vol 1, p 339-432.

De Kretser DM: The fine structure of the testicular interstitial cells in men of normal androgenic status. Cell Tiss Res 80: 594, 1967.

De Kretser, DM: Crystals of Reinke in the nuclei of human testicular interstitial cells. Experientia 24: 587, 1968.

De Kretser, DM: The regulation of male fertility: the state of the art and future possibilities. Contraception 9: 561, 1974.

De Kretser DM, Holstein AF: Testicular biopsy and abnormal germ cells. In: Human semen and fertility regulation in the male. Hafez ESE (ed), St. Louis, Mosby, 1976, ch 30.

De Kretser DM, Burger HG, Fortune D, Hudson B, Long AR, Paulsen CA, Taft HP: Hormonal, histological and chromosomal studies in adult males with testicular disorders. J Clin Endocr Metab 35: 392, 1972.

Dym M: The fine structure of the monkey (*Macaca*) Sertoli cell and its role in maintaining the blood-testis barrier. Anat Rec 175: 639, 970.

Dym M, Fawcett DW: The blood-testis barrier in the rat and the physiological compartmentation of the seminiferous epithelium. Biol Reprod 3: 308, 1970.

Fabbrini A, Hafez ESE: Testis-epididymis. In: Human reproduction: conception and contraception, Hafez ESE (ed), Hagerstown, Maryland, Harper and Row, 1980.

Fabbrini A, Re M, Conti C: Glycogen in normal human testis: a histological and histochemical study. J Endocr 43: 499, 1969.

Fawcett DW: Ultrastructure and function of the Sertoli cell. In: Handbook of physiology, sec 7: Endocrinology; vol 5: Male reproductive system, Greep RO, Astwood EB (eds), Baltimore, Williams and Wilkins, 1975.

Fawcett DW, Gilula NB, Aoki A: Recent observations on the organization of the seminiferous epithelium. Gumma Symp Endocr 13: 49, 1976.

Girgis SM, Hafez ESE: Evaluation of testicular biopsy. In: Techniques of human andrology, Hafez ESE (ed), Amsterdam, North-Holland Biomedical Press, 1977.

Heller CG, Clermont Y: Kinetics of the germinal epithelium in man. Recent Progr Hormone Res 20: 545, 575, 1964.

Heller CG, Leach DR: Quantification of Leydig cells and measurements of Leydig cell size following administration of human chorionic gonadotropin to normal men. J Reprod Fertil 25: 185, 1971.

Heller CG, Lalli MF, Pearson JE, Leach DR: A method for the quantification of Leydig cells in man. J Reprod Fertil 25: 177, 1971.

Hooker CW: The intertubular tissue of the testis. In: The testis, Johnson AD, Gomes WR, Vandemark NL (eds), New York, Academic Press, 1970, vol 1, p 483-550.

Johnson SV: Investigations into the feedback mechanism between spermatogenesis and gonadotropin level in man. In: The human testis, Rosemberg E, Paulsen CA (eds), New York, Plenum, 1970.

Nagano T, Suzuki F: Freeze-fracture observations on the intercellular junctions of Sertoli cells and of Leydig cells in the human testis. Cell Tiss Res 166: 37, 1976a.

Nagano T, Suzuki F: The postnatal development of the junctional complexes of the mouse Sertoli cells and revealed by freeze-fracture. Anat Rec 185: 403, 1976b.

Nelson WO, Bunge RG: The effect of therapeutic doses of nitrofurane (Furadantine) upon spermatogenesis in man. J Urol 77: 275, 1957.

Solari AJ, Tres LL: Ultrastructure and histochemistry of the nucleus during male meiotic prophase. In: The human testis, Rosemberg E, Paulsen CA (eds), New York, Plenum, 1970, p 127-138.

Vilar O, Paulsen CA, Moore DJ: Electron microscopy of the human seminiferous tubules. In: The human testis, Rosemberg E, Paulsen CA (eds), New York, Plenum, 1970, p 63-74.

Vilar O: Effects of cystostatic drugs on human testicular function. In: Male fertility and sterility, Mancini RE, Martini L (eds), New York, Academic Press, 1974, p 423.

3. GERM CELLS

LUCIA CASTELLANI-CERESA

1. INTRODUCTION

The seminiferous tubule is lined by a highly specialized epithelium, the germinal or seminiferous epithelium, which rests upon a thin basal lamina. In the
adult, the seminiferous epithelium is composed of
two main groups of cells, the nutrient and supporting elements (Sertoli cells) and the germinal or
spermatogenic cells. The germ cells constantly undergo changes in the continuous process of differentiation that leads to the mature spermatozoa.
The sequence of events by which spermatogonia are
transformed into spermatozoa is referred to as
spermatogenesis, which involves three processes
(Figure 1). The first is *spermatocytogenesis*, in which
spermatogonia undergo mitotic divisions to multiply themselves and become spermatocytes. The
reduction from the diploid to the haploid number of
chromosomes takes place during *meiosis*, in which
spermatocytes undergo two maturation divisions
and spermatids result. Cellular differentiation is
referred to as *spermiogenesis*; during this phase a
number of developmental events occur which lead to
the formation of mature spermatozoa.

In this chapter, the ultrastructure of spermatogonia and spermatocytes will be examined; spermiogenesis is handled in Chapter 4.

2. SPERMATOGONIA

The earlier germ cells in the adult testis are the
spermatogonia, which are in contact with the basal
lamina. Three spermatogonial types in man have
been identified using light microscopy (Clermont
1963, 1966a; Heller and Clermont 1964; Mancini et
al. 1960; Roosen-Runge and Barlow 1953): the dark
type A (AD), the pale type A (AP), and the B type.
Nuclear size and shape, density and staining of

chromatin, number and position of nucleoli, and
presence or absence of cytoplasmic glycogen are the
morphological features which distinguish these three
types. Electron microscopy has allowed the identification, in each cell of the seminiferous epithelium, of
particular subcellular characteristics, which were
impossible to determine by light microscopy. On the
basis of cytological data, obtained from both light
and electron microscopy, four types of spermatogonia have recently been described in man (Bustos-
Obregón et al. 1975; Clermont 1970; Rowley et al.
1971; Tres and Solari 1968; Vilar et al. 1970;
Wartenberg 1976). These are commonly listed by
using the alphabet; although there is some criticism
about this method (Vilar et al. 1970) in this chapter
the letters will be used, as they are in most of the
literature, to facilitate understanding (Figure 2).

The *A long (AL)* and *A dark (AD)* spermatogonia are flat cells, attached for a great extent to the
basal lamina (Figure 3). Many features are common
to these two types: the nuclei are more or less
regularly oval; one or two nucleoli are located
against the inner membrane of the nuclear envelope.
The nucleolus in these cells is composed only of a
granular region (nucleolonema). In the cytoplasm,
numerous granules of glycogen which are not present in the other types of spermatogonia are found.
The mitochondria contain a dense matrix with
tubular cristae, and they tend to aggregate in groups
close to the poles of the nucleus (Figure 4a);
furthermore, they are always absent from the region
near the basal lamina. In the flat type of human
spermatogonia, a crystalloid structure (Figure 4b),
crystalloid of Lubarsch (Lubarsch 1896), has been
described (Nagano 1969). The crystalloid of
Lubarsch is composed of many tubular elements
embedded in fine granular material, and each tubule

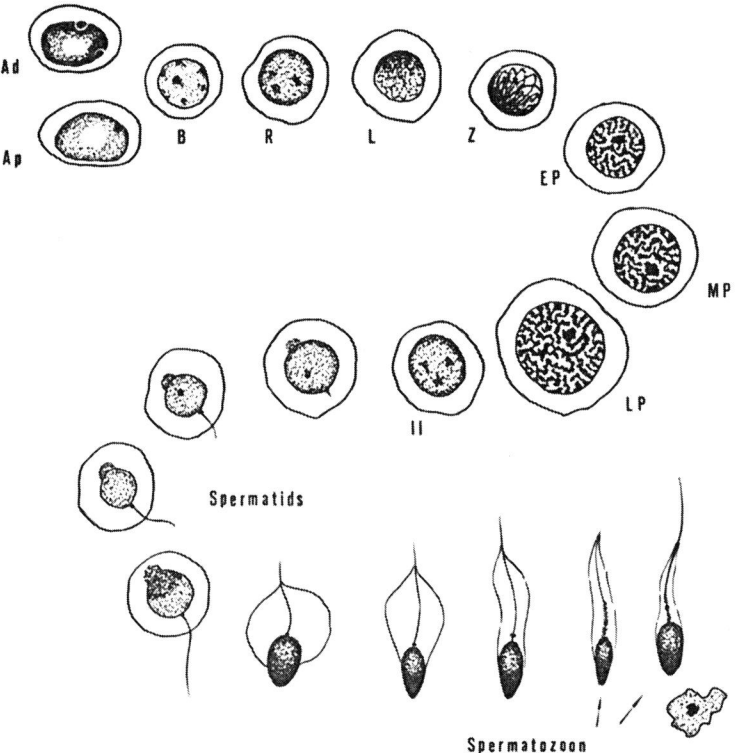

Figure 1. The main steps of spermatogenesis in man. Spermatogenesis begins with
the spermatogonia at the top left and terminates with a spermatozoon at the bottom
right. Labels: Ad: dark type-A spermatogonia; Ap: pale type-A spermatogonia;
B: type-B spermatogonia; R: preleptotene primary spermatocyte; L: leptotene
spermatocyte; Z: zygotene spermatocyte; EP: early pachytene spermatocyte; MP:
mid-pachytene spermatocyte; LP: late pachytene spermatocyte; II: secondary
spermatocytes. Spermatids are shown at various steps of spermiogenesis. A
spermatozoon is illustrated as seen from its lateral (left) and frontal (right) aspects.
A residual body is also shown. (Courtesy of Y. Clermont.)

is 80-120 Å in diameter. The tubules run parallel to
each other and are connected by dense material
forming lamellae (Nagano 1969). The main difference between the A-long and A-dark spermatogonia are: the A-dark type has a more regular outline
of the nuclear membrane and a more compact
nucleolus; it is the only germ cell in which a region
of rarefaction which corresponds to the nuclear
vacuole of light microscopy appears within the
nucleus. In the cytoplasm of the A-dark type, unlike
A-long, the mitochondria are sometimes joined by
strands of dense material (Figure 4c), similar to that
described by André (1962) in rat spermatogonia and
by Nagano (1969) in human spermatogonia.

The *A pale (AP)* spermatogonium is a large,
round cell, also attached to the basal lamina; it has a
nearly round nucleus, with pale chromatin (Figure
5a). A small nucleolus is found near the nuclear

periphery. The cytoplasm does not contain glycogen
granules, and it appears less dense than in the other
spermatogonia. Microtubules, which were present in
AL and AD types, are missing, and the crystalloid of
Lubarsch was never observed by us in this cell type,
although this structure has occasionally been found
even in more differentiated germ cells (Nagano
1969). The mitochondria, which are scattered
through the cytoplasm, are single or in groups of
only two elements, with platelike cristae. *B spermatogonium* has very little contact with the basal
lamina (Figure 5b); it shows a spheroid nucleus
containing chromatin granules of varying size distributed along the nuclear envelope or attached to
the nucleoli; one or more large, irregular nucleoli are
present and do not touch the nuclear membrane. The
mitochondria are single and scattered through the
cytoplasm. Neither glycogen granules nor crystal-

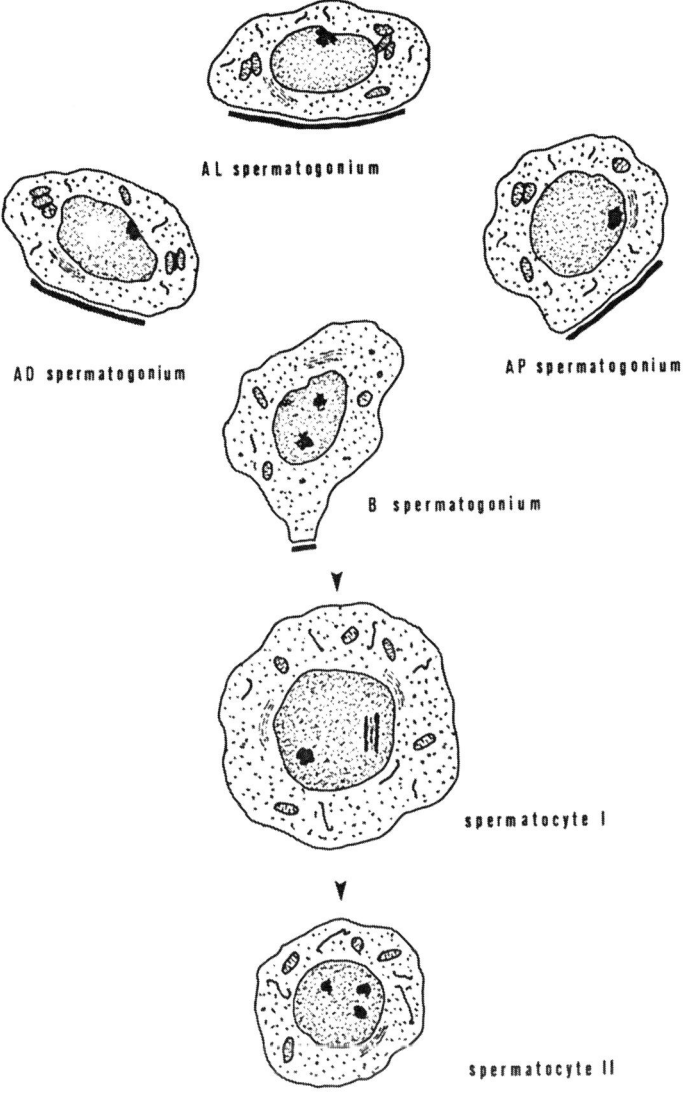

AL spermatogonium

AD spermatogonium

AP spermatogonium

B spermatogonium

spermatocyte I

spermatocyte II

Figure 2. Differentiation of germ cells from spermatogonium to spermatocyte II.

loid of Lubarsch are present.

On the basis of ultrastructural and histochemical studies, several bodies in the human spermatogonial nuclei have been described (Tres and Solari 1968). In the nucleus of the type-B spermatogonium, besides some nucleoli, there are flakes of chromatin, devoid of any definite structure. Five different types of bodies have been found in the nuclei of A-type spermatogonia: type I and I' bodies have the structural components of nucleoli; they are found in nuclei with a homogeneous and pale chromatin, which are devoid of vacuoles or other kinds of bodies. Type II bodies are the most frequent of all, and they are frequently found in nuclei with a central

vacuole; together with type III and V bodies, they are considered to be atypical nucleoli. Type IV bodies are small chromatin condensations. Although Tres and Solari (1968) found cell differences in the distribution of the nuclear bodies, these authors could not distinguish the different kinds of A gonia at the ultrastructural level.

It is of value at this point to note that the order in which the spermatogonia are described here (AL, AD, AP, B) is the same as that used in other studies carried out on the mode of renewal of spermatogonia. While these studies in many mammalian species are very numerous – see reviews by Leblond et al. (1963) and Roosen-Runge (1962) – very little

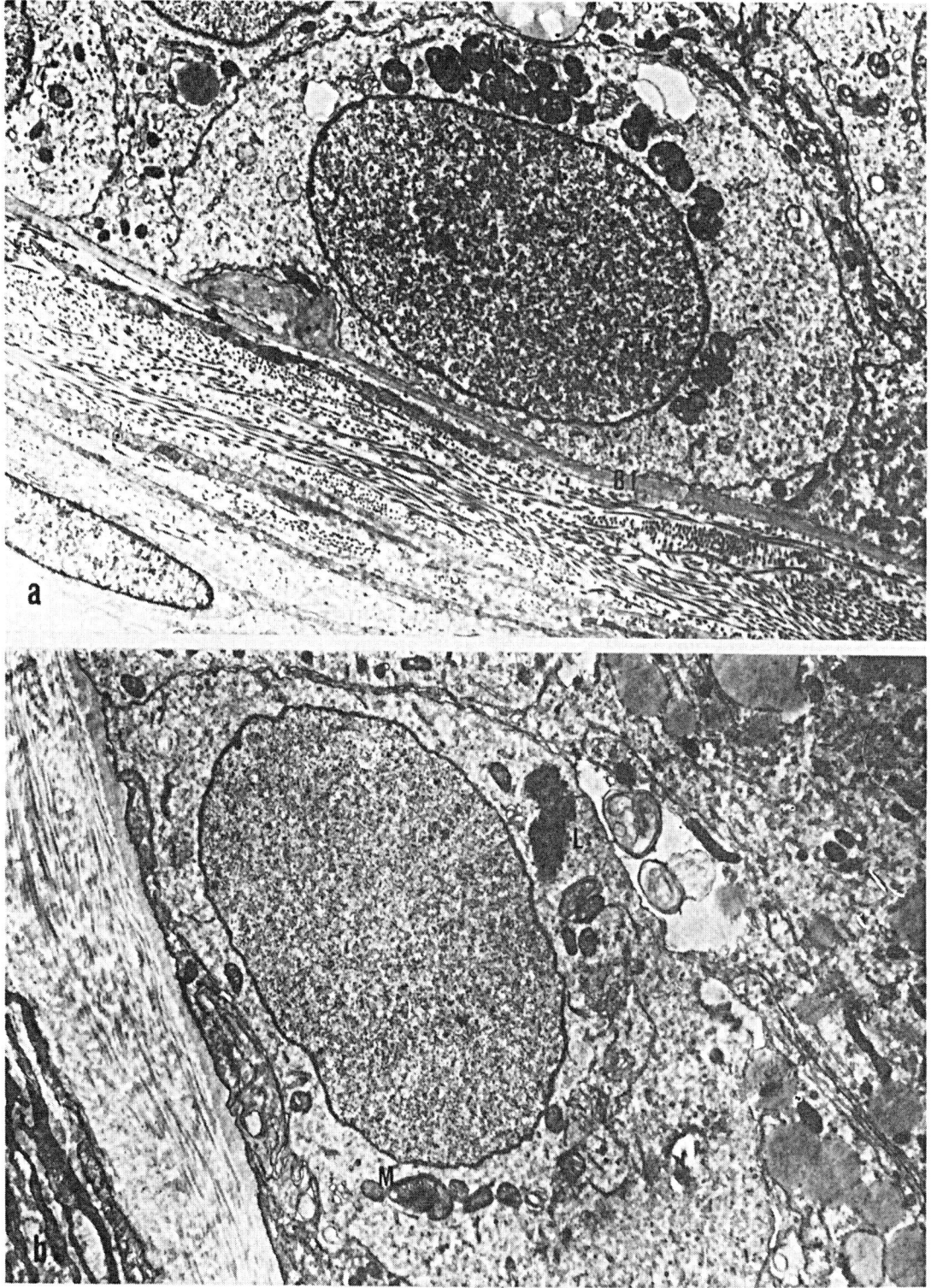

Figure 3. (a) AL-type spermatogonium, in contact with the basal lamina (Bl). The nucleoplasm is homogeneous. The mitochondria (M) are grouped and are located away from the basal lamina (× 7,200). (b) AD-spermatogonium. Mitochondria (M) are joined to each other. In the cytoplasm, a crystalloid of Lubarsch (L) is visible (× 9,200).

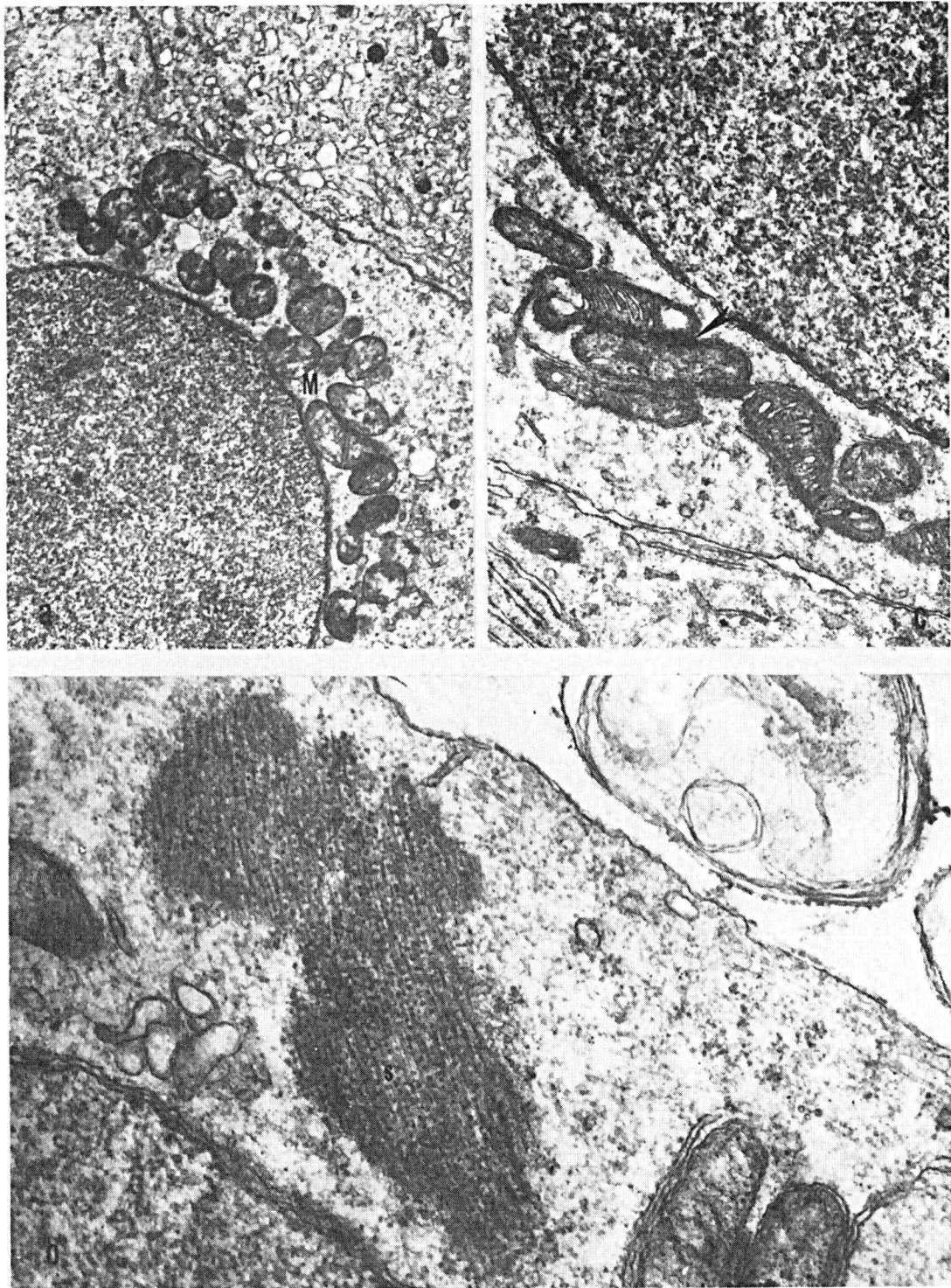

Figure 4. (a) Groups of mitochondria (M) in contact with the nucleus in an AL-spermatogonium (× 10,600). (b) Longitudinal section of the crystalloid of Lubarsch shown in Figure 3(b) at higher magnification. Electron-opaque spheres (s) are visible between the filaments (× 47,500). (c) AD-spermatogonium. Mitochondria (arrow) are joined by electron-opaque bars (× 25,000).

work has been done on man. The cellular progression from AD to AP to B was proposed on the basis of quantitative and topographical analysis of the various types of spermatogonia (Clermont 1966b, 1970). The addition of AL before AD was suggested by Rowley et al. (1971) on the basis of its ultrastructural characteristics (Table 1).

3. SPERMATOCYTES

Type-B spermatogonia divide only once before becoming spermatocytes (Ohno 1970) which represent the meiotic stage of the male germ cells.

3.1. Primary spermatocytes

The first cell originating from the last spermatogonial division is the *preleptotene* spermatocyte (Tobias 1956). The identification of the human preleptotene stage is not easy, owing to the close similarity of its subcellular characteristics to those of B spermatogonium. The main difference is that, unlike B spermatogonium, it is detached from the basal lamina; the ramifications of the Sertoli cell cytoplasm separate this spermatocyte from both the tubular limiting membrane and the neighbouring cells. This cell has been designated also as 'resting spermatocyte' (Leblond and Clermont 1952); however, during this stage, besides the replication of DNA, the preleptotene spermatocytes engage in intense transcriptional and translational activities, so that most of the enzymes and proteins needed during the following stages of spermiogenesis are synthesized by and stored in the cytoplasm of this cell. The cytoplasm of the primary spermatocytes presents uniform features throughout the course of meiosis: the mitochondria, in contrast to the regular morphology observed in the spermatogonia, appear to be swollen and show an irregular course of the cristae mitochondriales. With the exception of polysomes, which are more numerous than in other stages, little else is found in the ground substance. Nevertheless the nucleus undergoes remarkable changes through the various steps of prophase of the first maturation division, and five stages can be identified (Vilar 1973).

In the *leptotene* stage, the nucleus is characterized by the condensation of chromatin and the formation of fine chromosomal filaments. A small nucleolus,

often horseshoe-shaped, is present. Longitudinal pairing between two homologous chromosomes occurs in the *zygotene* stage (Figure 6a); a 'synaptinemal complex' (Figure 6b, c), which appears at the beginning of zygotene, has been described in human material (Fawcett 1956; Solari and Tres 1970; Westergaard and von Wettstein 1972). The synaptinemal complex appears as a plane, tripartite structure, composed of a central threadlike element lying equidistant from the pair flanking it, which joins homologous autosomal bivalents along their lengths (Moses 1968). Unlike autosomes, there is very little homology between the X and the Y chromosomes, and yet they must form a bivalent to assure the segregation of the X from the Y at the end of this first meiotic division. To bring the X and the Y chromosomes together, at the beginning of the zygotene stage a sex vesicle forms, where pairing is observed between the short homologous segments of both chromosomal cores (Solari and Tres 1970). At the beginning of *pachytene*, longitudinal pairing is completed, and genetic recombination due to an exchange of part of the chromatids between homologous chromosomes (crossing-over) occurs. The paired homologous chromosomes start to separate at the beginning of *diplotene*, but the separation is incomplete with chiasmata forming. In this stage, the synaptinemal complex virtually disappears. During the *diakinesis* stage, a progressive condensation of bivalents and a terminalization of chiasmata occur. The nuclear membrane disappears at the end of diakinesis and metaphase follows, in which the bivalents are arranged on an equatorial plane. During *anaphase*, the chromosomes, each of which consists of two chromatids held together by the unsplit centromere, migrate towards opposite poles of the cell. Cell division is often incomplete, and intercellular bridges can be seen between daughter cells. As a result of the first meiotic division, the nuclei of each daughter cell, or secondary spermatocyte, have an apparently haploid set of chromosomes (each chromosome is actually made up of two chromatids) recombined through crossing-over.

3.2. Secondary spermatocytes

The secondary spermatocytes (Figure 6d) are relatively small cells; their spherical nuclei contain some large chromatin granules and often are devoid of a

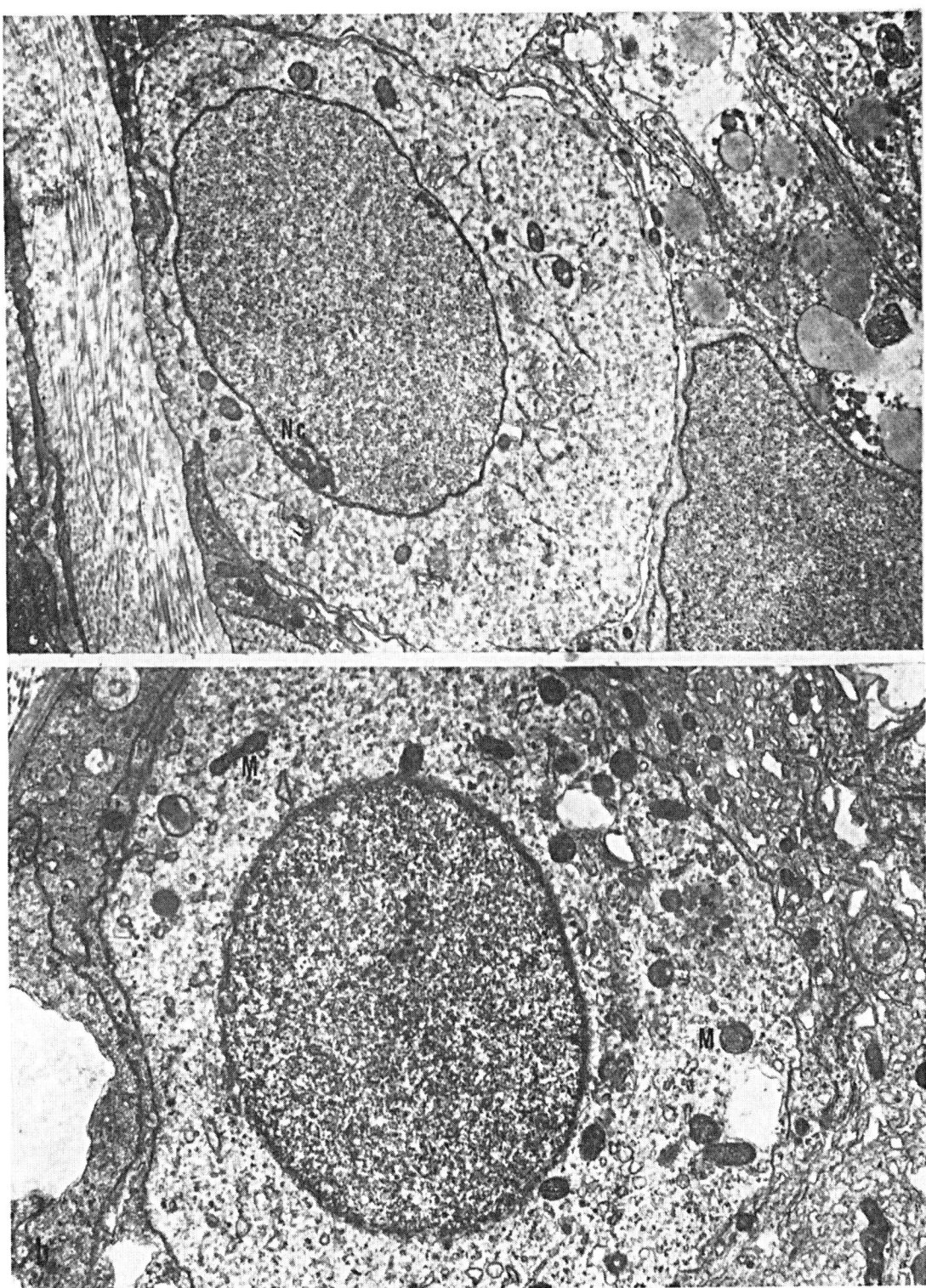

Figure 5. (a) AP-spermatogonium. A small nucleolus (Nc) is visible in a peripheral position. The cytoplasm appears slightly lighter than in the other spermatogonia. The contact with the basal lamina is reduced ($\times 8.800$). (b) B-spermatogonium. Mitochondria (M) are scattered throughout the cytoplasm. The contact with the basal lamina is minimal ($\times 10.800$).

Table 1. Cytological criteria of human spermatogonia (according to Rowley et al. 1971).*

Classification	AL long	AD dark	AP pale	B
Shape of cell	very flat	flat	rounded	pear-shaped
Attachment to basal lamina	~ 30 μm	wide	less wide	<2 μm
Nuclear shape	oval-irregular	oval-regular	spherical	spherical
Chromatin	homogeneous	granular, rarefaction	homogeneous	granular
Type of nucleolus	nucleolonema	nucleolonema	nucleolonema pars amorpha	nucleolonema pars amorpha
Position of nucleolus	peripheral	peripheral	peripheral	central
Type of mitochondria	tubular	tubular	cristae	cristae
Arrangements of mitochondria	groups with ER	groups with ER	pairs with bars	single
Glycogen	positive	positive	negative	negative

* From Wartenberg (1976, p. 126), by permission of the author.

nucleolus. These cells are seen infrequently and can easily be confused with young spermatids, which they resemble. After a brief interkinesis, without DNA replication, the secondary spermatocytes undergo the second meiotic division, which yields haploid spermatids. Theoretically, four spermatids should be produced for each primary spermatocyte; however, in man, some spermatocytes degenerate during the two maturation divisions (Clermont 1966a), and the ratio of spermatids to primary spermatocytes is 2.5 to 1.

The germ cells of infertile men, with infertility depending on several factors, have also been studied (Barham and Berlin 1974; Camatini et al. 1978; Castellani et al. 1978; Cotelli et al. 1976). Although many multinucleate cells were found and cellular degeneration was frequent, no significant difference from the norm was found in spermatogonia and spermatocytes.

4. CELL ASSOCIATION

The seminiferous epithelium is composed of a succession of different generations of cells; the most primitive germ cells, the spermatogonia, rest on the basal lamina, and the more differentiated cells are found at successively higher levels. In mammals, the cells of different stages are grouped in combinations of fixed composition, termed *cellular associations*. In any given area of the seminiferous epithelium, these cell associations appear in a fixed sequence, which repeats itself in time, and each cell association may be considered as a stage of a cyclic process,

called 'cycle of the seminiferous epithelium'. This cycle was defined as 'a complete series of cellular associations appearing successively in any one area of a seminiferous tubule' (Clermont 1966b). Various cytological and histological criteria can be used to identify and classify the typical cell associations. According to Clermont (1963), six well-defined stages can be recognized in man (Figure 7). These stages, however, are partly obscured by irregularities, leading to an apparently disordered arrangement of the various generations of a germ cell. One irregularity is caused by the fact that each stage occupies only small areas of the seminiferous tubule, so that more than one cell association may be seen in a cross-section of the tubule. Thus, the zones where cells can intermix are much more numerous than in other mammalian species, in which a tubular cross-section usually shows a single cell association (Heller and Clermont 1964).

Furthermore, one or two generations of germ cells can be absent from a given cell association. These, and possibly other irregularities, overshadow the actual organization of cell associations in man; however, man is not fundamentally different from other mammals, and the existence of a cycle of the seminiferous epithelium is now well established. The six typical associations are shown in Figure 7. The duration of the cycle of the seminiferous epithelium in man was estimated, using locally injected (^{3}H)-thymidine and radioautography (Heller and Clermont 1963, 1964), to be close to 16 days. The whole spermatogenesis in the adult extends over 4.6 cycles for a total of about 74 days.

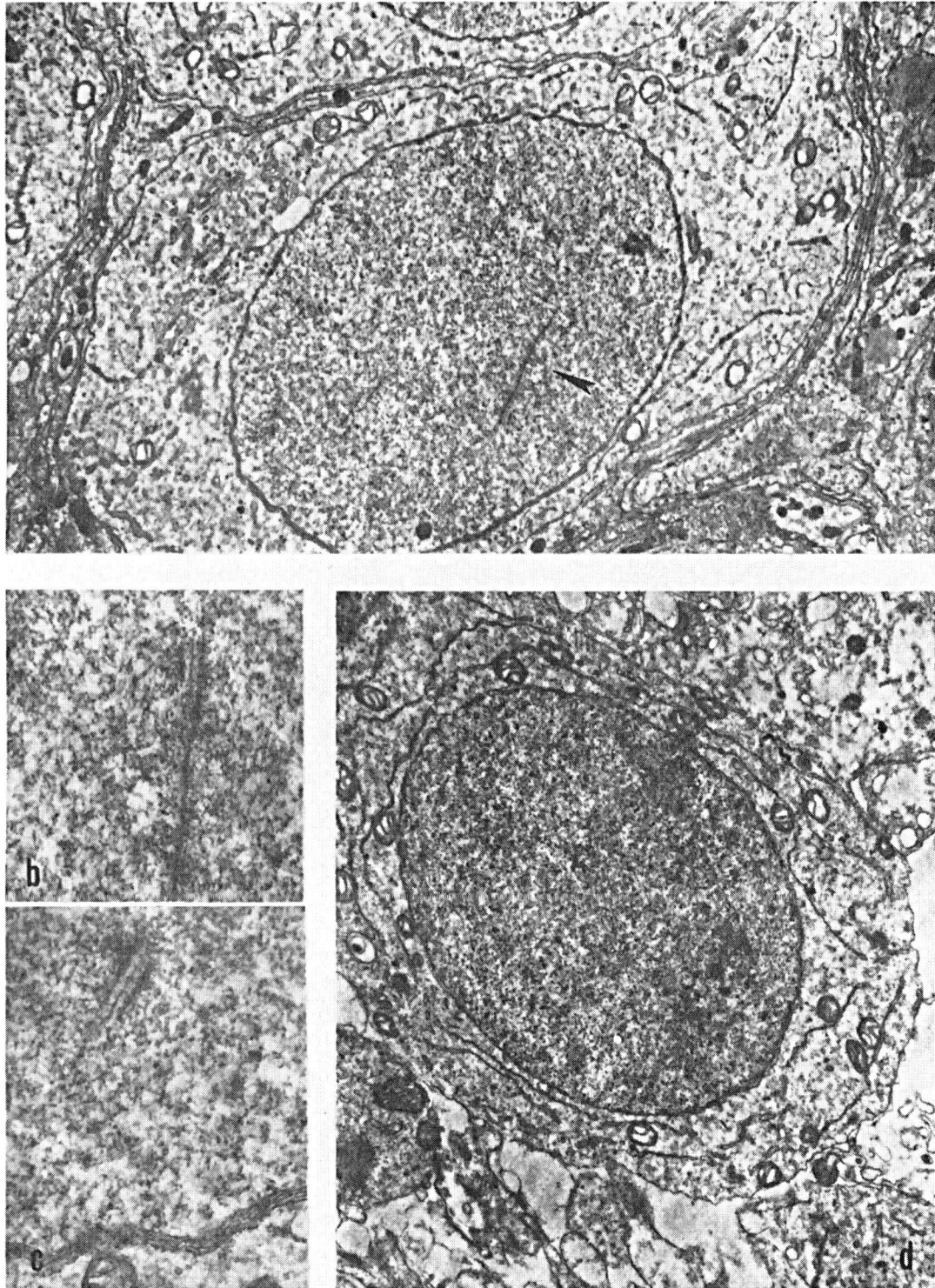

Figure 6. (a) Primary spermatocyte. In the nucleus. a synaptinemal complex (arrow) is visible (× 8,800). (b) Synaptinemal complex (× 24,000). (c) Synaptinemal complex (× 24,000). (d) Secondary spermatocyte (× 12,000).

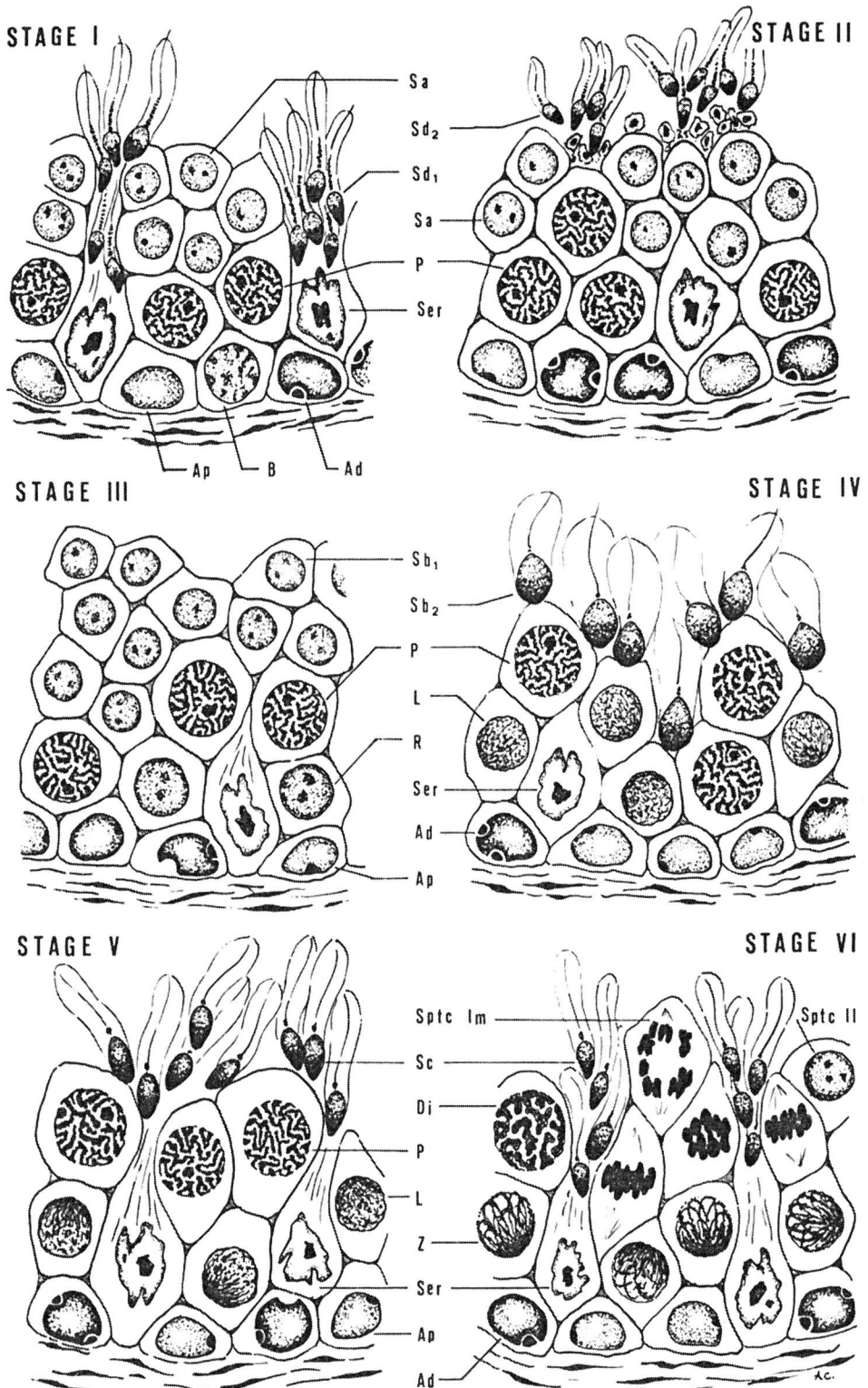

Figure 7. This six 'cellular associations' in the human seminiferous epithelium. These cell associations correspond to the stages of the cycle of the seminiferous epithelium. Legends: Ser: Sertoli nuclei; Ad and Ap: dark and pale type-A spermatogonia; B: type-B spermatogonia; R: resting (or preleptotene) primary spermatocytes; L: leptotene spermatocytes; Z: zygotene spermatocytes; P: pachytene spermatocytes; Di: diplotene spermatocytes; Sptc Im: primary spermatocytes in division; Sptc II: secondary spermatocytes in interphase; Sa, Sb1, Sb2, Sc, Sd1, Sd2: spermatids at various steps of spermiogenesis. (Courtesy of C.G. Heller and Y. Clermont.)

5. CONCLUSIONS

The various types of spermatogonia and spermatocytes are described on the basis of ultrastructural observations of their subcellular characteristics. A comparison was made of the data collected by electron microscopy and those obtained by light microscopy, and the classification used in previous works has been retained, with the exception of the AL type, which was not identified using light microscopy. However, in consideration of the cellular association, an ultrastructural analysis is not useful, and observations should be made on histological sections. The use of autoradiographic analyses of testicular biopsies from human volunteers allowed determination of the duration of the cycle of the seminiferous epithelium and the whole spermatogenesis in man.

ACKNOWLEDGEMENTS

The author thanks the staff of the electron microscopy laboratory for their technical assistance and Dr. A. Ceresa for the drawings. The research was supported by the Consiglio Nazionale delle Ricerche project 'Biology of Reproduction'.

REFERENCES

André J: Contribution à la connaissance du chondriome. J Ultrastruct Res, Suppl 3, 1962.

Barham SS, Berlin JD: Fine structure and cytochemistry of testicular cells in men treated with testosterone propionate. Cell Tiss Res 148: 159-182, 1974.

Bustos-Obregón E, Courot M, Flechon JE, Hochereau de Reviers M-T, Holstein AF: Morphological appraisal of gametogenetic process in mammals with particular reference to man. Andrologia 7(2): 141-163, 1975.

Camatini M, Faleri M, Franchi E: Testicular biopsy of secretory azoospermia: electron and light microscopic analysis. Arch Androl 1: 281-289, 1978.

Castellani L, Chiara F, Cotelli F: Fine structure and cytochemistry of the morphogenesis of round-headed human sperm. Arch Androl 1: 291-297, 1978.

Clermont Y: The cycle of the seminiferous epithelium in man. Am J Anat 112: 35-52, 1963.

Clermont Y: Spermatogenesis in man: a study of the spermatogonial population. Fertil Steril 17: 705-721, 1966a.

Clermont Y: Renewal of spermatogonia in man. Am J Anat 118: 509-524, 1966b.

Clermont Y: Dynamics of human spermatogenesis. In: The human testis. Rosemberg E, Paulsen CA (eds), New York, Plenum, 1970, p 47-61.

Cotelli F, Della Morte E, Gambacorta M: Aspetti ultrastrutturali atipici della azoospermie. Cong Soc Ital Urol 49, 1976.

Fawcett DW: The fine structure of chromosomes in the meiotic prophase of vertebrate spermatocytes. J Biophys Biochem Cytol 2(4): 403-406, 1956.

Heller CG, Clermont Y: Spermatogenesis in man: an estimate of its duration. Science 140: 184-185, 1963.

Heller GC, Clermont Y: Kinetics of the germinal epithelium in man. Recent Progr Hormone Res 20: 545-575, 1964.

Leblond CP, Clermont Y: Definition of the stages of the cycle of the seminiferous epithelium in the rat. Ann NY Acad Sci 55: 548-573, 1952.

Leblond CP, Steinberger E, Roosen-Runge EC: Spermatogenesis. In: Mechanisms concerned with conception, Hartman CG (ed), Oxford, Pergamon, 1963.

Lubarsch O: Über das Vorkommen krystallinischer und krystalloider Bildungen in den Zellen des menschlichen Hodens. Virchows Arch Path Anat 145: 316-338, 1896.

Mancini RE, Narbaitz R, Lavieri JC: Origin and development of the germinative epithelium and Sertoli cells in the human testis: cytological, cytochemical, and quantitative study. Anat Rec 136: 477-489, 1960.

Moses MJ: Synaptinemal complex. Ann Rev Genet 2: 363-412, 1968.

Nagano T: The crystalloid of Lubarsch in the human spermatogonium. Cell Tiss Res 97: 491-501, 1969.

Ohno S: Morphological aspects of meiosis and their genetical significance. In: The human testis, Rosemberg E, Paulsen CA (eds), New York, Plenum, 1970, p 115-125.

Roosen-Runge EC: The process of spermatogenesis in mammals. Biol Rev 37: 343-377, 1962.

Roosen-Runge EC, Barlow FD: Quantitative studies on human spermatogenesis I: spermatogonia. Am J Anat 93: 143, 1953.

Rowley MJ, Berlin JD, Heller CG: The ultrastructure of four types of human spermatogonia. Cell Tiss Res 112: 139-157, 1971.

Solari AJ, Tres LL: Ultrastructure and histochemistry of the nucleus during male meiotic prophase. In: The human testis, Rosemberg E, Paulsen CA (eds), New York, Plenum, 1970, p 127-137.

Tobias PV: Chromosomes, sex-cells and evolution in a mammal, London, Percy, Lund, Humphries, 1956.

Tres LL, Solari AJ: The ultrastructure of the nuclei and the behaviour of the sex chromosomes of human spermatogonia. Cell Tiss Res 91: 75-89, 1968.

Vilar O: Spermatogenesis. In: Human reproduction: conception and contraception, Hafez ESE, Evans TN (eds), New York, Harper and Row, 1973, p 12-37.

Vilar O, Paulsen CA, Moore DJ: Electron microscopy of the human seminiferous tubules. In: The human testis. Rosemberg E, Paulsen CA (eds), New York, Plenum, 1970, p 63-74.

Wartenberg H: Comparative cytomorphologic aspects of the male germ cells, especially of the 'gonia'. Andrologia 8(2): 117-130, 1976.

Westergaard M, Wettstein D von: The synaptinemal complex. Ann Rev Genet 6: 71-108, 1972.

4. ULTRASTRUCTURE OF SPERMIOGENESIS IN NORMAL AND PATHOLOGICAL TESTIS

MARINA CAMATINI

1. SPERMIOGENESIS IN THE HUMAN SEMINIFEROUS TUBULE

The spermatids which derive from the division of the secondary spermatocytes undergo a complex morphogenetic process. The newly formed spermatids have a centrally located spherical nucleus with a well-developed Golgi zone nearby, numerous mitochondria, and a pair of centrioles. Spermiogenesis involves marked differentiation of all these cellular structures. The cytological changes of human spermatids have been examined and described in numerous light and electron microscopic publications (Fawcett and Burgos 1956, Schultz-Larsen 1958, Horstmann 1961, Roosen-Runge 1962, Clermont 1963, Heller and Clermont 1964, Fawcett 1965, De Kretser 1969, Pedersen 1969, Burgos et al. 1970, Vilar et al. 1970, Vilar 1970, Horstmann 1970, Pedersen 1972, Pedersen 1974) and an impressive amount of work has been done in this field. This review of human spermiogenesis aims to follow the cellular components during their morphological changes at ultrastructural level, starting from their initial constitution and continuing through to the mature form. Since the current terminology concerns individual aspects of the cell, then in this chapter the sequence of events will be considered in subsequent sections each of which will follow the morphogenesis of the individual components: the acrosome, the nucleus, and the tail.

1.1. The acrosome

The Golgi apparatus, next to the nucleus, appears well organized and is associated with numerous vesicles, containing small granules responsive to Schiff periodic acid staining (PAS) and frequently referred to as proacrosomic vesicles (Figure 1a, b). The Golgi apparatus is the most evident working system of this period, which is known as the 'Golgi phase'. The vesicles coalesce in a progressively larger structure to form the acrosomal vesicle (Figure 1c); the granular material gathers in a zone adhering to the inner surface of the vesicle while the remaining area appears electron transparent. The precision of the underlying mechanism, responsible for the specialization of that region of the nuclear membrane subjacent to the acrosomal vesicle, is the starting point for the subsequent extension of the vesicle over the nucleus (Figure 2a, b). It is not clear whether the specialization of the membrane results from an interaction between the nucleus and the Golgi apparatus, or whether it is an independent event controlled by the nucleus. The position of the acrosome establishes the anterior pole of the spermatid. The acrosomal vesicle becomes progressively flattened and expands over the anterior two-thirds of the nucleus. The shaping of the acrosome is not dependent upon externally-applied forces (Fawcett et al. 1971) and its morphogenesis apparently depends upon intrinsic factors. The acrosomal material becomes distributed in a uniform manner and at the end of this process the flattened vesicle, filled with the homogeneous electron-dense material, covers the anterior half of the ovoid nucleus (Figure 2b). The cytoplasm between the acrosome and the cell membrane shifts caudally and also the Golgi apparatus leaves the surface of the acrosome and moves back. The outer membrane of the acrosomal cap comes into contact with the inner layer of the plasma membrane. After the acrosomal cap is fully formed, there is a reorientation of the anterior pole of the nucleus toward the base of the seminiferous tubule; elongation and condensation of the nucleus itself occur (Figure 2c, d). The freeze-fracture technique usefully illustrates the sequence of these events (Figure 3).

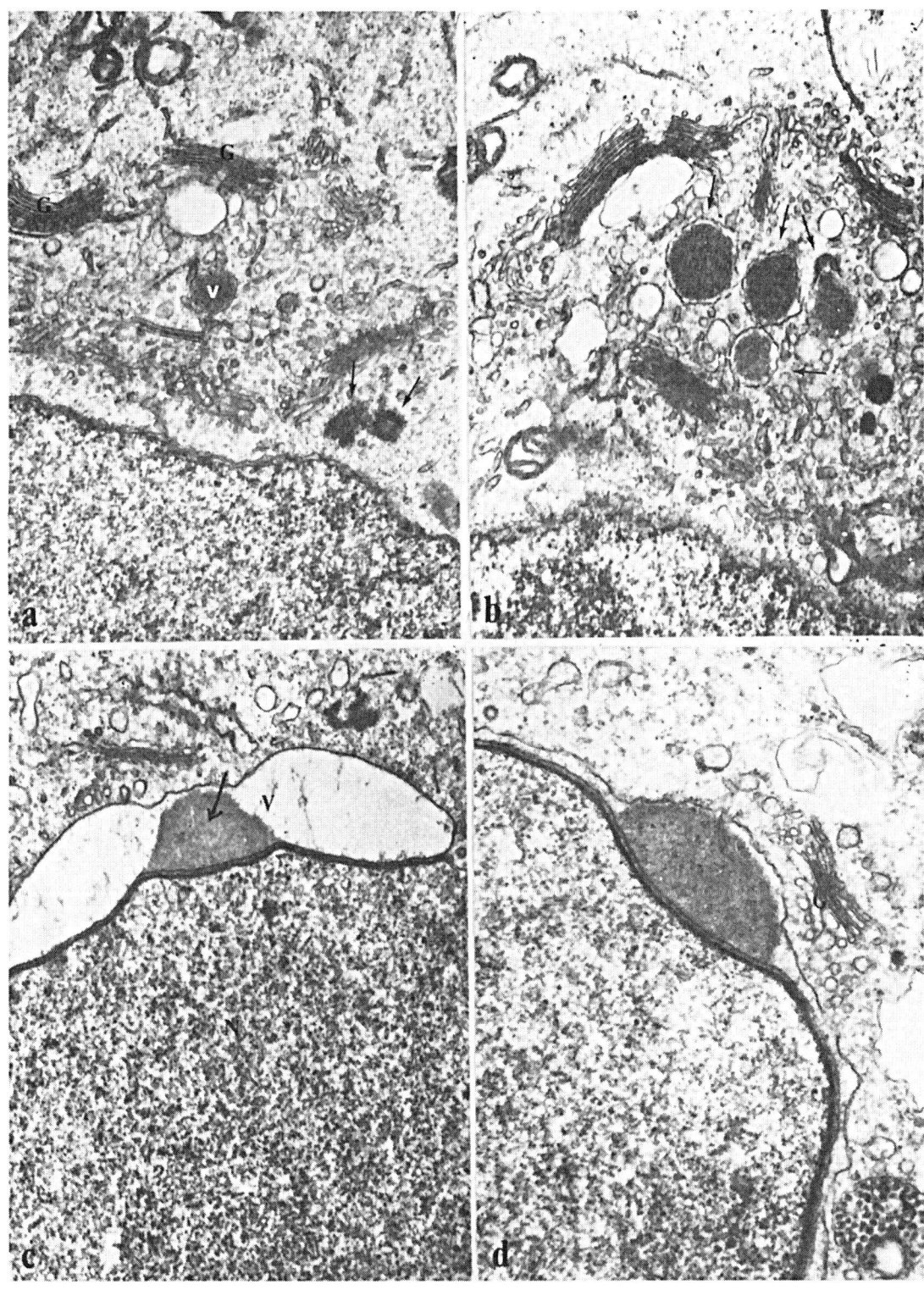

Figure 1. Successive stages of acrosomal vesicle formation. (a) Golgi phase: Googi apparatus (G) and proacrosomal vesicles (V) are evident; the pair of centrioles (arrows) lies near the Golgi complex (× 22,000). (b) Golgi phase: proacrosomal granules (arrows) are enclosed in vesicles (× 22,000). (c) Cap phase: the acrosomal vesicle (V), derived by the fusion of small vesicles, covers one pole of the nucleus (N); granular content is arrowed (× 16,000). (d) Cap phase: the acrosome has extended over the nucleus, while the Golgi apparatus (G) appears reduced (× 22,000).

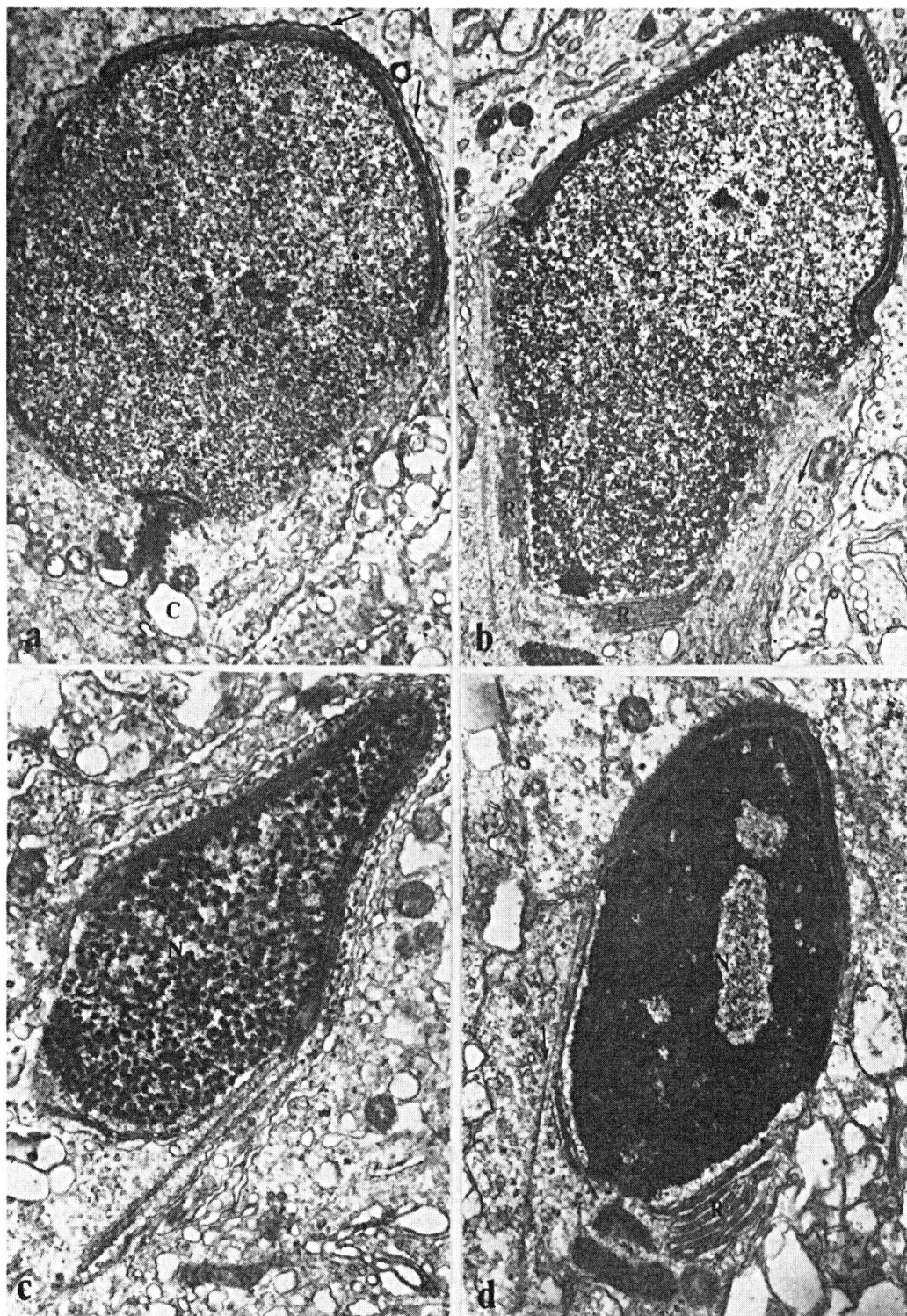

Figure 2. Shaping of the head. (a) Beginning of spermatid elongation: caudal displacement of cytoplasm brings the plasma membrane into close apposition to the acrosomal cap (arrows); the flagellar channel (C) is forming (× 15,000).

(b) With the completion of acrosomal cap (A), nuclear condensation begins; Microtubules (arrows) appear tangential to the caudal portion of the nucleus; R = redundant nuclear membranes (× 15,000). (c) The nucleus (N) changes shape and increases condensation (× 15,000). (d) Aspect of the head of a late spermatid: N = nucleus; arrows = microtubules; R = redundant nuclear membranes (× 15,000).

1.2. The nucleus

The oval nucleus of the early spermatid is characterized by a moderate electron-dense karyoplasm and occupies a central position. Its movement to an eccentric position takes place at the same time as the spreading of the acrosome cap over its anterior pole. The chromatin undergoes extensive reorganization, while the nucleus takes on the characteristic shape. A ring of microtubules (manchette microtubules) polymerize in the cytoplasm surrounding the nucleus; they start from the zone subjacent the posterior acrosomal cap and extend into the postnuclear cytoplasm (Figure 2b, c). During this process, spermatid elongation proceeds, and chromatin condenses in granular masses (Figure 2c) which coalesce to form a homogeneous electron-dense mass (Figure 4a). The relation between chromatin condensation and chromosomes remains unknown. These changes in nuclear shape, volume and position have been clearly described in the studies of Clermont (1963), Horstmann (1961), Fawcett (1971) and De Kretser (1969). The nuclear volume is markedly reduced and the head, during the elongation process, becomes firstly pear-shaped, then flattened in a plane parallel to the long axis of the cell. According to some researchers the microtubules are involved in the shaping of the nucleus and represent the extrinsic factors responsible for the final shape of the head. This assertion is difficult to demonstrate, as there is a great diversity in specific shape both of mammalian sperm head and in human sperm. Abnormalities in head development are frequent, and the manchette is always present with the same arrangement. The manchette participates in spermatid elongation with transport of cytoplasm to the caudal region of the cell, and this is its demonstrated function and direct involvement. The nuclear envelope collapses and in the caudal region exhibits considerable folding, where it is termed the 'redundant nuclear membranes' (Figure 2d) and contains nuclear pores. This sequence corresponds to the chromatin condensation in a fully compact form, with the extrusion of portions of nuclear membrane with the transparent content of the nucleus.

The acrosome and the nucleus form the head of the spermatid (Figure 3d; Figure 4a and 7). The nucleus contains the haploid genoma and presents a compact aspect, except in the apical and basal region where electron-transparent areas are present. Between the nucleus and the acrosome (anterior segment) there is a thin space filled with electron-dense substance which also surrounds the terminal portion of the nucleus (equatorial segment), covered only by the plasma membrane.

1.3. The axial filament

The early spermatid possesses a pair of centrioles, which lie at right angles to each other close to the Golgi complex (Figure 1a). The centrioles migrate to the opposite pole (Figure 2a) during the cap phase of acrosome formation, so that the still round spermatid exhibits the adluminal pole of the nucleus covered by the acrosomal cap and the opposite area with a small infolding of the nuclear envelope, where the centrioles migrated. The centriole oriented parallel to the longitudinal axis of the spermatid constitutes the basal body of the flagellum and is termed the distal centriole; the perpendicular one is referred to as the proximal centriole, which occupies a groove in the caudal nuclear envelope called the 'implantation fossa' (Figure 2a; Figure 4a, b). A thickness of the outer nuclear membrane is present in this region and is called the 'basal plate'. The longitudinal centriole gives rise to the axial filament, which develops within the spermatid cytoplasm (Figure 5b). The distal centriole disappears during spermiogenesis; the proximal centriole persists in the mature sperm.

A portion of the axial filament projects from the cell surface, covered by a layer of cytoplasm and by the plasma membrane, and is therefore situated in a cylindrical cytoplasmic channel, the 'flagellar canal', which anteriorly is delimited by the invaginated sleeves of the cell membrane at the annulus (Figure 5a, b). This structure is formed by dense material, which extends to the inner surface of the plasma membrane. The outer dense fibers have began to develop in the flagellum along the outer aspect of each doublet of the axoneme (Figure 5a; Figure 4c). Meanwhile the circumferential elements of the fibrous sheet appear in the portion of the flagellum distal to the flagellar canal. In close opposition to the centrioles the striated columns form; at this time the neck region has differentiated (Figure 4b).

During tail elongation, in the cylindrical cytoplasmic channel, distal to the annulus, an enlarged cytoplasmic area appears (Figure 6). This area,

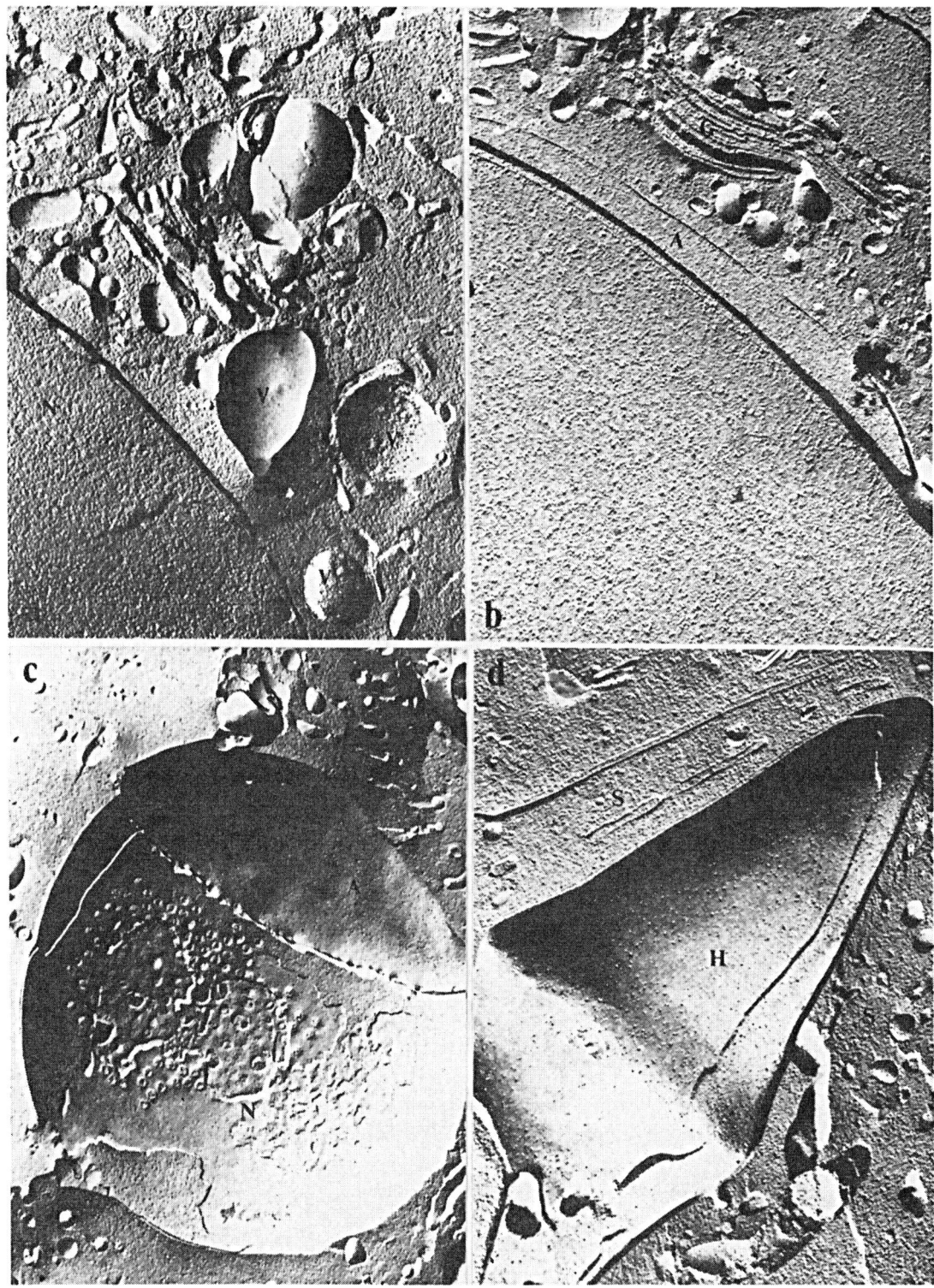

Figure 3. Freeze-fracture aspect of human spermiogenesis. (a) Golgi phase: N = nucleus; V = acrosomal vesicle (× 33,000). (b) Acrosomal cap formation (A); G = Golgi apparatus (× 31,000). (c) Early spermatid: A = acrosome; N = nucleus (× 15,000). (d) Late spermatid: H = head; S = Sertoli cell (× 31,000).

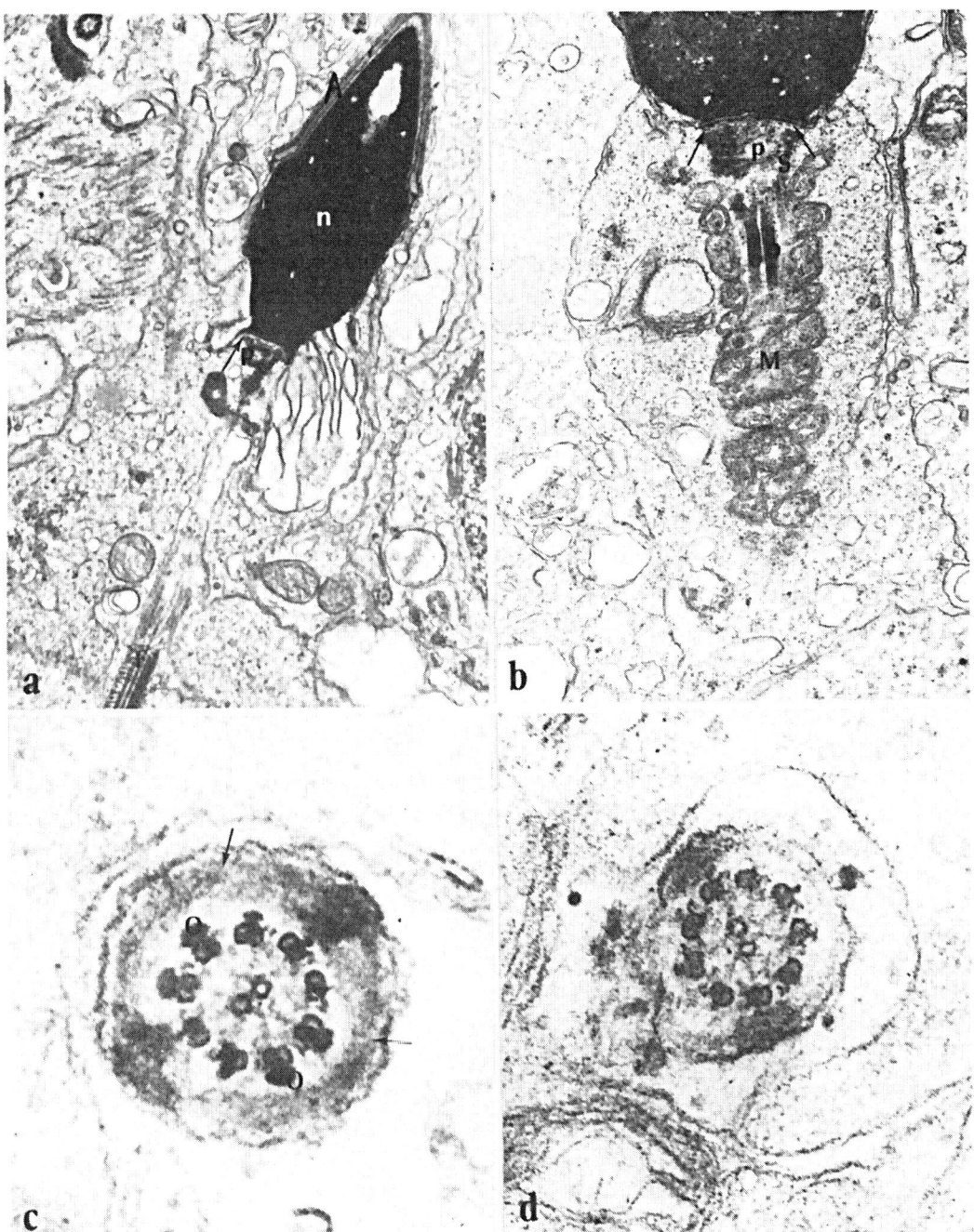

Figure 4. (a) Longitudinal section of a late spermatid: n = nucleus; A = acrosome; F = flagellum; arrow: basal plate;
p = proximal centriole (× 12,000). (b) Neck region: arrows = basal plate; p = proximal centriole; S = striated columns;
o = outer fibers; M = mitochondrial sheet (× 20,000). (c) Transverse section of the distal portion of the principal piece:
the outer fibers (0) are evident; arrows = fibrous sheet (× 96,000). (d) Transverse section through the end piece (× 95,000).

surrounding the periphery of the doublets, is filled
with helically arranged microtubules (Figure 5c)
which constitute the 'spindle-shaped body'. Some
authors (Wartenberg and Holstein 1975) suggest
some functional connection between this structure
and the formation of the fibrous sheet, while others

(Fawcett and Phillips 1969a) do not see any micro-
tubular structure proximal to the fibrous sheet. This
structure migrates distally and disappears, while the
annulus moves caudally and the mitochondria arrange themselves around the axoneme to form the
mitochondrial helix of the middle piece (De Kretser

1969, Wartemberg and Holstein 1975, Bustos-Obregón 1975) (Figure 6, late spermatid; Figure 5d).

So the developed tail is constituted of: *the neck
region*, characterized by the basal plate, the implantation fossa with the proximal centriole, and the
connecting piece constituted of nine cross-striated
columns derived from the distal centriole (Fawcett
1970); *the middle piece* comprising the proximal
portion of the axoneme, surrounded by the mitochondrial sheet, and the annulus, demarcating this
region from *the principal piece*, the intermediate
portion of the flagellum, enwrapped by the fibrous
sheet; and *the end piece*, the short distal portions
comprising the doublets surrounded only by the
plasma membrane.

2. SPERMIATION

The entire process of spermatid differentiation takes
place in the recesses of Sertoli cells. During the
course of spermiogenesis there occurs a changing
relationship between the developing spermatids and
the Sertoli cells. The young spermatids are placed
along the lateral aspect of the cells, while the mature
spermatids occupy the luminal position (Figure 7).
Sertoli-spermatid junctional specializations are
established during the earliest stages of spermiogenesis, and are characterized by grouped thin
filaments underlined by a single fenestrated cisterna
of smooth endoplasmic reticulum (Fawcett 1970,
Dym and Fawcett 1970, Ross 1976). The cytoplasmic processes of Sertoli cells with these specializations conform to the morphogenesis of the sperm
head and are maintained to the end of the maturation phase. During the last developmental period the
spermatids are displaced towards the lumen (Figure
7). The mechanism responsible for the release of
sperm is not well known. It has been studied in
numerous mammals (Ross 1976, Sapsford 1969,
Fawcett and Phillips 1969b, Fouquet 1974) and it
involves two separate events. The first step is the
extrusion of the head from the Sertoli cells. The
Sertoli cell filaments contain actin (Toyama 1976)
and are possibly involved in the release phenomenon. It has been demonstrated that the lack of these
filaments and of smooth endoplasmic reticulum in
the ectoplasmic Sertoli cell regions results in a
retention of the spermatids (Dym and Madhwa Raj
1977). Following the sperm head release, complete
disengagement from the epithelium involves the

separation of the thin stalk connecting the neck
region of the spermatid to its residual body. The
residual bodies are retained within the tubule wall by
Sertoli cell processes (Fawcett and Phillips 1969b).

3. SPERMIOGENESIS DEFECTS IN PATHOLOG-
ICAL HUMAN TESTIS

Malformations of spermatozoa are frequent in man
and defects of spermiogenesis within a relatively
narrow range are described for normal fertile men.
These abnormalities do not affect fertility when they
occur occasionally.

Testicular biopsy of infertile patients may reveal
developmental anomalies of one component of the
sperm cell, i.e. the acrosome, the nucleus or the tail
(Holstein 1975). Morphological aberrations may be
primarily founded early in spermatogenesis, e.g. by
the genetic constitution, or they may be acquired
later during sperm maturation.

3.1. Acrosomal malformations

Reports on acrosomal malformations (Holstein et
al. 1973, Holstein 1976, Matano 1971, Camatini,
Franchi and Faleri 1978, Camatini, Chiara et al.
1978) indicate that developmental anomalies are
extremely frequent and appear during the Golgi
phase (Camatini, Franchi and Faleri 1978, Camatini, Chiara et al. 1978, Camatini et al. 1979). The
abnormalities may have several patterns: the most
frequent are aberrant vesicles, which extend over the
nucleus to form deformed head caps (Figure 6). Also
frequent are multinucleated spermatids, which show
the same acrosome (Figure 6). The acrosomal vesicle
is also frequent in young spermatids, giving rise to
'round-headed sperm' (Holstein et al. 1973, Schirren
et al. 1971, Baccetti et al. 1977 and Chapter 3 of this
volume). Further development of the vesicle does
not take place and it has been suggested that when
sperm are released into the tubule, the vesicle is left
behind and digested by the Sertoli cells.

3.2. Abnormal morphogenesis of the nucleus

Normally spermatids equipped with distorted acrosomal cap give rise to sperm with abnormal head
morphology (Figure 6). The apical area of the
nucleus, surrounded by distorted cap, adapts to the

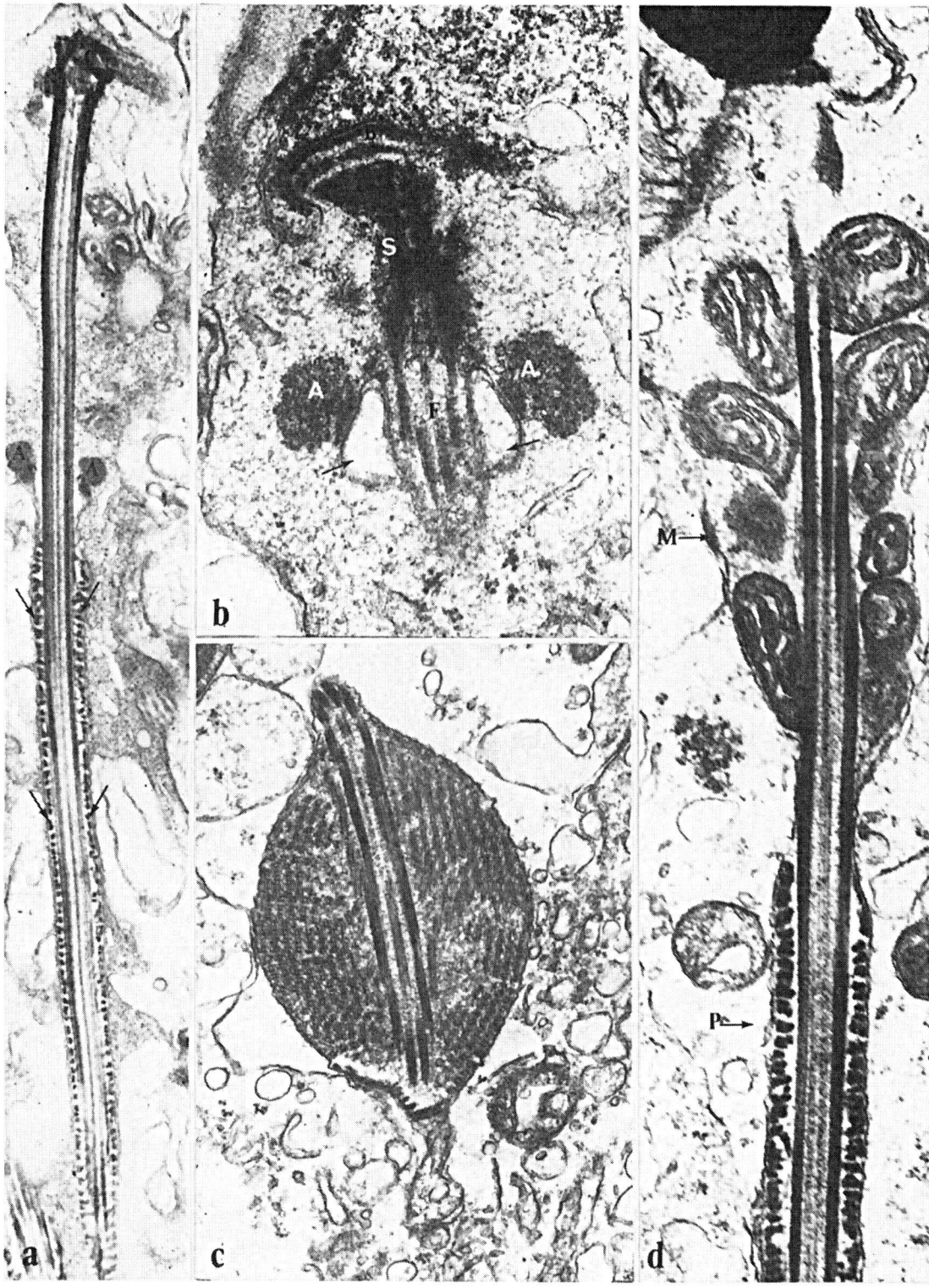

Figure 5. Axial filament formation in longitudinal section. (a) The flagellum has lengthened and fibrous sheet (arrowed) is present around the axoneme: A = annulus; C = proximal centriole; S = striated columns (× 17,000). (b) Implantation fossa: B = basal plate; F = flagellum; S = striated columns; A = annulus; arrow = flagellar channel (× 47,000). (c) Spindle-shaped body with helically-arranged microtubules (× 36,000). (d) Aspect of the middle (M) piece and principal (P) piece (× 39,000).

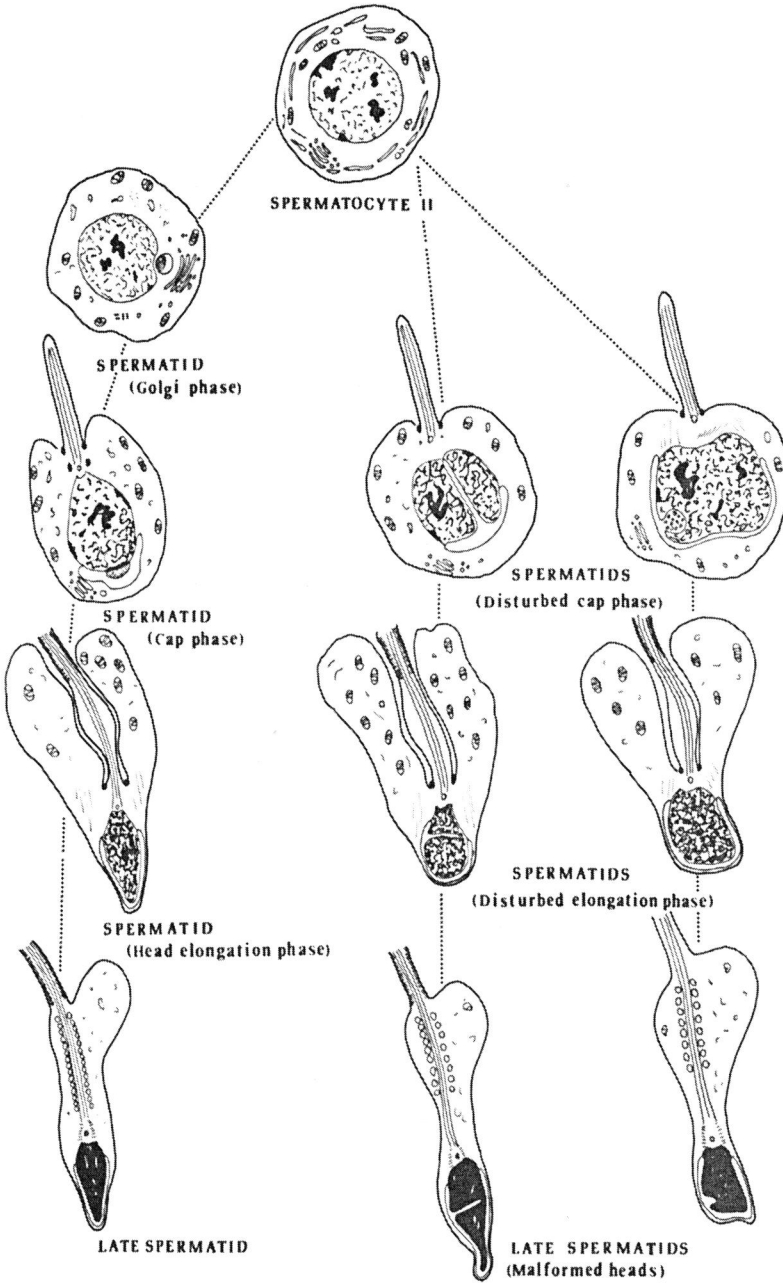

Figure 6. Differentiation of human spermatids in normal and pathological forms. The most common abnormal aspects during the morphogenesis of the head are illustrated in the centre and at right of the figure. These aspects may be compared with the normal morphogenesis, at left of the figure.

same deformation. Chromatin condensation in these cases proceeds in a normal manner, but even the completion of this process may be delayed.

The presence of coarse chromatin indicating immaturity affects fertility (Ross et al. 1973, Lacy et al. 1974). This defect has been frequently described and corresponds to an arrest in chromatin conden-

sation during the morphogenesis of the nucleus. The appearance of the manchette microtubules does not differ significantly from normal spermatids in these cases, thus confirming that the sperm head is largely determined by genetically controlled proteins and DNA aggregation during chromatin condensation.

The spermiogenesis of round-headed sperm re-

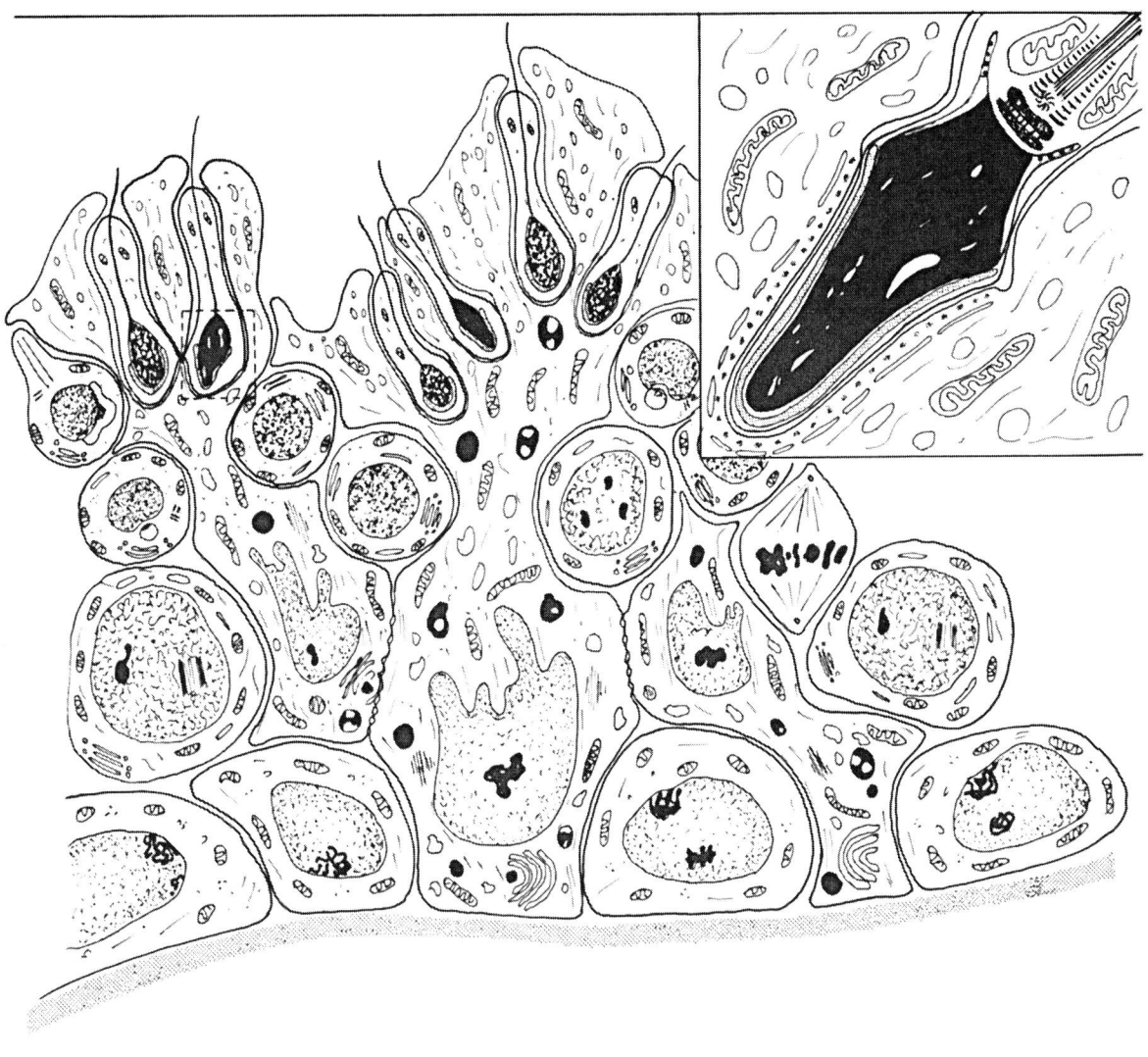

Figure 7. The processes of spermatogenesis, spermiogenesis and spermiation in a segment of a human seminiferous tubule. Spermatogonia occupy a basal compartment below the occluding junctions between Sertoli cells. Spermatocytes and early spermatids occupy deep niches of the supporting cells. Late spermatids are placed in apical recesses. *Inset:* relationship between the head of a late spermatid and the surrounding Sertoli cell (redrawn from Leeson and Leeson 1970).

veals the presence of disordered bundles of microtubules around the nucleus which tend to maintain the nucleus in the shape which it has in early spermatids (see Chapter 3). The formation of multinucleated spermatids has been described in men treated with testosterone and they could be formed by enlargement of the cytoplasmic bridges known to connect large numbers of developing sperm cells (Dym and Fawcett 1970).

3.3. Abnormal tail formation

Specific tail defects from subfertile men, presenting, for example, a middle piece with abnormal morphology and loss or excess of the outer sheath of fibers, have been described (Ross et al. 1973, Ross et al. 1971, Pedersen et al. 1971).

It has been demonstrated that these abnormalities are present during the maturation of sperm within the seminiferous tubules. The most striking abnormality, first described by Afzelius et al. (1975)

and Pedersen and Rebbe (1975) concerns the total immotility of sperm which lack arms on the doublets; the same feature was found in all stages of spermatid formation.

Short-tailed sperm (Baccetti et al. 1975) are characterized by the presence of two abnormal axonemes, with disorganized doublets. The presence of double-tailed sperm has also been described.

It is significant that normally only one component of the early spermatid develops in an abnormal way.

Malformed heads presents normal flagellar ultrastructure and development, and ejaculated sperm with such structure are motile despite the degree of abnormalities of the head.

These observations suggest the idea that the development of the sperm head may be presumed to be under the control of a group of genes distinct from those mediating flagellar development events. Such a view is further substantiated by Hollander (1976).

ACKNOWLEDGEMENTS

I thank the staff of the Comparative Anatomy Laboratory, particularly Dr. E. Franchi for completing the drawings. I am also grateful to Dr. F. Clementi for the use of freeze-fracture apparatus. Research performed under Consiglio Nazionale delle Ricerche project, 'Biology of Reproduction'.

REFERENCES

Afzelius BA, Eliasson R, Johnsen O, Lindholmer C: Lack of dynein arms in immotile human spermatozoa. J Cell Biol 66: 225-232, 1975.
Baccetti B, Burrini A, Pallini V, Renieri T, Rosati F, Menchini-Fabris GF: The short-tailed human spermatozoa: ultrastructural alterations and dynein absence. J Submicr Cytol 7: 349-359, 1975.
Baccetti B, Renieri T, Rosati F, Selmi MG, Casanova S: Further observations on the morphogenesis of the round-headed human spermatozoa. Andrologia 9: 255-264, 1977.
Burgos MH, Vitale-Calpe R, Aoki A: Fine structure of the testis and its functional significance. In: The testis, Johnson AD, Gomes WR, Vandemark NL (eds), New York, Academic Press, 1970, p 551-649.
Bustos-Obregón E, Courot M, Flechon JE, Hochereau de Reviers M-T, Holstein AF: Morphological appraisal of gametogenesis: spermatogenetic process in mammals with particular reference to man. Andrologia 7: 141-163, 1975.
Camatini M, Chiara F, Franchi E, Bellone L: Acrosomal cap abnormalities of spermatids from infertile men. In: Recent progress in andrology, Fabbrini A, Steinberger E (eds), London, Academic Press, 1978, p 402-408.
Camatini M, Franchi E, Faleri M: Ultrastructure of acrosomal malformations in men with obstructive azoospermia. Arch Androl 1: 203-209, 1978.
Camatini M, Franchi E, Faleri M: Ultrastructure of spermiogenesis in men and congenital absence of the vasa deferentia. Arch Androl 3, 93-99, 1979.
Clermont Y: The cycle of the seminiferous epithelium in man. Am J Anat 112: 35-51, 1963.
Dym M, Fawcett DW: The blood-testis barrier in the rat and the physiological compartmentation of seminiferous epithelium. Biol Reprod 3: 308-326, 1970.
Dym M, Madhwa Raj HG: Response of adult rat Sertoli cells and Leydig cells to depletion of luteinizing hormone and testosterone. Biol Reprod 17: 676-696, 1977.
Fawcett DW: The anatomy of the mammalian spermatozoon with particular reference to the guinea pig. Cell Tiss Res 67: 279-296, 1965.

Fawcett DW: A comparative view of sperm ultrastructure. Biol Reprod, suppl 2: 90-127, 1970.
Fawcett DW, Anderson WA, Phillips DM: Morphogenetic factors influencing the shape of the sperm head. Dev Biol 26: 220-251, 1971.
Fawcett DW, Burgos MH: Observations on the cytomorphosis of the germinal and interstitial cells of the human testis. Ciba Found Colloq Ageing 2: 86-99, 1956.
Fawcett DW, Leak LV, Heideger Jr PM: Electron microscopic observations on the structural components of the blood-testis barrier. J Reprod Fertil, suppl 10: 105-122, 1970.
Fawcett DW, Phillips DM: Fine structure and development of the neck region of the mammalian spermatozoon. Anat Rec 165: 153-184, 1969a.
Fawcett DW, Phillips DM: Observations on the release of spermatozoa and on changes in the head during passage through the epididymis. J Reprod Fertil, suppl 6: 405-418, 1969b.
Fouquet JP: La spermiation et la formation des corps résidus chez le hamster: rôle des cellules de Sertoli. J Microscopie 19: 161-168, 1974.
De Kretser DM: Ultrastructural features of human spermiogenesis. Cell Tiss Res 94: 477-505, 1969.
Heller CG, Clermont Y: Kinetics of the germinal epithelium in man. Recent Progr Hormone Res 20: 545-575, 1964.
Hollander WF: Hydrocefalic-polydactyl, a recessive pleiotropic mutant in the mouse and its location in chromosome 6. Iowa St J Res 51: 13-23, 1976.
Holstein AF: Morphologische Studien an abnormen Spermatiden und Spermatozoen des Menschen. Virschows Arch Path Anat 367: 93-112, 1975.
Holstein AF: Ultrastructural observations on the differentiation of spermatids in man. Andrologia 8: 157-165, 1976.
Holstein AF, Schirren C, Schirren CG: Human spermatids and spermatozoa lacking acrosomes. J Reprod Fertil 35: 489-491, 1973.
Horstmann E: Elektronmikroskopische Untersuchungen zur Spermiogenese beim Menschen. Cell Tiss Res 54: 68-89, 1961.
Horstmann E: Structure of caryoplasm during the differentiation of spermatids. In: Morphological aspects of andrology, Berlin, Grosse, 1970, p 24-28.

Lacy D. Pettit AJ, Pettit JM, Martin BS: Application of scanning electron microscopy to semen analysis of the sub-fertile man utilising data obtained by transmission electron microscopy as an aid to interpretation. Micron 5: 135-173, 1974.

Leeson TS, Leeson CR: Histology. 2nd ed. Philadelphia, Saunders Company, 1970, p 450.

Matano Y: Ultrastructural study on human binucleate spermatids. J Ultrastruct Res 34: 123-134, 1971.

Pedersen H: Ultrastructure of the ejaculate human sperm. Cell Tiss Res 94: 542-554, 1969.

Pedersen H: Further observations on the fine structure of the human spermatozoon. Cell Tiss Res 123: 305-315, 1972.

Pedersen H: The human spermatozoon. Danish Med Bull 21 (suppl 1), 1974.

Pedersen H, Rebbe H: Absence of arms in the axoneme of immotile human spermatozoa. Biol Reprod 12: 541-544, 1975.

Pedersen H, Rebbe H, Hammen R: Human sperm fine structure in a case of severe asthenospermia-necrospermia. Fertil Steril 22: 156-167, 1971.

Roosen-Runge EC: The process of spermatogenesis in mammals. Biol Rev 37: 343-377, 1962.

Ross A, Christie S, Edmond P: Ultrastructural tail defects in the spermatozoa from two men attending a subfertility clinic. J Reprod Fert 32: 243-251, 1973.

Ross A, Christie S, Kerr MG: An electron microscope study of a tail abnormality in spermatozoa from a subfertile man. J Reprod Fertil 24: 99-103, 1971.

Ross MH: The Sertoli cell junctional specialization during spermiogenesis and spermiation. Anat Rec 186: 79-104, 1976.

Sapsford CS, Clare AR, Cleland KW: Ultrastructural studies on maturing spermatids and on Sertoli cells in the bandicoot *Perameles nasuta* Geoffroy (Marsupialia). Aust J Zool 17: 195-292, 1969.

Schirren CG, Holstein AF, Schirren C: Über die Morphogenese rundköpfiger Spermatozoen des Menschen. Andrologia 3: 117-125, 1971.

Schultz-Larsen J: The morphology of the human sperm. Acta Path Microbiol Scand, suppl 128, 1958.

Toyama Y: Actin-like filaments in the Sertoli cell junctional specializations in the swine and mouse testis. Anat Rec 186: 477-492, 1976.

Vilar O: Histology of the human testis from neonatal period to adolescence. In: The human testis. Rosemberg E, Paulsen CA (eds). New York, Plenum, 1970, p 95-111.

Vilar O, Paulsen CA, Moore DJ: Electron microscopy of the human seminiferous tubules. In: The human testis. Rosemberg E, Paulsen CA (eds). New York, Plenum, 1970, p 63-74.

Wartemberg H, Holstein AF: Morphology of the 'spindle-shaped body' in the developing tail of human spermatids. Cell Tiss Res 159: 435-443, 1975.

5. ACROSOMAL FORMATION AND MALFORMATION

Shirley Siew, Philip Troen and Howard R. Nankin

1. SIGNIFICANCE OF THE ACROSOME

The acrosome is a highly specialized membrane-enclosed, subcellular organelle, which is unique to the male reproductive system. Its nomenclature is derived from the Greek *akron* - extremity, top or summit - and *soma* - body - as it is normally situated at the anterior extremity, top or summit of the spermatozoon, where it occupies the space between the plasmalemma and the nuclear envelope. The inner acrosomal membrane is in juxtaposition to the nuclear membrane and the acrosome spreads over the anterior pole of the nucleus to cover it like a cap.

The inception of its formation from the Golgi apparatus of the spermatid ushers in the last phase of spermatogenesis-spermiogenesis. In its further development, it constitutes one of the prominent hallmarks of spermiogenesis and this fact was used by Clermont and Leblond (1955) in their delineation of human spermiogenesis into twelve steps. The acrosome is an essential attribute of the mature spermatozoon, for in its absence, penetration of the ovum cannot take place, as it produces the enzymes that facilitate the movement of the spermatozoon through the extracellular matrix of the cumulus and the corona cells and the penetration of the zona pellucida. However, it is a deciduous structure because in order for its enzymes to be liberated, the bulk of the outer acrosomal membrane and the overlying plasmalemma have to be shed permanently from the cell.

2. HUMAN SPERMIOGENESIS WITH REFERENCE TO THE DEVELOPMENT OF THE NORMAL ACROSOME

The third and final phase of spermatogenesis, spermiogenesis, is concerned with the transforma-tion of the spermatid into the spermatozoon. At the end of the second phase, spermatids are formed as a result of the second maturation division of the secondary spermatocytes. Owing to the incomplete nature of cytokinesis after the early spermatogonial divisions, the spermatids are still connected by intercellular bridges and form clusters of cells in the innermost, adluminal zone of the tubule. Cytoplasmic extensions of the Sertoli cells come into close apposition to the spermatids, leaving an intercellular space of 200-250 Å.

The individual spermatid is a spherical or polygonal cell, measuring 9 μm, which is about half the size of the primary spermatocyte. The spermatid nucleus is comparatively large - 6 μm. It is rounded and is situated in the centre of the cell. The chromatin is pale and finely granular. Like the secondary spermatocyte, the spermatid has a haploid number of chromosomes. In the cytoplasm, the mitochondria are small; they tend to be distributed in a layer close to the cell membrane. Their centres are comparatively electron-lucent due to peripheral margination of the cristae. The Golgi apparatus is prominent: it is situated close to one pole of the nucleus and shows parallel arrays of membranes around the periphery, surrounding an interior mass of vesicles. Between the Golgi and the nucleus, there is a small pair of centrioles (Figure 1).

There is no further cell division after the formation of the spermatid. In order for it to develop into the spermatozoon, it has to undergo a complicated metamorphosis, the basic features of which are the elaboration of a nuclear cap (acrosome) from the Golgi apparatus, alteration in the configuration of the nucleus and condensation of its chromatin, formation of a motile flagellum, and extensive shedding of cytoplasm.

Clermont and Leblond (1955) applied the PA Schiff technique in their light microscopic studies,

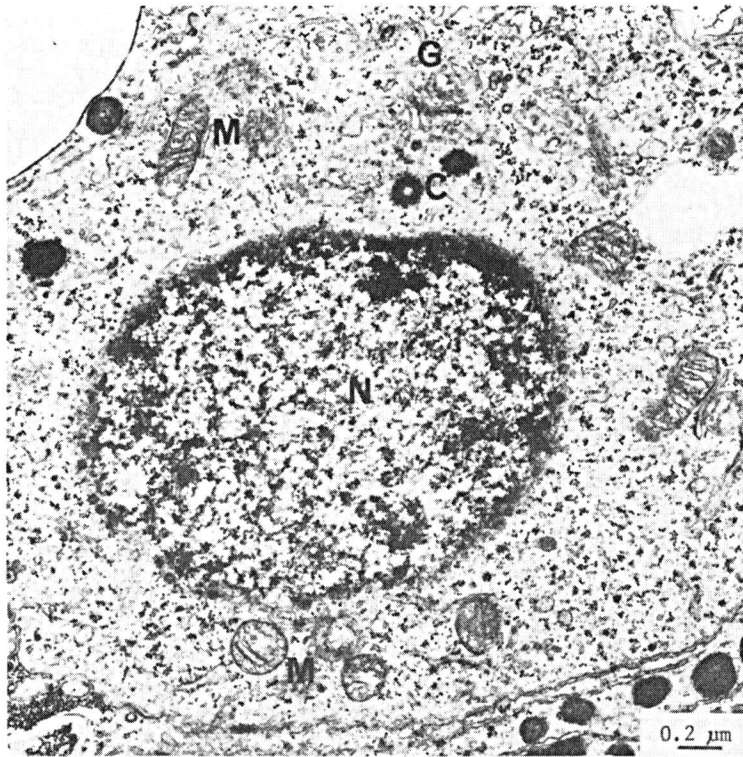

Figure 1. Early stage of spermatid formation. C: centrioles; G: Golgi apparatus; M: mitochondria; N: nucleus.

primarily to demonstrate the acrosome, because of the PA Schiff positivity of its contents. By this means they were able to delineate twelve steps of spermiogenesis, which were divided into three phases:

1. The Golgi phase, during which the acrosomic granule was formed in the Golgi zone (this consisted of the first three steps);

2. The cap phase (steps 4-7) dealing with the formation of the head cap over the nucleus;

3. The acrosomic and maturation phase (steps 8-12).

Clermont (1963) used the morphological changes of the spermatid nucleus to identify the steps of spermiogenesis, which he subdivided into four main groups, *Sa-Sd.* De Kretser (1969) has correlated Clermont's basic light microscopic classifications with transmission electron microscopic findings in order to elucidate the stages of human spermiogenesis at the ultrastructural level.

The first, or *Sa*, stage, corresponds to the Golgi phase. It commences with a localized grouping of the Golgi membranes, often into a concentric configuration, and the development within a series of the vesicles of small proacrosomal granules (Figure 2).

This is followed by the aggregation of the small proacrosomal granules into a single large acrosomal granule which is contained in an acrosomal vesicle (Figure 3). The acrosomal vesicle comes into progressively closer apposition to the pole of the nucleus until the inner acrosome membrane becomes adherent to the outer aspect of the nuclear membrane. This marks the anterior pole of the nucleus. The Golgi apparatus is still in close association with the acrosomal vesicle and continues to contribute small vesicles to it. However, the centrioles leave the acrosomal pole and begin to migrate caudally (Figure 4).

The next stage is the Sb_1 stage. It consists of the cap phase and the acrosomal phase. In the cap phase, the acrosomal granule remains centrally placed, but the acrosomal vesicle spreads over the anterior pole of the nucleus and forms the head cap (Figure 5). Thereafter, in the acrosomal phase, the acrosomal granule spreads into the head cap and fills it. This gives rise to the acrosomal cap, which covers approximately one third of the nucleus (Figure 6). After the formation of the acrosomal cap has been completed, the Golgi leaves the anterior pole of the

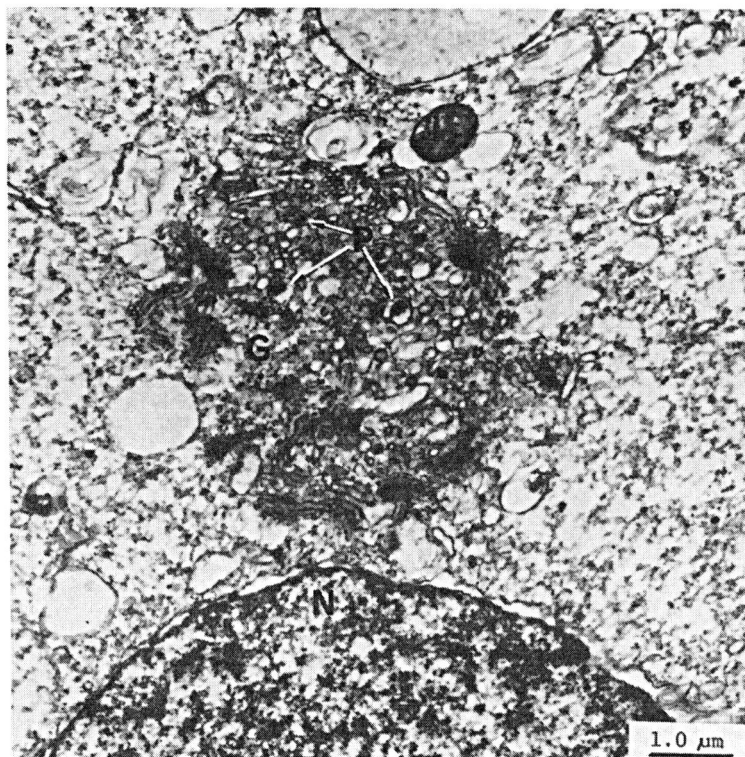

Figure 2. Golgi phase: *Sa* stage of spermiogenesis. G: Golgi apparatus; N: nucleus; P: proacrosomal granules.

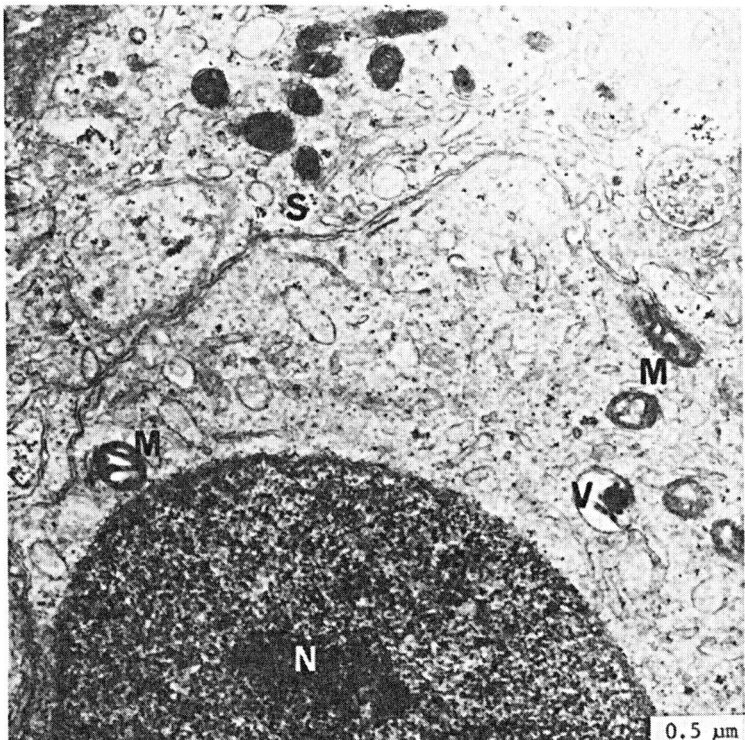

Figure 3. Formation of acrosomal vesicle. M: mitochondria with electron-lucent centres; N: nucleus; S: Sertoli cell cytoplasm; V: acrosomal vesicle containing large acrosomal granule.

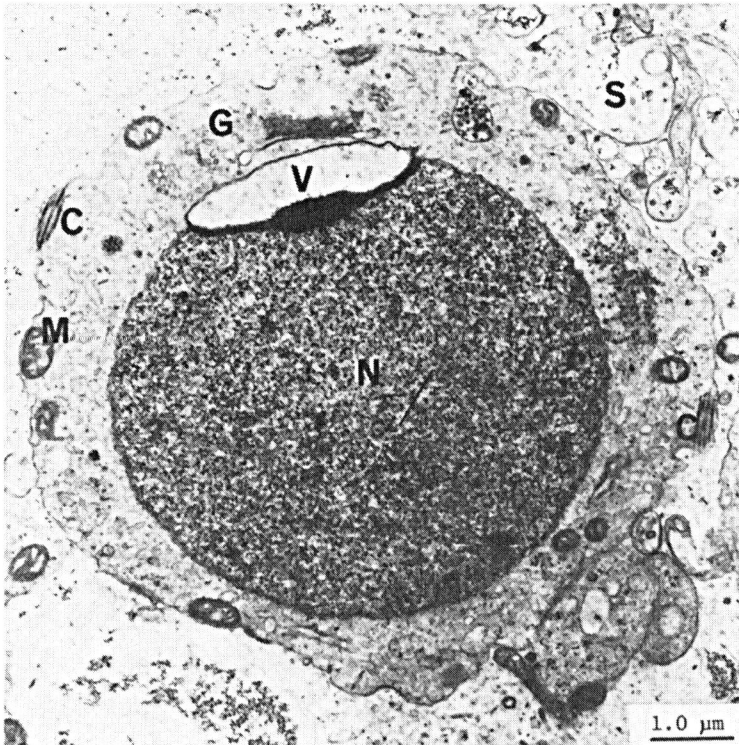

Figure 4. Apposition of acrosomal vesicle to nucleus. C: centrioles in longitudinal section; G: Golgi apparatus; M: mitochondria, arranged around periphery of cell and showing electron-lucent centres; N: nucleus; S: Sertoli cell cytoplasm; V: acrosomal vesicle with central granule.

cell and begins its migration to the postnuclear cytoplasm.

In the Sb_2 stage, the Golgi has migrated out of the supranuclear region, and the nucleus moves anteriorly to an eccentric position. There is an alteration in its shape as it becomes progressively more elongated and pear-shaped. With the forward movement of the nucleus, the outer acrosomal membrane comes into close apposition to the inner layer of the cell membrane.

The maturation phase is characterized by changes in the nuclear chromatin. In the Sc stage, markedly electron-dense granules, measuring 250-350 Å appear diffusely throughout the nucleus. But in the posterior portion of the nucleus, they are concentrated in the central zone, leaving a clear space between them and the nuclear membrane (Figure 7).

In the next, Sd, stage, the granules become larger, 700-1000 Å, and the nucleus diminishes in size. In the final, Sd_2 stage, the granules coalesce into a homogeneous, dense mass. The head is arrow-shaped in one plane and spatulate in the other (Figure 8).

In the mature human spermatozoon, the anterior two-thirds to three-quarters of the nucleus are covered by the acrosome, which is a relatively uniform structure, without any apical projection. In its distal portion, the acrosome tapers to end in a narrow condensed plaque, which is known as the equatorial segment. The acrosome lies in the space between the nuclear envelope and the cell membrane. Its inner membrane is in close apposition to the nuclear membrane throughout the entire extent of the cap. The outer acrosomal membrane is closely applied to the plasmalemma at the anterior tip of the cell. On either side of this central area, the plasma membrane balloons away from the acrosome, but remains equidistant to it over the circumference of the head. It reestablishes contact with the acrosome when it reaches the equatorial segment. In this region, a permanent union develops between the acrosomal and plasma membranes. The cell membrane, overlying the acrosome, encloses a compartment which contains fluid, cytosol, but it has no cytoplasmic organelles as all of these have moved caudally into the postnuclear cytoplasm.

Morphologically, the acrosomal contents are

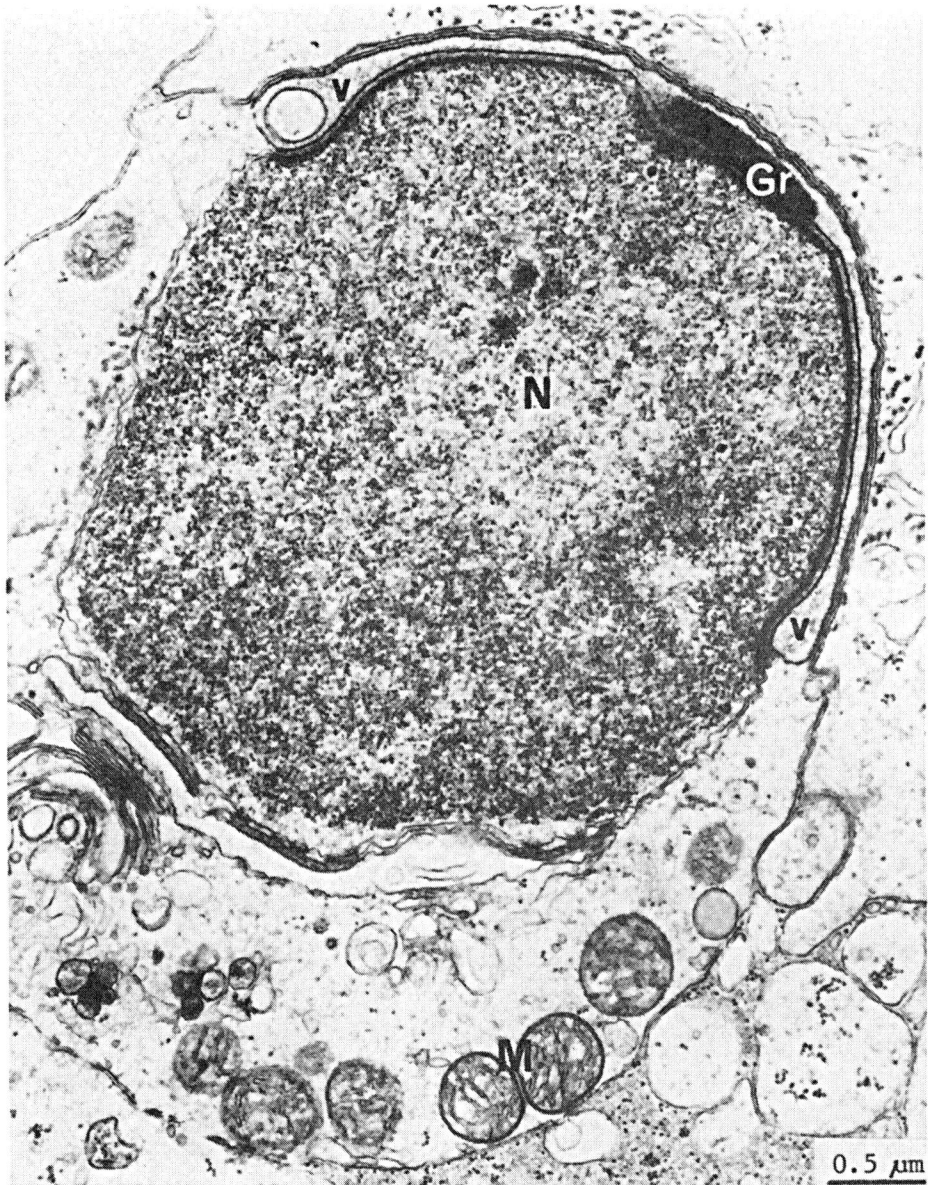

Figure 5. Cap phase: *Sb* stage of spermiogenesis with spread of acrosomal vesicle (v) over the anterior pole of the nucleus. Gr: central acrosomal granule within acrosomal vesicle; M: mitochondria; N: nucleus; V: acrosomal vesicle.

homogeneous and of medium electron density. Their appearance is relatively amorphous. Histochemically, it was apparent on light microscopy that the acrosome was rich in carbohydrate or glycoprotein as it gave a positive periodic acid Schiff reaction. As has been mentioned above, this staining property was used by Clermont and Leblond (1955) in their original delineation of the twelve steps of spermiogenesis. The biochemistry of the acrosome is becoming more complex with the isolation of an increasing number of enzymes. This ever-growing list includes hyaluronidase; acrosin - a trypsin-like protease; an enzyme with neuraminidase activity, aryl sulfatase; and a corona-penetrating enzyme which depolymerizes and disperses the matrix between the corona cells (Gordon 1977; Pedersen 1972; Yanagimachi and Teichman 1972). On this basis, the acrosome is considered to be a membrane-enclosed secretory granule which contains potent enzymes of lysosomal nature. Biochemically, the equatorial

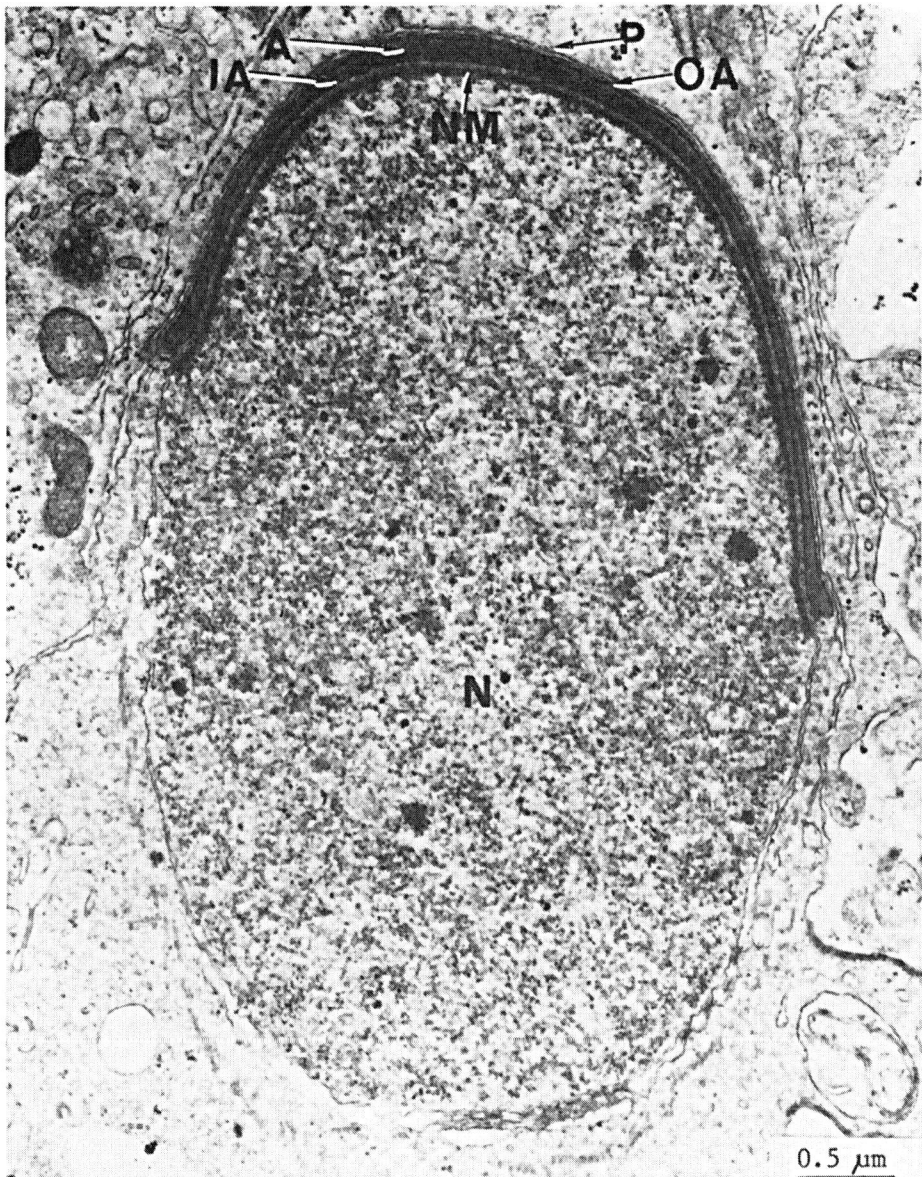

Figure 6. Acrosomal phase of spermiogenesis. A: Acrosomal granule has spread into the head cap and is filling it; IA: inner acrosomal membrane; OA: outer acrosomal membrane; NM: nuclear membrane; N: nucleus; P: plasma membrane.

segment differs from the rest of the acrosome in that it has been shown to lack enzyme activity (Yanagimachi and Teichman 1972).

Within the male genital tract, the acrosomal enzymes are inhibited by seminal plasma, in particular, by its decapacitation factor (Williams et al. 1967) which binds to the sperm. Upon reaching the female genital tract, the sperm are released from the decapacitation factor. This is the process whereby the spermatozoa become capacitated.

As a specific response to the presence of the ovum, capacitated spermatozoa undergo the acrosome reaction. In essence, this is a process of exocytosis. Initially, the outer acrosomal membrane fuses at multiple points with the overlying plasma membrane. Numerous openings are produced through which the acrosomal enzymes are liberated. The outer acrosomal membrane and the accompanying plasmalemma are shed permanently from the cell except in the region of the equatorial segment where

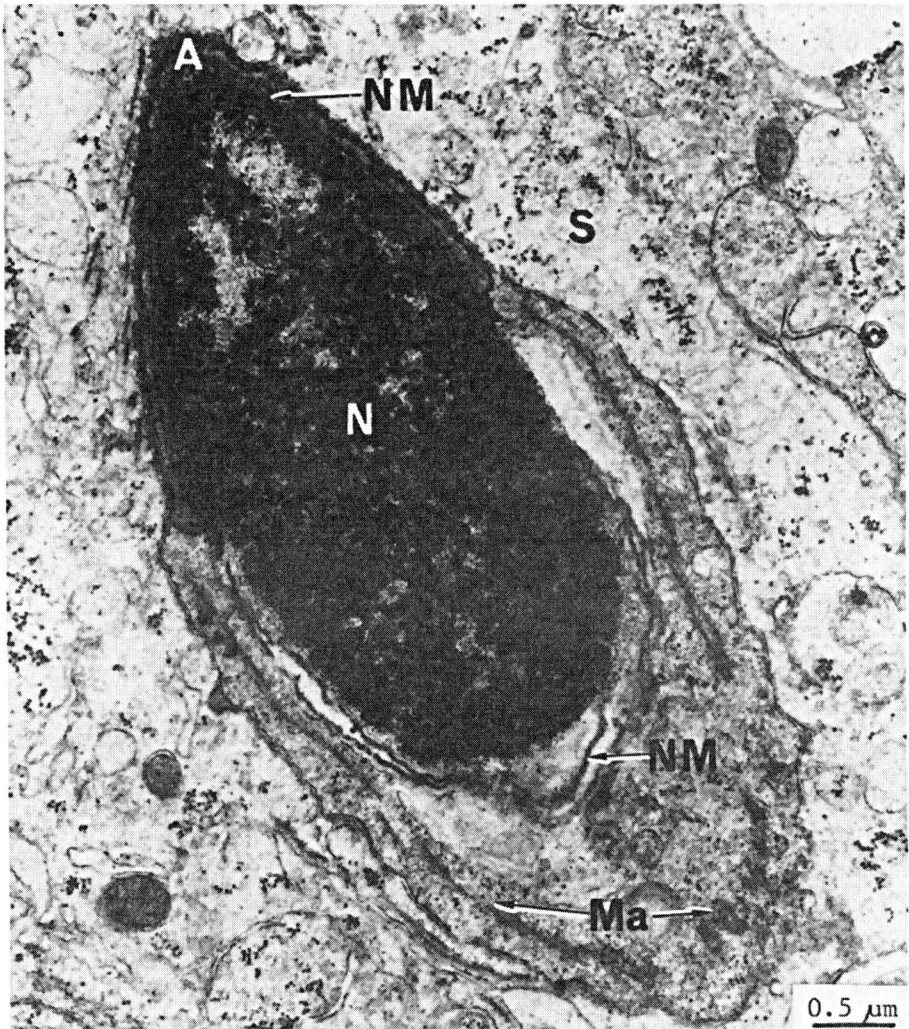

Figure 7. Sc stage of spermiogenesis showing condensation of nuclear chromatin. A: acrosome; Ma: manchette; N: nucleus; NM: nuclear membrane; S: Sertoli cytoplasm.

a firm union had been established between these two layers. The rest of the anterior portion of the nucleus remains covered only by the inner acrosomal membrane, which then forms the surface membrane of the cell in this region.

3. ABNORMALITIES OF ACROSOMAL FORMATION

Abnormalities of acrosomal formation may be associated with abnormal development of the spermatids. In the normal course of events, after the division of the secondary spermatocyte gives rise to spermatids, karyokinesis is completed before cytokinesis. Although the cells do not separate and remain linked by cytoplasmic bridges, there is separation of the cytoplasmic organelles, each nucleus having a distinct Golgi apparatus in relation to it, so that acrosome formation proceeds independently around the respective nuclei. As a rule, related contiguous spermatids tend to be at the same level of development. Figure 9 demonstrates several abnormal features. There is a very wide cytoplasmic bridge which has resulted in a binucleate cell. Nuclear division has been unequal in that there is marked disparity in size between the two nuclei. In both instances, a Golgi apparatus is present in close proximity to the nuclear membrane and/or acrosomal vesicle. A more advanced stage of development is seen on the left-hand side. The centriole has moved away from the Golgi and is situated peripherally, close to the cell membrane. The acrosomal

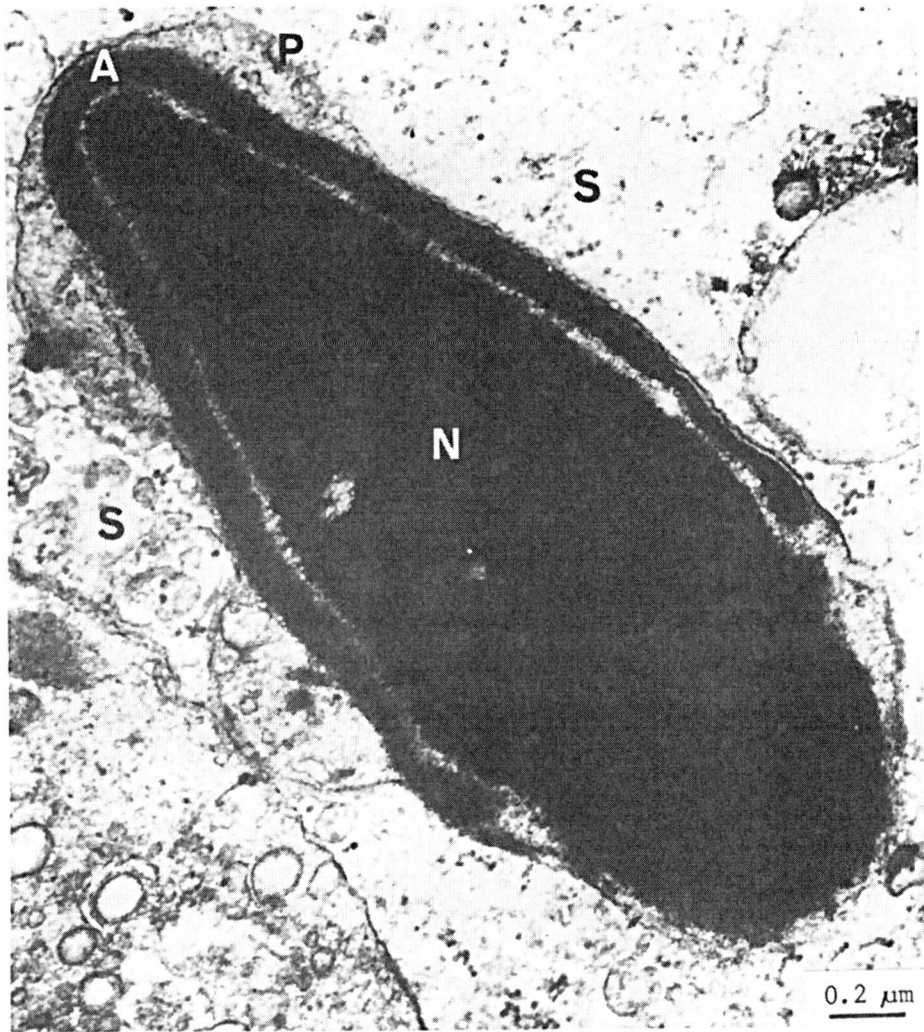

Figure 8. Sd₂ stage of spermiogenesis. A: acrosome; N: nucleus; P: plasma membrane; S: Sertoli cytoplasm.

granule has spread into the head cap. The nucleus is more pyriform with attenuation of it at the acrosomal pole. There has been lateral rather than forward migration of the nucleus and the outer membrane of the acrosomal cap on the left-hand side has come into close apposition with the nuclear membrane of the nucleus on the right. This nucleus is still spheroidal. A Golgi apparatus is present at its anterior pole and there is a centriole on the periphery of the Golgi. There is a small, flat acrosomal vesicle in close apposition to the nucleus but there is no acrosomal granule.

Another binucleate form is seen in Figure 10. There is a single Golgi apparatus, equidistant from the two nuclei. In such a case, a single acrosome will be formed in apposition to both nuclei (Figure 11).

In Figure 12, four nuclei share one acrosome.

Maturation of such multinucleate spermatids will give rise to spermatozoa with grossly deformed heads.

Complete absence of the acrosome has been documented by Pedersen and Rebbe (1974) and Holstein et al. (1973) in their investigation of ejaculates of infertile males, whose spermiograms consisted exclusively of round-headed or globular-headed spermatozoa. By means of transmission electron microscopy, these authors demonstrated that all such spermatozoa were devoid of acrosomes. While it is possible that aplasia of the acrosome may occur due to absolute failure on the part of the anlage, i.e., the Golgi apparatus, concurrent examination of the testicular biopsies in one of these series

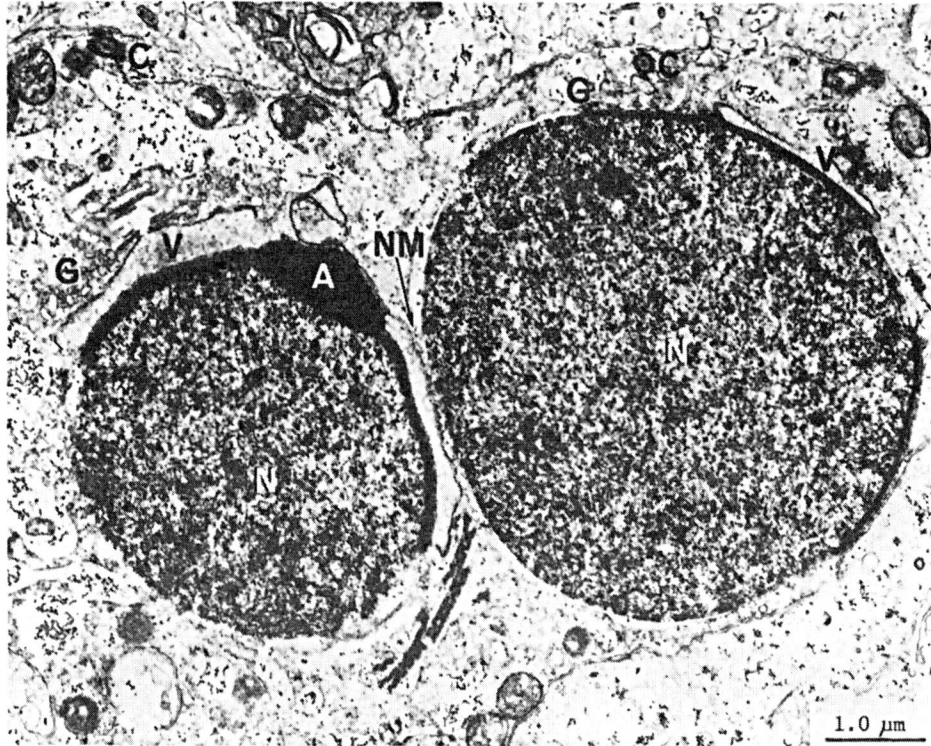

Figure 9. Binucleate spermatid. A: acrosomal granule spreading into head cap; C: centrioles; G: Golgi apparatus; NM: nuclear membrane; N: nuclei; V: acrosomal vesicles.

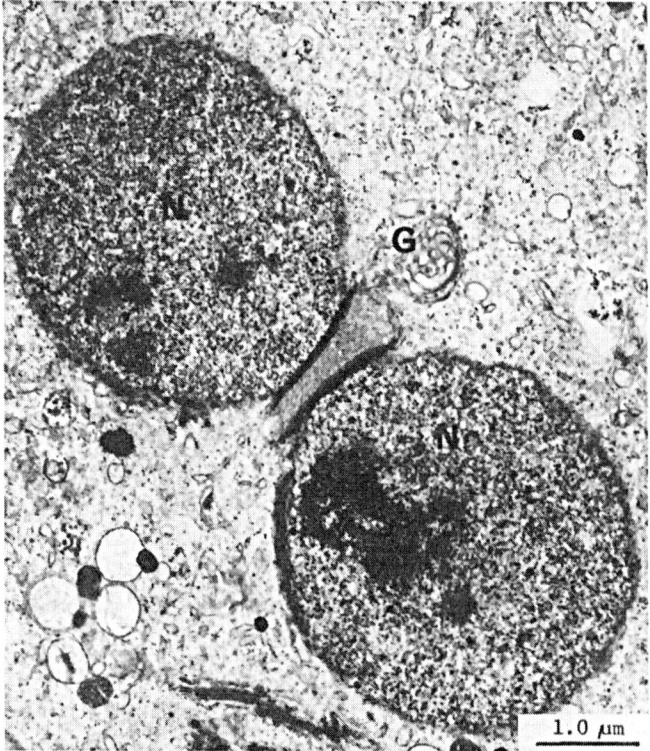

Figure 10. Binucleate spermatid with single Golgi apparatus. G: Golgi apparatus; N: nuclei.

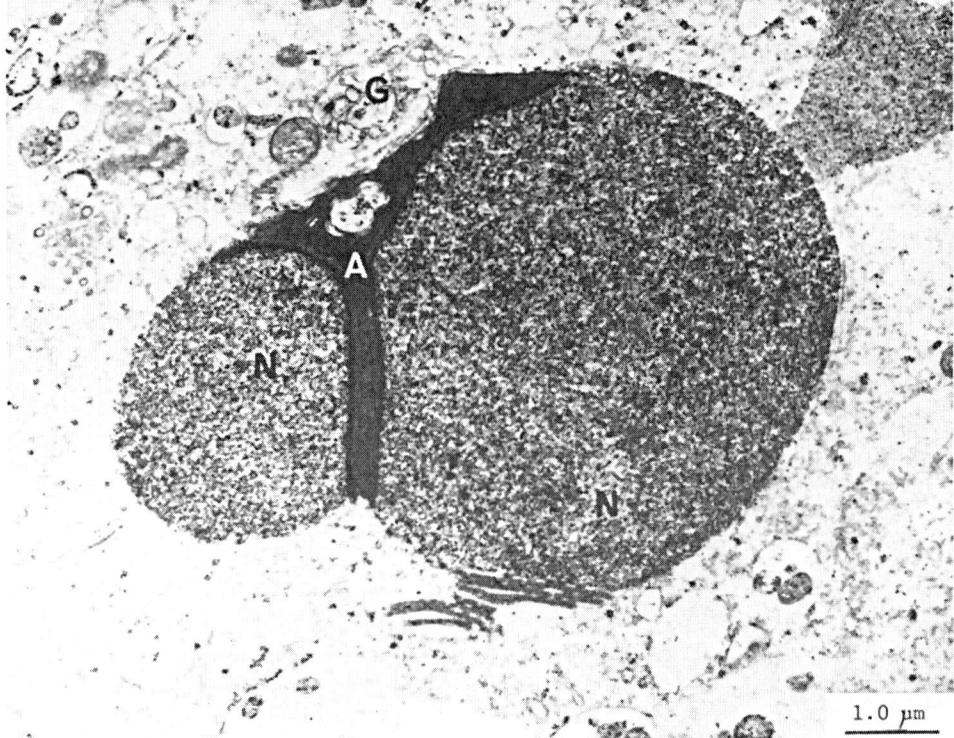

Figure 11. Binucleate spermatid with single acrosome. A: acrosome; G: Golgi apparatus; N: nuclei.

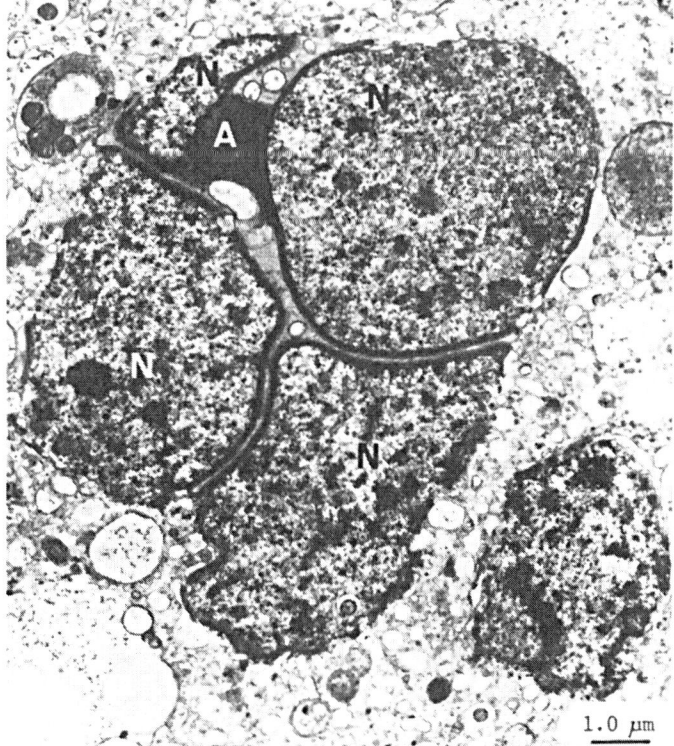

Figure 12. Multinucleate spermatid with common acrosome. A: acrosome; N: nuclei.

(Holstein et al. 1973) showed defective development of the acrosome with failure to establish contact with the spermatid's nucleus. Within the maturing spermatid, there are varying degrees of this abnormality, including increasingly wider separation of the cap from the nuclear membrane (Figure 13) while it is still placed within the environs of the nucleus and its shape follows the general outline of the anterior pole. There is flaring away from the nucleus in the equatorial region in contradistinction to the normal intimate apposition of the equatorial segment. Also, there is failure of formation of the postacrosomal sheath. In more severe forms, the acrosomal development bears no relationship to the nucleus and the acrosome is found as a detached independent structure elsewhere in the cell. Upon maturation of the spermatid, the abnormal acrosome is shed and it is incorporated into a Sertoli cell (Holstein et al. 1973).

It is of interest to note that the absence of the acrosome in these cases was associated with malformation of the sperm head as round-headed or globular-headed spermatozoa were observed. It is not clear what influence the acrosome has on the shape of the sperm head. In their discussion of

morphogenetic factors, which influence the shape of the sperm head, Fawcett et al. (1971) considered that genetically controlled protein and DNA aggregation determined the modelling of the chromatin and wondered whether filaments of the Sertoli cells could also play a part in shaping the head.

In lesser degrees, the lack of apposition of the acrosome to the nuclear membrane may involve only a portion of it. This may take place at any point in its course, leading to focal widening of the subacrosomal space and the formation of a subacrosomal vesicle. When this focal detachment occurs at the apex, it results in the formation of an apical segment (Figure 14).

Vesicles may be present in relation to the external surface of the acrosome and lead to its malformation. In Figure 15 a vesicle is seen at the acrosomal pole. It has invaginated into the acrosomal cap, which has splayed out on either side of the vesicle, giving rise to two anterior cornual projections of the acrosome. There is depression of the subjacent pole of the nucleus.

Vesicles may also be present within the acrosome. Figure 16 shows a vesicle at the anterior pole. It has

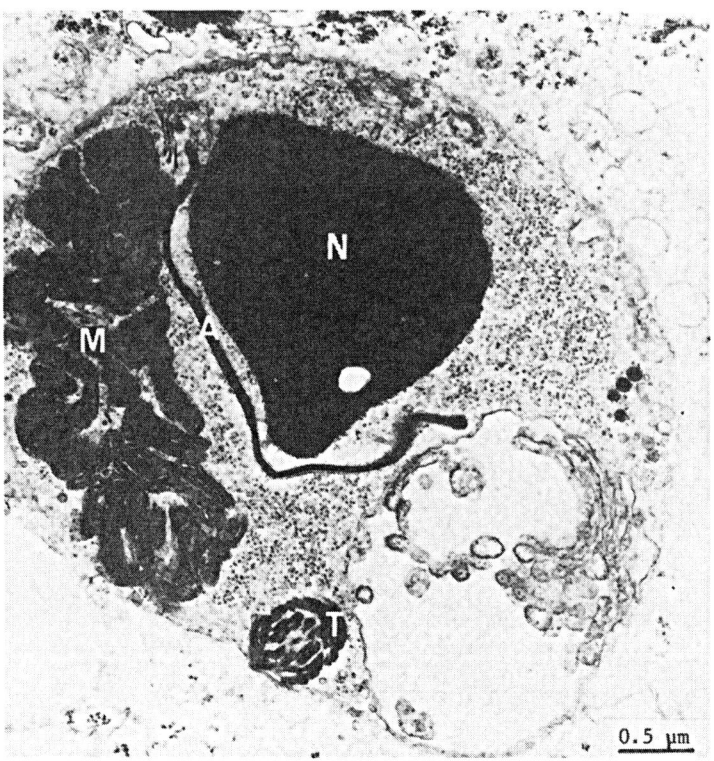

Figure 13. Abnormal spermatid with lack of apposition of acrosome to nucleus.
A: acrosome; M: mitochondria; N: nucleus; T: tail, transverse section.

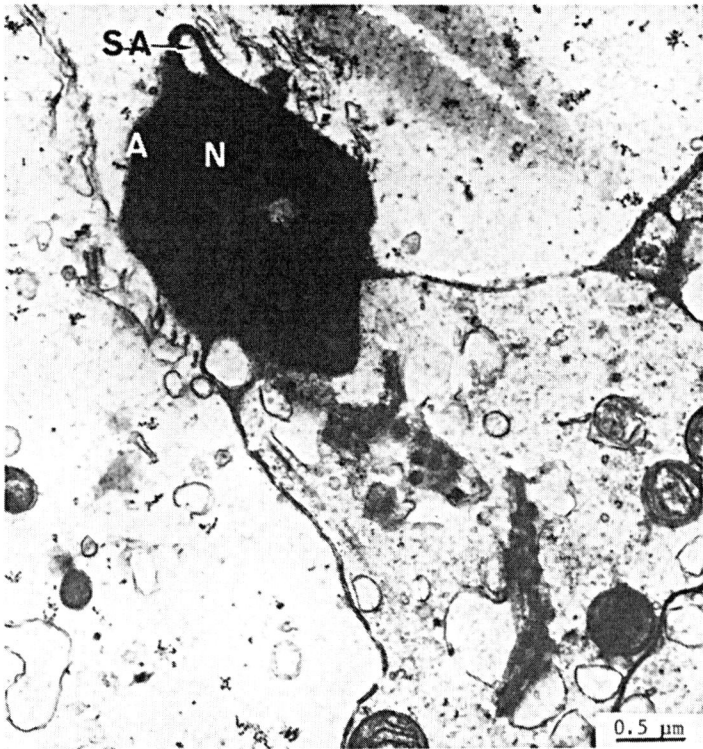

Figure 14. Subacrosomal vesicle with formation of apical segment. A: acrosome; N: nucleus; SA: subacrosomal vesicle.

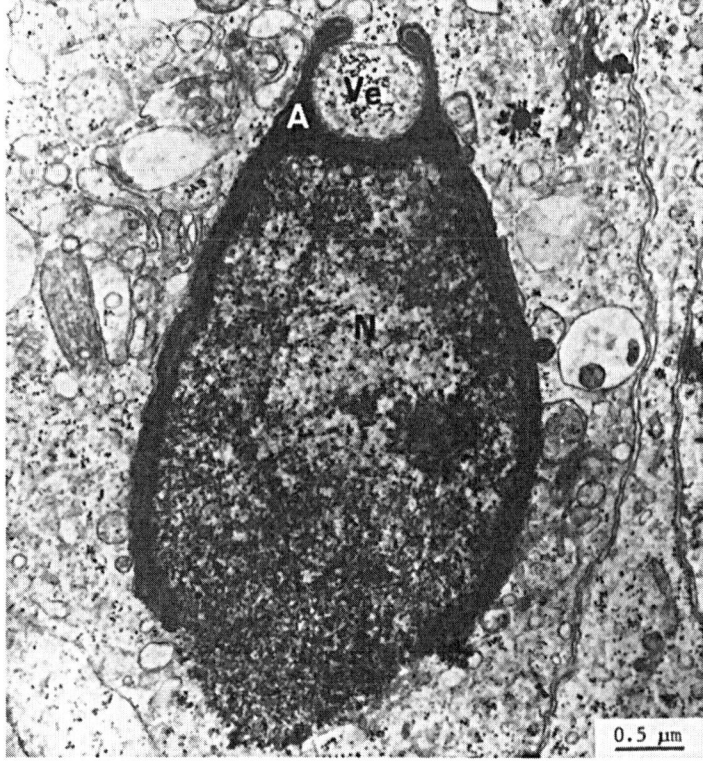

Figure 15. Abnormality of acrosome with bicornuate anterior projection. A: acrosome; N: nucleus; Ve: cytoplasmic vesicle.

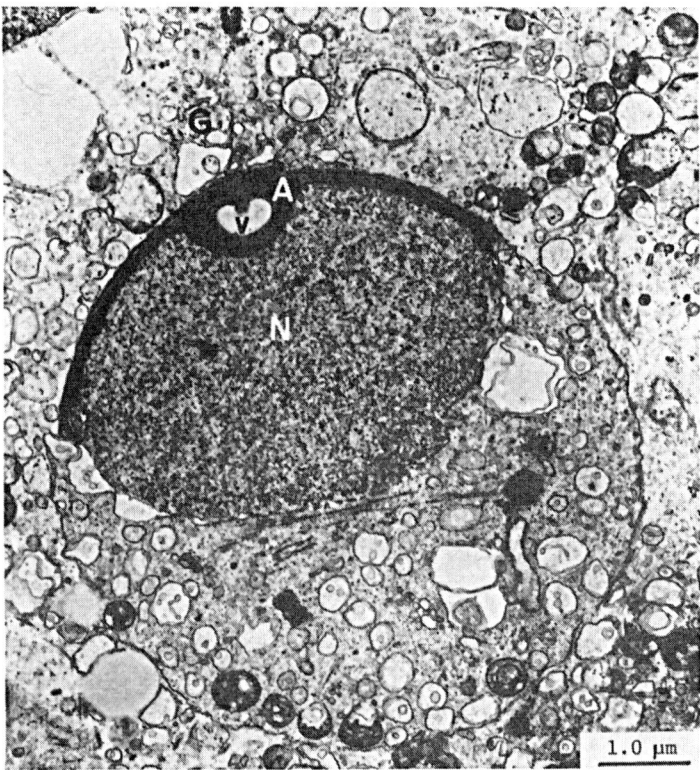

Figure 16. Vesicle within acrosome. A: acrosome; G: Golgi apparatus; N: nucleus; V: vesicle.

led to downward displacement of the acrosome with marked indentation of the nucleus.

Protrusions of the acrosome may also occur if there is disruption of the acrosomal membranes. In Figure 17 there is disruption of a portion of the inner acrosomal membrane with invagination of the acrosomal contents into the nucleus. In addition, there is a focal loss of the outer acrosomal membrane with outward protrusion of the contents. This area is surrounded by phagocytic vacuoles of the neighbouring Sertoli cell. It has been shown that there may be phagocytosis of abnormal spermatids by the Sertoli cells (Siew et al. 1977). It is not known what role release of the acrosomal contents and enzymes may play in such intracellular phagocytosis of the spermatid.

The acrosomal vesicle is derived from the confluence of small pro-acrosomal granule-containing vesicles of the Golgi apparatus. Should there be lack of fusion, the acrosome will be made up of a series of knoblike structures, resembling a string of beads (Figure 18).

There may be inadequate formation or hypoplasia of the acrosome. Once the acrosomal cap is formed,

it covers about one third of the nucleus, but it extends over two thirds to three quarters in the mature spermatozoon. In Figure 19 the manchette has been formed and there is caudal migration of the mitochondria but the acrosomal cap covers only the summit of the nucleus which is about one quarter of its circumference.

It has been pointed out (Figure 9) that an acrosomal vesicle may be formed and may be attached to the nuclear membrane, but that it may contain no acrosomal granule. There may be well-marked ballooning of such vesicles – a more advanced degree of development is shown in Figure 20. The nucleus shows the features of the Sd_2 stage: it is arrow-shaped and there has been condensation of the chromatin into coarse, electron-dense granules. It is surmounted by an extensive acrosomal vesicle which is mostly electron-lucent and shows a paucity of granular material.

4. DISCUSSION

The acrosome reaction is an essential prerequisite to

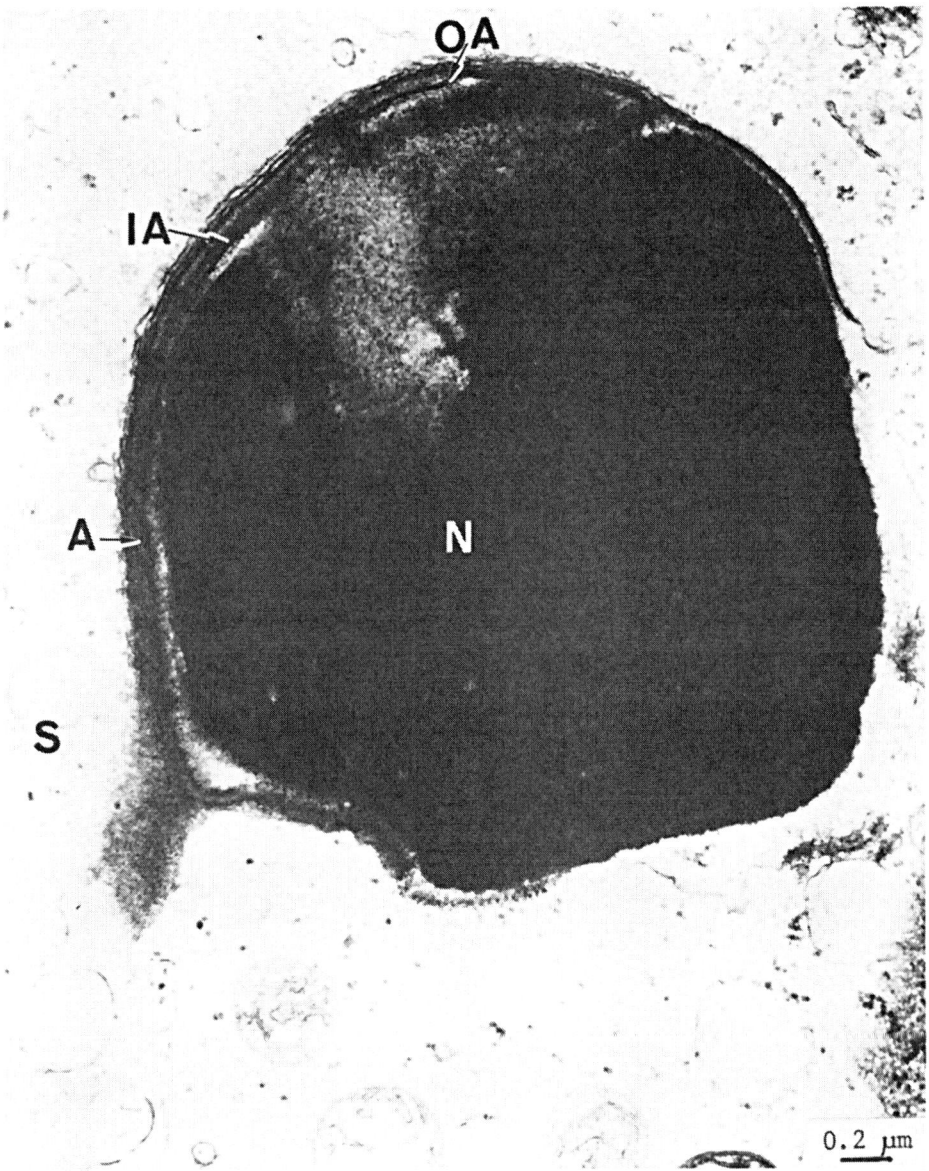

Figure 17. Disruption of acrosomal membranes. A: acrosome; IA: inner acrosomal membrane; OA: outer acrosomal membrane; N: nucleus; S: Sertoli cytoplasm.

the fertilization of the ovum. Any abnormalities of the acrosome that may impair, impede or interfere with this reaction will not allow fertilization to occur and will be associated with infertility. Therefore, it is not surprising that the percentage of acrosomal abnormalities is considerably higher in cases of male infertility (Siew et al. 1977; Camatini et al. 1978) than in the normal (Roosen-Runge 1973). Ultrastructural studies of testicular biopsies in male infertility have shown that there is phagocytosis of abnormal acrosomes (Holstein et al. 1973) and entire malformed spermatids (Siew et al. 1977) by the Sertoli

cells. In the latter instance, there is removal of some abnormal forms before they can be liberated from the tubule into the sperm and examination of the ejaculate would not give a true reflection as to the incidence of their formation.

In some types of acrosomal abnormalities, there is disruption of the acrosomal membranes with release of the contents (Figure 17). It is not known whether the decapacitation factor of the seminal plasma functions within the seminiferous epithelium nor whether the acrosomal enzymes may be activated there. Normally, there is protection against activa-

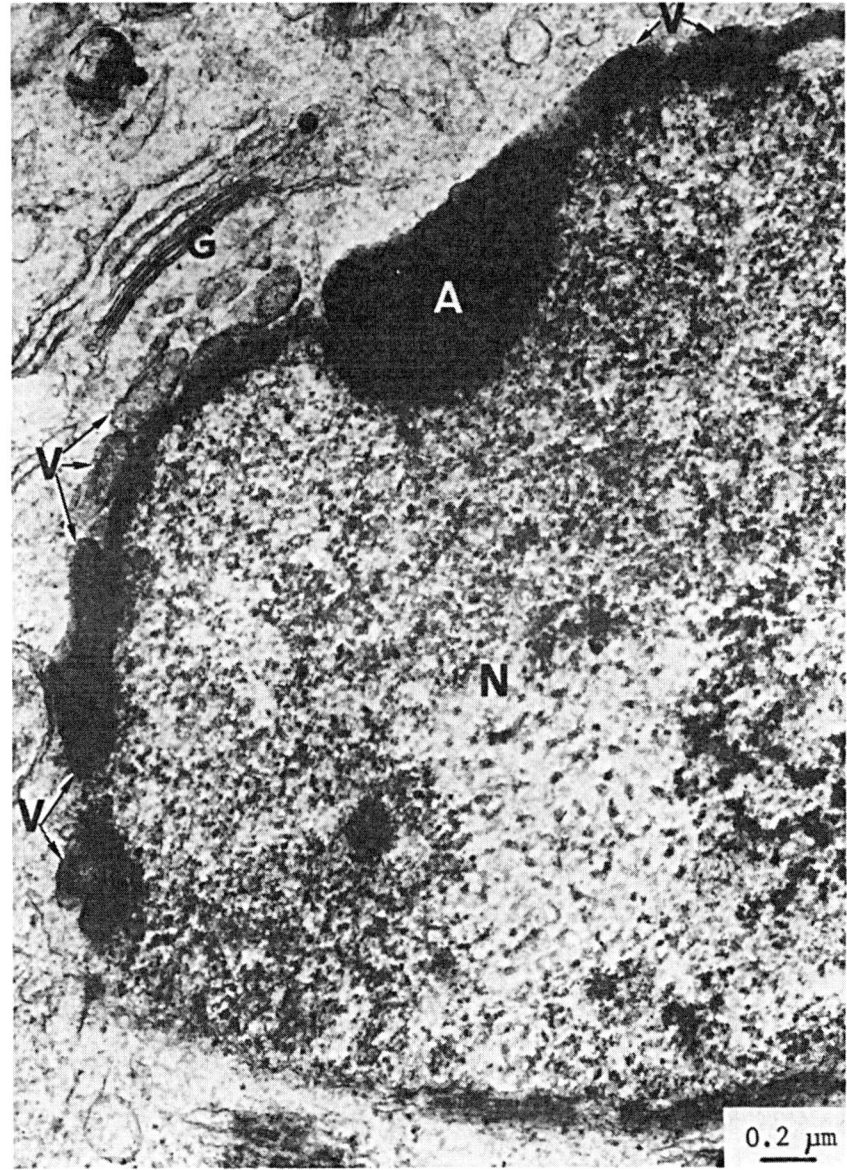

Figure 18. Lack of fusion of proacrosomal vesicles into a single acrosomal vesicle. A: acrosomal granule; G: Golgi apparatus; N: nucleus; V: multiple acrosomal vesicles in apposition to nuclear membrane.

tion of these lysosomal enzymes as this would result in a self-destructive process. However, the possibility has to be borne in mind that this may occur in malformation.

A brief account has been given of the maturation of the spermatid from the *Sa-Sd* stages with respect to the formation of the acrosome and the concomitant nuclear changes. The final result is an arrow-shaped, electron-dense nucleus which tapers anteriorly, at the acrosomal pole. It is covered by the acrosome, which is in close apposition to the nucleus and follows its contour for two thirds to three quarters of the nuclear circumference.

In spermatids which show abnormalities of acrosome formation, there is usually a loss of the normal correlation between the stage of development of the acrosome and the maturation of the nucleus. An example of such disparity is demonstrated in Figure 20, where acrosome formation is at the *Sb*, or head cap phase, but the nucleus is well into the Sd_2 stage. Figures 13, 14, and 17 show varying degrees of acrosomal abnormalities but there has been dense aggregation of the nuclear chromatin. The fact that acrosomal malformation may not affect the con-

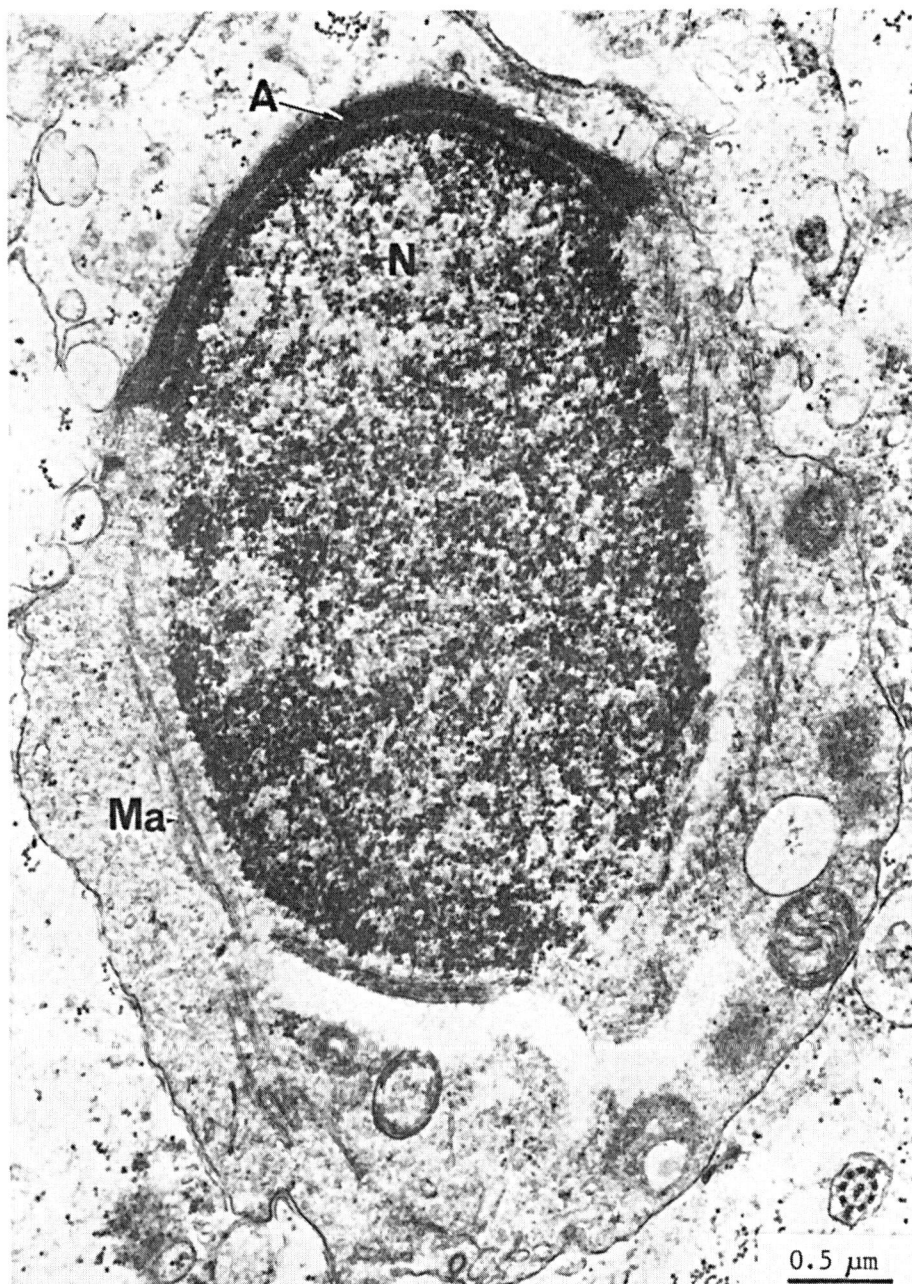

Figure 19. Hypoplasia: inadequate formation of acrosome. A: acrosome; Ma: manchette; N: nucleus.

densation of nuclear chromatin has been stressed by Camatini et al. (1978) in their study of testicular biopsies in men with obstructive azoospermia. In their series, abnormalities of the acrosome were not accompanied by other evidence of malformation of the spermatid.

In our ultrastructural studies of testicular biopsies of oligospermiac males who showed no systemic nor cytogenetic abnormalities (Siew et al. 1977) there were some instances of more severe degrees of malformation involving practically all aspects of spermatid maturation. This gave rise to grossly distorted, bizarre forms (Figure 13). In this micrograph, in addition to the lack of apposition of the acrosome to the nuclear membrane and the lack of formation of the postacrosomal sheath, there has not been a caudal but an anterior migration of the cytoplasm. The bulk of the mitochondria are grouped laterally and anteriorly to the nucleus and have assumed the lengthened rodlike appearance of

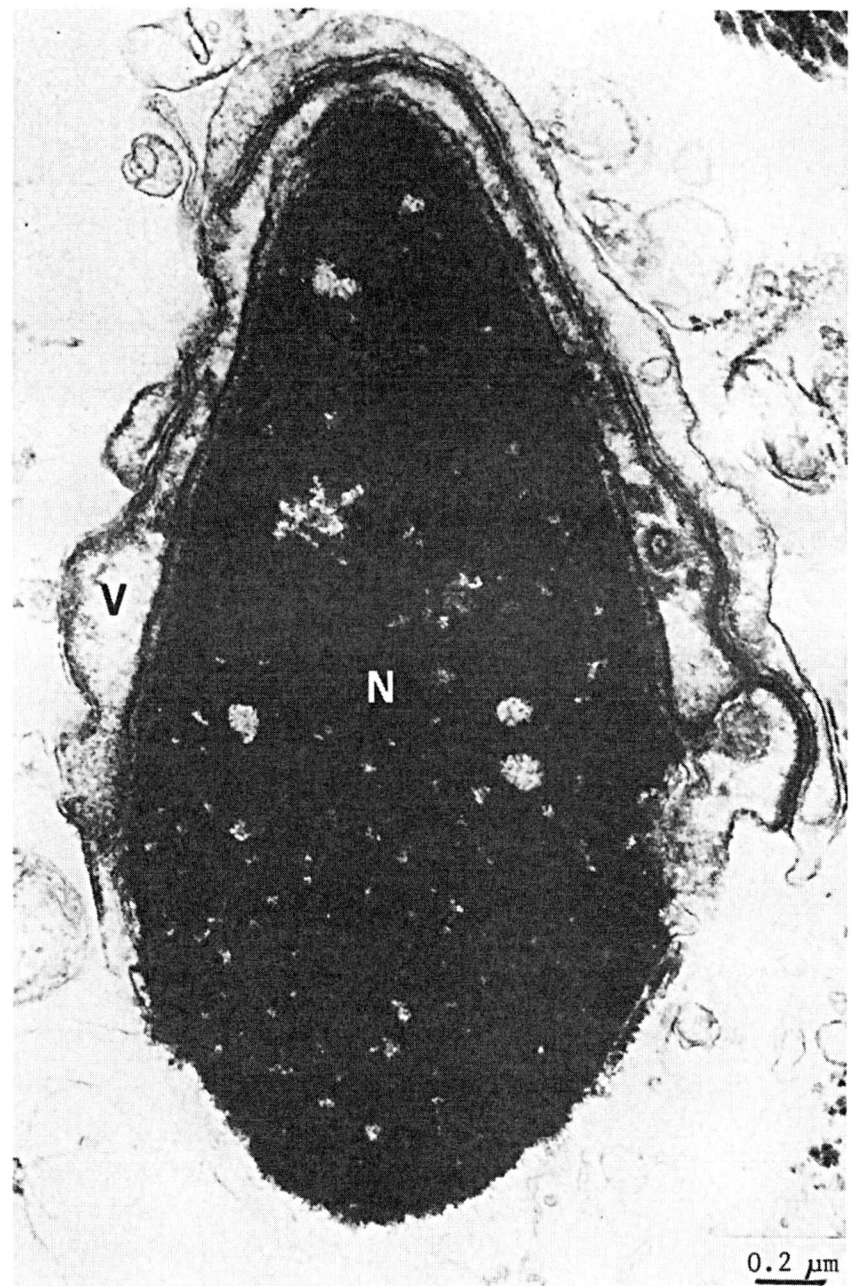

Figure 20. Lack of acrosomal granule in vesicle. N: Sd_2 stage nucleus; V: acrosomal vesicle showing
paucity of granule material.

those in the tail helix. A transected portion of the
principal piece is present at the anterior pole of the
cell. The presence of these tail elements in the
anterior compartment of the cell has interfered with
the anterior migration of the nucleus. So, despite its
pyriform shape and the dense aggregation of the
nuclear chromatin, the nucleus is situated in the
caudal area of the cell.

The cases reported by Pedersen and Rebbe (1974)
showed some nuclear abnormalities, abnormal
arrangement of the mitochondria, and tubular
derangement in the axoneme, in addition to the
absence of an acrosome and a postacrosomal sheath.
Holstein et al. (1973) found no pathological alterations in the nuclei of the spermatids insofar as the
condensation of the karyoplasm was concerned, but

the nuclear shape had remained spherical and the spermatozoa were round-headed.

It would appear that if the developmental defect is restricted to the Golgi apparatus, then the acrosomal abnormality would be the sole finding and that the formation of a normal acrosome is not required for nuclear condensation. However, in many of the spermatids with acrosomal malformation the nuclei do not undergo the tapering in shape and the anterior migration. Such spermatids mature into round-headed or globular-headed spermatozoa.

Although it is not known what effect the acrosome has upon the shape of the sperm head, as long as it is in juxtaposition to the nuclear membrane there is an association between alteration of nuclear and acro-somal morphology.

Fawcett et al. (1971) considered that the close investment of the maturing spermatids by the cyto-plasmic extensions of the Sertoli cells could play a part in the moulding of the nuclear shape. In normal spermiogenesis, the spermatids are clustered in the adluminal compartment of the tubule. In our ex-perience of testicular biopsies of infertile males, we have observed, on occasion, that the spermatids were found in the deeper layers of the seminiferous epithelium. It is possible that in such a situation there is a departure from the normal tissue tension exerted upon the spermatid with loss of normal nuclear moulding.

ACKNOWLEDGEMENT

This work was supported, in part, by Grant T-87, Health, Research and Services Foundation, Pittsburgh, Pennsylvania 15219.

REFERENCES

Allison AC, Hartree EF: Lysosomal enzymes in the acrosome and their possible role in fertilization. J Reprod Fertil 21: 501, 1979.

Camatini M, Franchi E, Faleri M: Ultrastructure of acrosomal malformations in men with obstructive azoospermia. Arch Androl 1: 203, 1978.

Clermont Y: The cycle of the seminiferous epithelium in man. Am J Anat 112: 35, 1963.

Clermont Y, Leblond CP: Spermiogenesis of man, monkey, ram and other mammals as shown by the 'periodic acid Schiff' technique. Am J Anat 96: 229, 1955.

De Kretser DM: Ultrastructural features of human spermio-genesis. Z Zellforsch 98: 477, 1969.

Fawcett DW, Anderson WA, Phillips DM: Morphogenetic factors influencing the shape of the sperm head. Dev Biol 26: 220, 1971.

Gordon M: Cytochemical analysis of the membranes of the mammalian sperm head. In: Male reproductive system. Yates R, Gordon M (eds), New York, Masson, 1977, p 15.

Holstein AF, Schirren C, Schirren CG: Human spermatids and spermatozoa lacking acrosomes. J Reprod Fertil 35: 489, 1973.

Pedersen H: The acrosome of the human spermatozoon: a new method for its extraction and an analysis of its trypsin-like enzyme activity. J Reprod Fertil 31: 99, 1972.

Pedersen H, Rebbe H: Fine structure of round-headed human spermatozoa. J Reprod Fertil 37: 51, 1974.

Roosen-Runge EC: Germinal cell loss in metazoon spermio-genesis. J Reprod Fertil 35: 339, 1973.

Siew S, Troen P, Nankin HR: Ultrastructural studies of human testicular biopsies in infertility. In: Male reproductive system. Yates R, Gordon M (eds), New York, Masson, 1977, p 79.

Williams WL, Abney TO, Chernoff HN, Dukelow WR, Pinsker MC: Biochemistry and physiology of decapacitation factor. J Reprod Fertil, suppl 2: 11, 1967.

Yanagimachi R, Teichman RJ: Chemical demonstration of acrosomal proteinase in mammalian and avian spermatozoa by a silver proteinate method. Biol Reprod 6: 87, 1972.

6. PERITUBULAR TISSUE

E. BUSTOS-OBREGÓN

1. INTRODUCTION

Regaud (1901) demonstrated in the rat that the seminiferous tubules were enveloped by epithelioid cells, polygonal in shape, and well delineated by silver impregnation.

This boundary tissue has been considered to be comparable to the connective tissue tunica propria of mucous membranes and is one of the three major compartments making up the structural organization of the mammalian testis. It will be seen later in this chapter that there is an interaction between the intratubular compartment (comprised of germinal and Sertoli cells) and the peritubular compartment. The latter represents the notable structure in contact with the extratubular compartment, of which the vascular, lymphatic, interstitial and Leydig cell components are the most relevant subcompartments.

By the beginning of this century, it was also noted that certain dyes were excluded from the seminiferous tubules (Bouffard 1906; Ribbert 1914) although this phenomenon was not studied in detail until 1962 (Goldacre and Sylvén 1962). In spite of the anatomical disposition mentioned above, and by analogy to the 'blood-brain barrier', this exclusion was at first assumed to be localized in the walls of the capillaries of the testis (Kormano 1967). However, a systematic study on the possible sites of the 'blood-testis barrier' led to the conclusion that it was situated at the specialized cell-to-cell junctions of the Sertoli cells within the seminiferous tubule (Fawcett et al. 1970). A partial barrier is also represented by the cells in the peritubular tissue and by the seminiferous tubule basal membrane, which in some species may be multifolded (Bustos-Obregón 1976).

A detailed analysis of the peritubular tissue considered as part of the blood-testis barrier is to be found in Chapter 7.

2. DEFINITIONS AND TERMINOLOGY

The peritubular tissue, which has been termed lamina propria of the seminiferous tubules (Bustos-Obregón and Holstein 1973), limiting membrane (Clermont 1958), boundary tissue (Lacy and Rotblat 1960), and peritubular layer (McCord 1970), comprises 'the classic basement membrane or basal lamina plus a framework of fibers and cells which give support to the germinal epithelium' (Burgos et al. 1970).

The intercellular materials and fibers are those found in connective tissue. The cells of the boundary tissue, which in many species do not constitute a homogeneous population (Fawcett 1973), have been characterized and variously named by different authors.

Thus, Fawcett et al. (1969) have coined the name of 'myoid' cells to emphasize the ultrastructural similarities between these cells and smooth muscle cells. The topographical arrangement of the cells has also led to the use of the names such as interlamellar cells (Clermont 1958) or peritubular cells (Ross 1967; McCord 1970). In human material, the peritubular cells are commonly called contractile cells (Ross and Long 1966) and sometimes considered as a special kind of fibroblast, myofibroblast (Bock et al. 1972).

3. HUMAN PERITUBULAR TISSUE

3.1. Development

Shortly after birth, human testicular biopsies reveal a basal membrane composed of an inner, electron-lucid thin zone and an outer, thicker, electron-opaque layer. Few collagen fibers can be seen near this area (Hadžiselimović and Seguchi 1975).

The tubules are surrounded by one or two layers of fibroblasts. The fibroblasts of the inner and outer layer differ mostly in their nuclear morphology but in none of them is there any cytoplasmic structure that would allow identification of these cells as contractile elements.

Around puberty, as shown in biopsy from a 13-year-old boy, the basal membrane becomes multi-layered and displays frequent 'knobs' or infoldings toward the seminiferous epithelium. The collagen zone is wider and exhibits an organized packing of the fibers. The peritubular cells arrange themselves in many layers. Those closest to the tubules display the ultrastructure typical of myoid (contractile) cells to be described later. The outer layers, facing the interstitial space, are composed of rather typical fibroblasts.

Differentiation of the peritubule in man occurs then postnatally and much later than in laboratory animals. In the rat, filaments responsible for contractility and histochemically demonstrable phosphatases are present by two weeks after birth (Kormano and Hovatta 1972) when the seminiferous tubules begin to contract. All these parameters reach their full expression around puberty (i.e. in the 40-day-old rat).

Ultrastructural specialization of both cellular and noncellular components of the peritubular tissue is reached even earlier in some farm animals. In the ram, clear signs of morphological differentiation appear only three weeks after sexual differentiation (i.e. by 54 days postcoitum). A few days after birth, the overall organization of the peritubule is essentially similar to the aspect found in sexually mature animals (Bustos-Obregón and Courot 1974).

3.2. Normal structure in the adult

The lamina propria of the normal, adult seminiferous tubule, consists of a 800 Å-thick basement membrane, applied to the basal surface of Sertoli and germinal cells. Some invaginations ('knobs') are occasionally seen.

Outwardly, layers of fibroblast-like (contractile, myoid) cells (usually around six) alternate with intercellular spaces, where collagen bundles run, either longitudinally or circularly to the tubules (Figure 1).

The contractile cells are elongated and their cytoplasmic profiles, often 1 μm or less in thickness,

are difficult to study in any detail by light microscopy.

Bundles of 80 Å filaments, particulary abundant in the periphery of the cell and anchored to dense areas subjacent to the plasma membrane, are the distinctive cytoplasmic differentiation of the contractile cells. In addition, Furuya et al. (1977) have more recently demonstrated 100 Å filaments and chemically characterized the thin (80 Å) filaments as actin (or actin-like) in nature, since they form characteristic arrowhead complexes when incubated with heavy meromyosin. Similar cytochemical observations have been made in boar and mouse testes.

The exact nature of the 100 Å filaments has not been as yet clearly established for this or any other cell type. It has been suggested that these filaments are part of the cytoskeleton (Cook 1976).

In the vicinity to the surface of the contractile cells, numerous microvesicles are found. Mitochondria and glycogen granules are scattered in the cytoplasm. The rough endoplasmic reticulum is scarce, but quite often large lamellar zones of smooth membranes are found (Figure 2).

In sections tangential to the tubular wall, the stellate shape of the contractile cells can be seen, with expansions of neighbouring cells coming closer to one another. In these areas, a thickening under the plasma membrane is also observed (Figure 2). Though the intercellular space in no instance was found to be narrower than 100 Å, it may be speculated that these areas represent 'gap junctions'. Cells practically identical to the peritubular cells have been described in the human testicular capsule (Langford and Heller 1973). A 'gap junction', with a 50 Å space between cells, has been claimed to represent a zone with low electrical resistance, related to the propagation of cell contraction of the whole system. Since the contractions of the seminiferous tubules involve large segments of their length, it seems reasonable to assume that many myoid cells contract synchronously (Roosen-Runge 1951; Suvanto and Kormano 1970).

The 100 Å-thick cytoplasmic filaments are generally found in a perinuclear position; they are often curled and sometimes form a loose network. Myosin-like thick filaments have not been found in peritubular cells (Furuya et al. 1977).

The nucleus is elongated, with an irregular outline, with chromatin clumps, mainly located against the nuclear membrane. Most cells are surrounded by

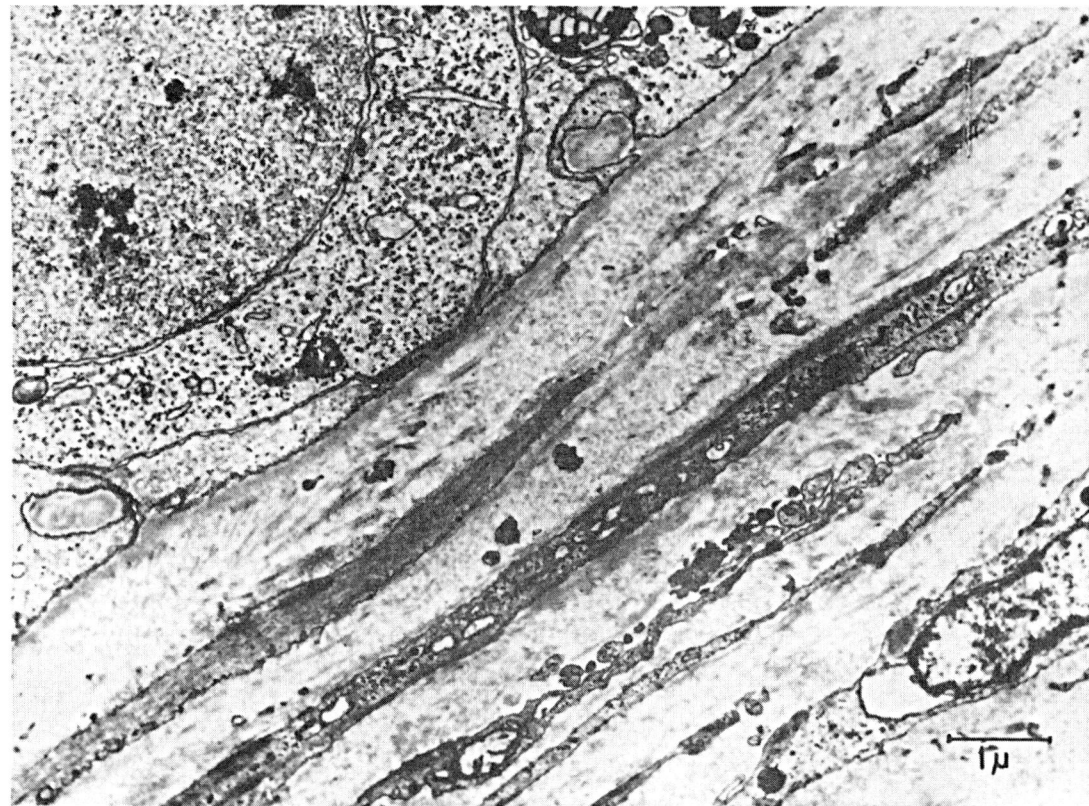

Figure 1. Lamina propria of normal (adult) seminiferous tubule. Note one infolding ('knob') of the basal membrane into the epithelium. Alternate layers of intercellular material (mostly collagen) and elongated myoid cells are seen. The cells are partially enveloped by a cell coat (Bustos-Obregón and Holstein 1973).

an incomplete cell coat.

Most of the intercellular spaces are occupied by collagen fibrils; in some places a basement membrane-like material or a microfibrillar component (most probably unrelated to elastic elements) appears quite conspicuously.

The outermost layer of peritubular cells lacks the morphological traits of contractile cells and more resembles fibroblasts. According to our observations on the development of the peritubular tissue in the ram (Bustos-Obregón and Courot 1974) and to the suggestions advanced by Eigel (1973) in a work on kinetics of the peritubular cells in newborn rats, the outer cell layer may correspond to the renewing compartment of the boundary tissue.

2.3. Pathological structural patterns

Maximal thickening of the seminiferous tubule lamina propria observed in light microscopy usually corresponds to a marked damage of the seminiferous epithelium, clinically expressed either as azoospermia or severe oligozoospermia.

Detailed knowledge of pathological changes can only be appreciated by electron microscopy. Better light microscopical results can be obtained from μm thin sections of plastic-embedded biopsies (Mihatsch 1973), allowing more accurate diagnoses and eventual ultrastructural analysis of the same material.

Three major changes can be seen in pathological ultrastructure:

1. *Thickening and bi- or multilayered aspect of the seminiferous tubule basal membrane, which shows infoldings or knobs of variable shapes and depth of invagination into either the Sertoli cells or the spaces between Sertoli and germinal cells.* These knobs probably result from infoldings of the basement membrane due to the loss (or absence) of germinal cells. This situation corresponds to types B and C of basement membrane modifications described by Furuya (1975), precisely in cases of hypospermato-

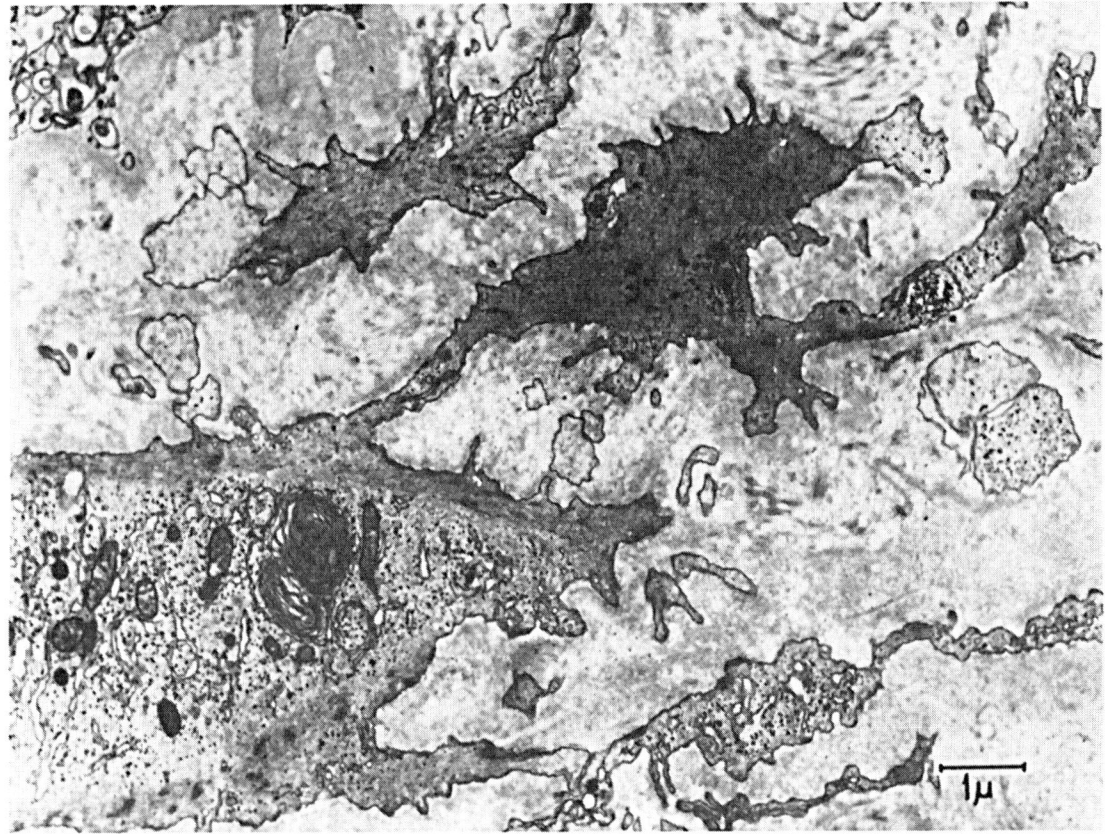

Figure 2. Tangential section to one layer of contractile cells. Narrow spaces exist between some cell expansions. Note the abundance of peripherally located bundles of filaments and the array of smooth membranes in concentric whirls (Bustos-Obregón and Holstein 1973).

genesis and Sertoli cell-only syndrome. Type D is, in our experience, not a clear entity but it is described as corresponding also to germ cell aplasia.

2. *Increased intercellular material, which corresponds more often to increased deposition of collagen and less frequently to areas with abundant cell-coat-like material or microfibrillar elements.* The distribution of collagen permits identification of two morphological patterns. In one case, the layer adjacent to the basement membrane has increased collagen areas (Figure 3); the other layers may remain practically unchanged. In the other, widening due to collagen deposition is found in any of the layers more peripherally located (Figure 4). In all cases, collagen tends to form bundles or even large islands, whose disposition may even resemble that of tendon.

Since no cell element other than well-differentiated, typical contractile cells is found in these areas, it may be postulated that these cells synthesize collagen and that they export it to the intercellular

space with variable polarity, either towards the seminiferous tubule aspect or towards the opposite side. Thus, the two patterns outlined above are likely to emerge (Figure 5).

It seems well established that the contractile cells of the human testis are of mesenchymal origin (De la Balze et al. 1960) and that they behave as multi-functional mesenchymal elements which synthesize all the extracellular components. A similar situation has been claimed to occur with the smooth muscle cells of the aortic media (Wissler 1967).

Preliminary unpublished results in our laboratory have demonstrated incorporation of tritiated pro-line into the peritubular cells of cat testis twenty minutes after intratesticular injection. The radio-autographical reaction can be detected, with variable intensity, in animals two weeks, two months and fourteen months old. There seems to be no difference in uptake between the inner and the outer myoid cells.

3. *Changes in the contractile cells, which can be*

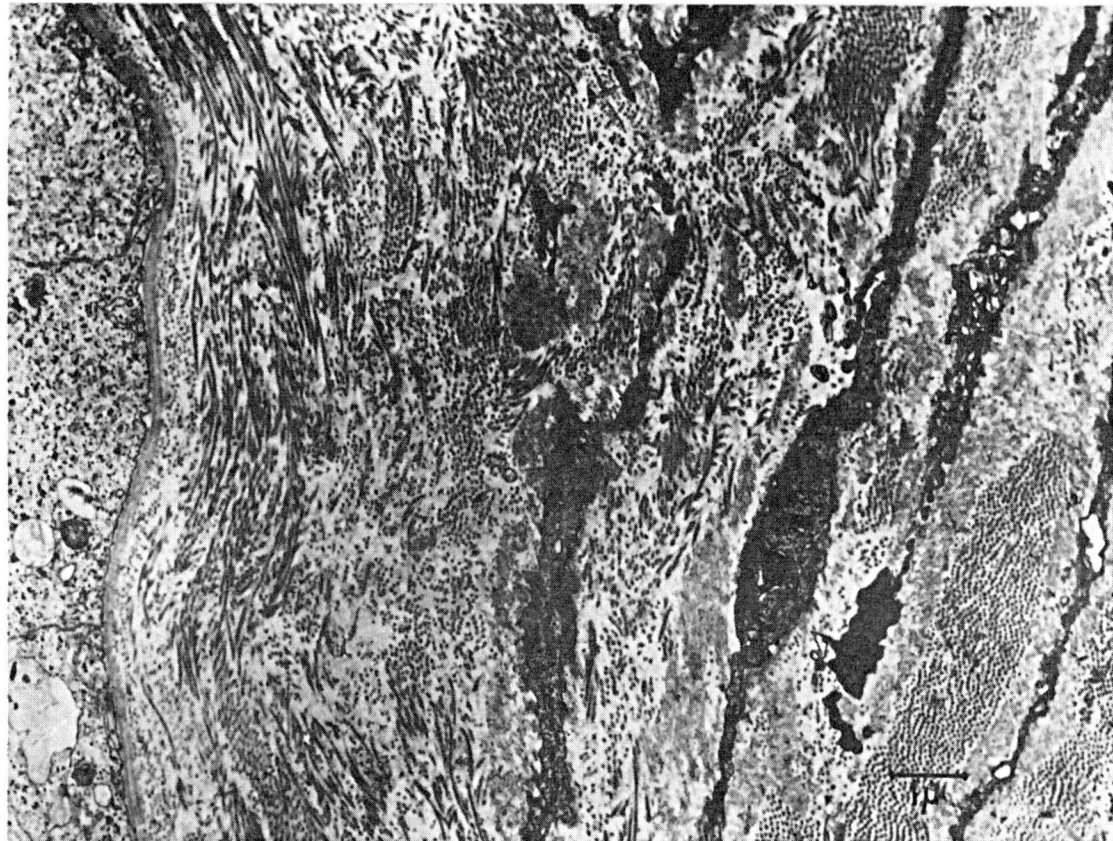

Figure 3. Thickened lamina propria, with a wide collagen zone between the seminiferous tubule basement membrane and the first layer of myoid cells (see Figure 5, *centre*, for diagrammatic representation of this topography). Sample corresponds to a case of primary hypergonadotrophic hypogonadism (Bustos-Obregón and Holstein 1973).

very minor, such as appearance of lipid or glycogen deposits in the cytoplasm, up to a dedifferentiation that reverts the aspect of the myoid cells towards a rather undifferentiated fibroblast. Extreme dedifferentiation can be obtained in adult animals either by blocking the peripheral effects of androgens (as by treating animals with cyproterone acetate) or by eliminating gonadotrophic action, as observed in hypophysectomized rams – Figure 6 (Bustos-Obregón and Courot 1974).

4. COMPARATIVE ANATOMY OF THE PERITUBULAR TISSUE

An important body of literature concerned with the blood-testis barrier has tangentially elaborated on the structure of the peritubular tissue (for a review, see Setchell and Waites 1975; and Neaves 1977).

Only rather recently, a survey of the ultrastructural patterns of the lamina propria of mammalian seminiferous tubules consisting of the most common laboratory animals, some farm animals and man, has been published (Bustos-Obregón 1976). The basement membrane may be a typical one or present infoldings (human) or be split into two layers (human pathology, normal structure for rabbit and boar) or even be multilayered (with as many as eight to ten layers, in adult goat, ram and bull).

The myoid cells can form one layer (rat, mouse, guinea pig) or many layers (up to five or six: man, monkey). Figure 7 is a summary of the four main structural patterns for the seminiferous tubule lamina propria in the cases we have investigated.

In large mammals, where several layers of myoid cells seem to be the rule, the cells closest to the seminiferous tubules are typical contractile cells. There appears to be a gradient of differentiation, so that in the more peripheral layers there is a progressive diminution of the 80 Å cytoplasmic filaments

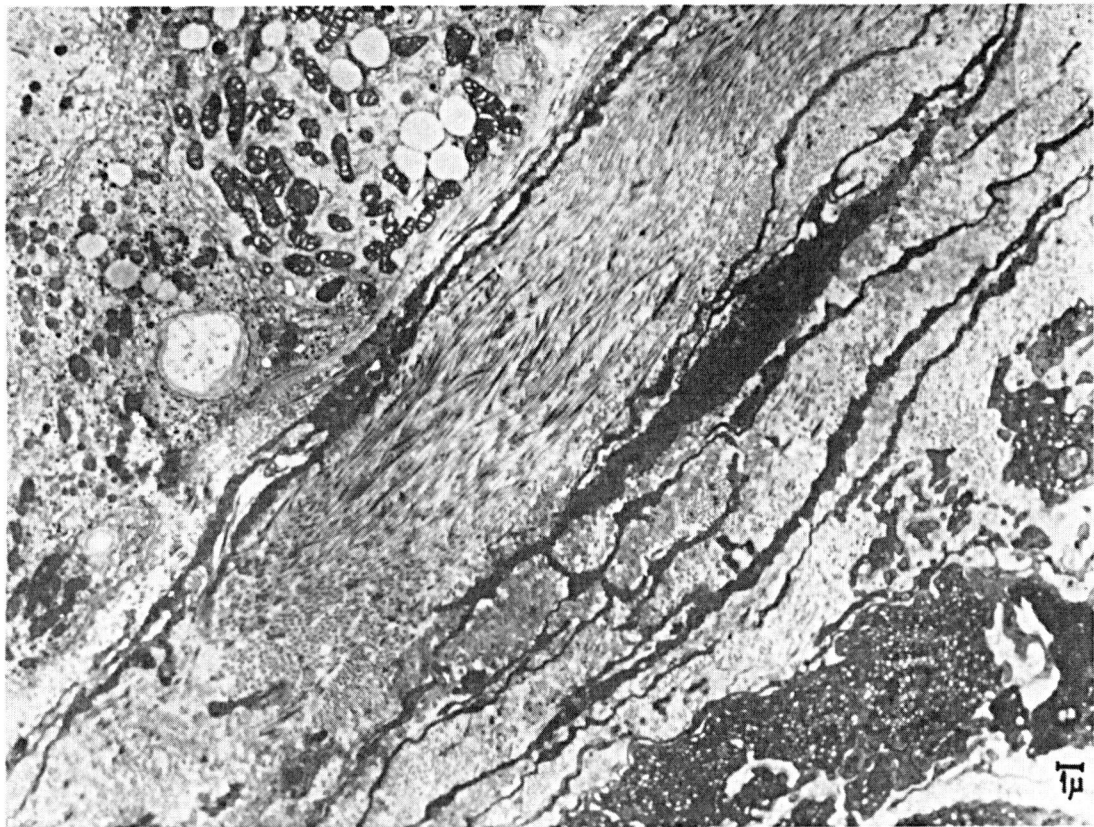

Figure 4. A case similar to Figure 3 (see Figure 5, *right,* for its diagram). The thickening is due to increased collagen deposition in the third intercellular layer (Bustos-Obregón and Holstein 1973).

and the cells resemble fibroblasts. This fact is of interest since in newborn animals the peritubular cells are a rather homogeneous population of mesenchymal origin. When testes of newborn mice are transplanted into testes of adult normal and hypophysectomized animals, it is found that myoid cell differentiation depends upon normal pituitary function and is mediated, at least in part, by androgen (Bressler and Ross 1972). Since only those cells immediately adjacent to the seminiferous tubule acquired myoid characteristics, Bressler and Ross (1972) postulated that the hormonal effects were not acting directly upon these cells, but most probably acted via the Sertoli cells, and that these, in turn, induced differentiation in the adjacent peritubular cells. This interpretation agrees with the topographical cell gradient of myoid differentiation observed in many species (Bustos-Obregón 1976) and clearly discussed by Fawcett (1973). In the ram, however, we have observed a certain degree of morphological differentiation of the peritubular

cells as soon as the first third of pregnancy, when the cellular components of the seminiferous cords are gonocytes and Sertoli cell precursors. In this case, the differentiation of the lamina propria components seems independent of the hormonally controlled events that will take place later, affecting the differentiation of the intratubular cells (Courot 1967).

In view of the different ultrastructural patterns displayed by the peritubular tissue in mammals, it seems advisable to extend its histophysiological analysis to a larger number of experimental animals. Many primates have an organization of the peritubular tissue similar to man (Flechon et al. 1976) and thus, a number of observations on the blood-testis barrier (using electron-opaque tracers) have been made in monkeys (Dym 1973; Dym and Cavicchia 1977).

It may be of interest to consider that the structure of the lamina propria in the cat is identical to that of man (Bustos-Obregón and López 1976), its devel-

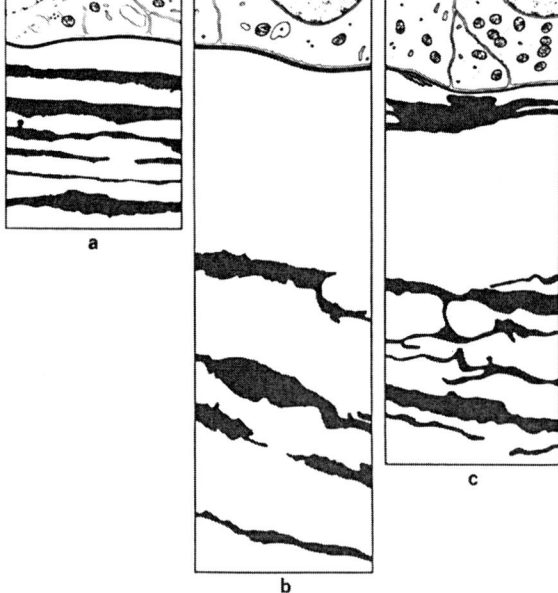

Figure 5. Left: schematic representation of the normal relationship between the seminiferous epithelium (*top*) and the boundary tissue of the seminiferous tubules – the contractile cells are shown as dark areas and the intercellular spaces as light zones between them; *centre:* thickened lamina propria of the seminiferous tubule where the basement membrane (dark line at top) is far removed from the first layer of contactile cells; *right:* a second mode of thickening of the boundary tissue; the intercellular space that is widened is not that in direct contact with the basement membrane of the epithelium – note some areolar areas between the contractile cells, where collagen bundles can be found (Bustos-Obregón 1974).

opmental steps also being similar (Figure 8). This situation offers a good experimental model to study cell functions in the peritubular tissue, that is, synthetic abilities of the myoid cell and renewal behaviour of the outermost, fibroblast-like peritubular cells, as previously discussed.

Many other fields still await a more complete analysis in this area, such as tracer experiments designed to follow the transit of biologically significant molecules across this boundary or endocrine control of pathological changes in the altered lamina propria of the seminiferous tubules.

5. ENDOCRINE FACTORS AND MYOID CELL DIFFERENTIATION

As emphasized before, morphological differentiation of the myoid cells can take place very early in development as in the ram (Figure 9). In this case, by the first third of pregnancy some mesenchymal

peritubular cells begin to elongate, redistribute their cytoplasmic organelles and exhibit bundles of filaments underneath the plasma membrane (Bustos-Obregón and Courot 1974). This situation is found three weeks after sexual differentiation, at a time when there is some LH activity in the fetal pituitary (Dubois and Mauleon 1969); hence, not only maternal but fetal hormones may play a role. Moreover, testosterone is elaborated very early by the fetal testis of the sheep (Attal 1969).

Already by the first week after birth in the ram, the noncellular component of the tunica propria is formed by eight to ten lamellae, those closer to the seminiferous tubule basement membrane being well defined, of a mature aspect, whereas those closer to the first myoid cell layer are loosely organized, as if recently laid out by cellular activity. The cellular component is by now typical contractile cells, fibroblasts being located only at the periphery of the peritubular tissue. Basically, the same aspect is found in the adult ram (Figure 10).

As shown in Figure 6, hypophysectomy induces deposit of lipids in the cytoplasm of adult animals. This effect can be prevented by the administration of LH, FSH or testosterone to the animal.

A similar lipid deposition differentiation and the occurrence of numerous multivesicular bodies in the myoid cell cytoplasm can be found in normal animals injected with cyproterone acetate (Figure 6).

Curiously enough, in the newborn cat, although there are well-differentiated Leydig cells, no signs of myoid cell differentiation can be seen. In contrast with other species, however, abundant collagen zones are found (Bustos-Obregón and López 1976). Only by two months after birth can a clear differentiation of the contractile cells in the cat be recognized.

The relationships between the myoid cells, the ability of this layer to contract, and the appearance of histochemically demonstrable phosphatase activities related to cell contraction, have been systematically analyzed in the rat (Kormano and Hovatta 1972). The same group has studied the in-vitro characteristics of rat seminiferous tubule contractility (Hovatta 1972a), and elucidated many aspects of the myoid cell physiology and development (Hovatta 1972b).

Nevertheless, much remains to be discovered in this regard as well as in the endocrine modulation of myoid cell function in normal and pathological conditions.

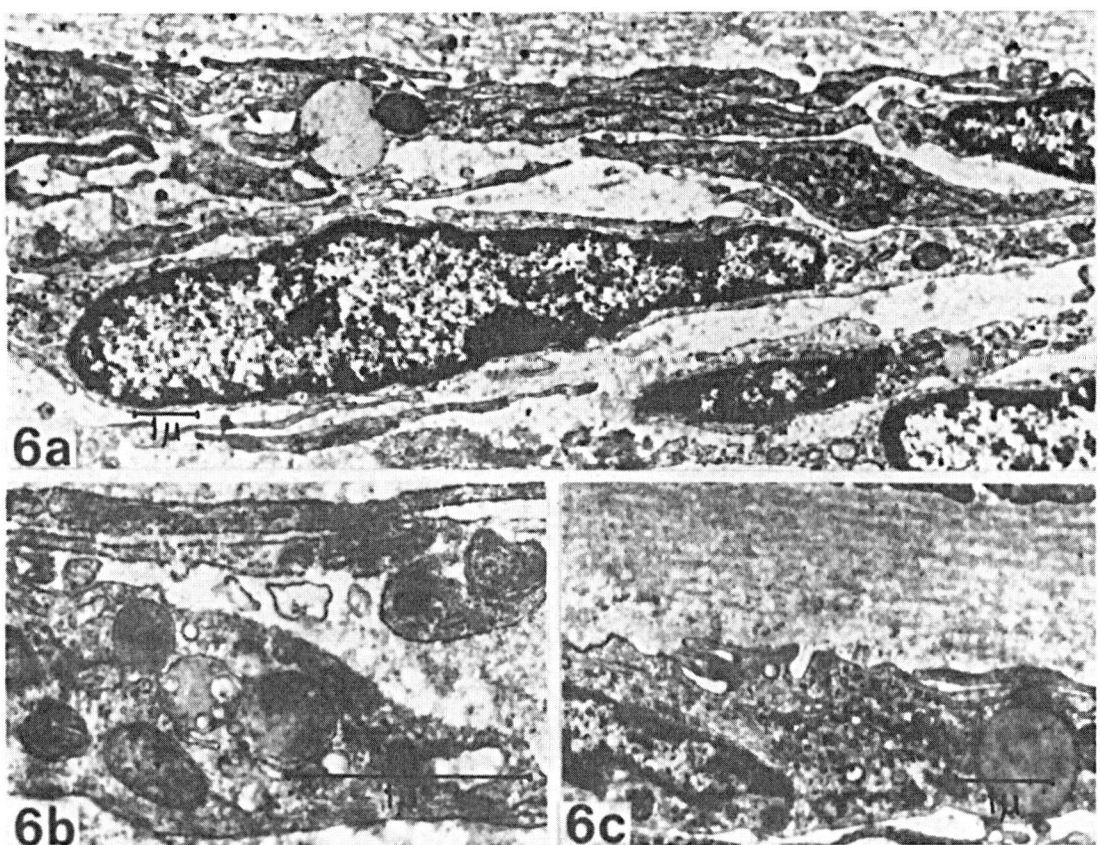

Figure 6. (a) Lamina propria of a lamb, two months after hypophysectomy. Lipid inclusions of different sizes and aspects can be seen in the cytoplasm of some contractile cells. Other cells as well as the noncellular component remain unchanged. (b, c) Lamina propria of normal animals treated for 15 days with cyproterone acetate: (b) lipid inclusion and multivesicular bodies are seen inside one contractile cell; (c) lipid inclusion and a hypertrophic Golgi zone are found in another contractile cell. In both the noncellular component remains unmodified (Bustos-Obregón and Courot 1974).

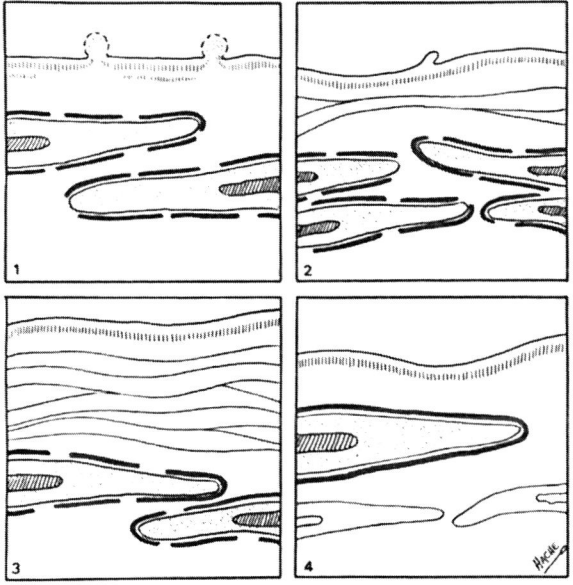

Figure 7. (1) The ultrastructural pattern of the seminiferous tubule lamina propria in man, monkey, stallion, dog and cat. The infoldings of the basal cell surface, followed by the epithelial basement membrane and its partial duplication are characteristic of human material. The contractile cells are disposed in several layers, as for diagrams 2 and 3, where they also present an incomplete cell coat. (2) Ultrastructural pattern of boar and rabbit lamina propria. Basement membrane-like material is found split into two and sometimes more layers. (3) Multi-layered basement membrane-like material, showing eight, ten or more lamellae, characteristic of goat, ram and bull lamina propria. (4) Lamina propria in rodents, as described for the rat: one layer of contractile cells, exhibiting a continuous cell coat (Bustos-Obregón, 1976).

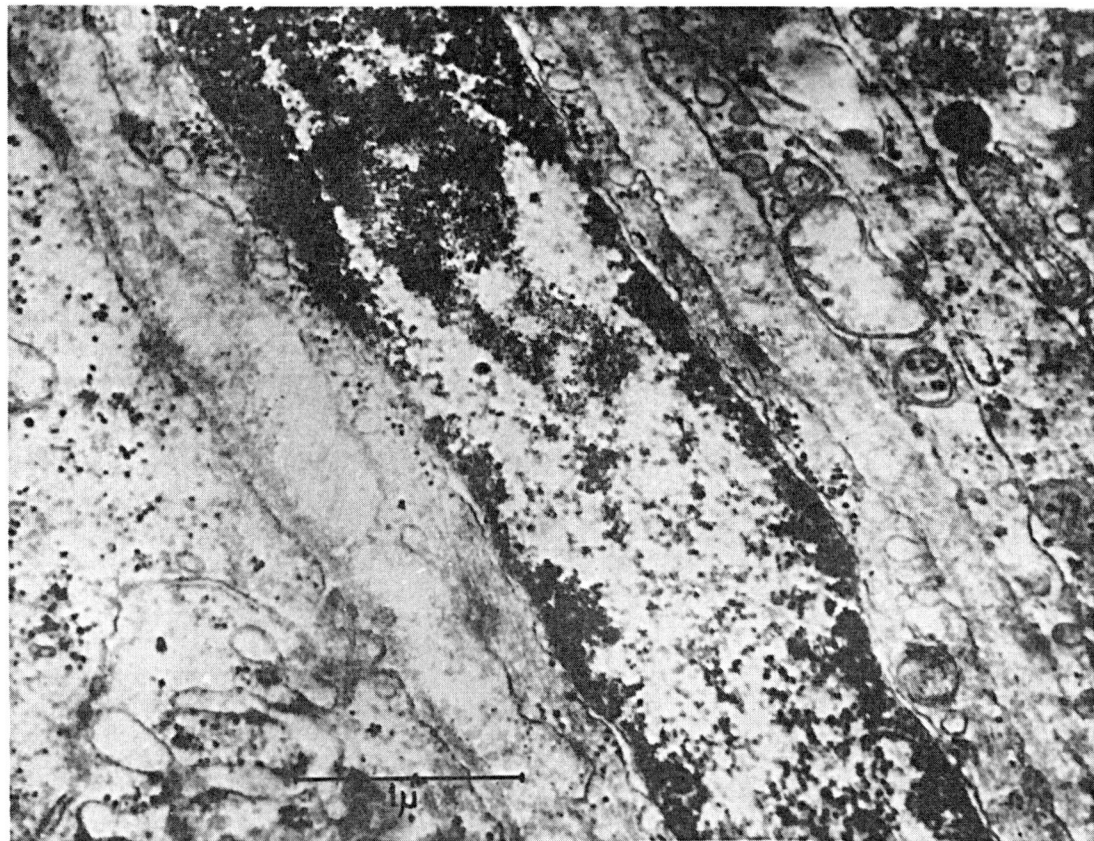

Figure 8. Lamina propria of seminiferous tubule in the adult cat. Note the striking resemblance to the human peritubular tissue, with alternating layers of noncellular material and contractile cells.

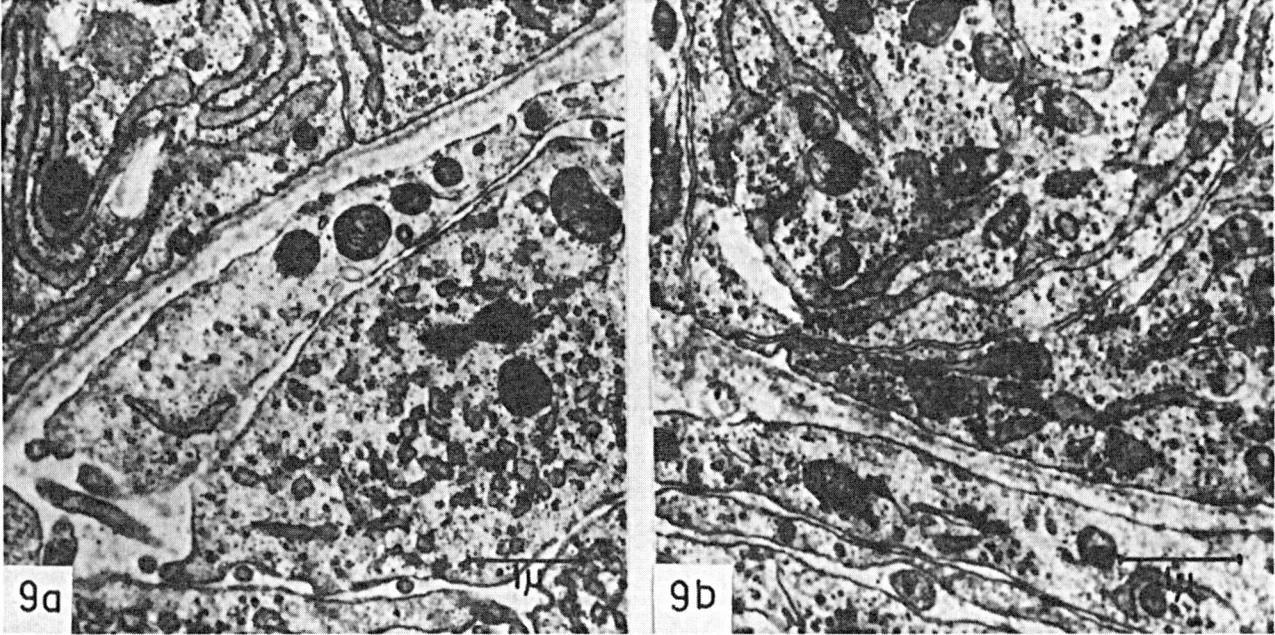

Figure 9. (a) Lamina propria of the seminiferous tubules of lamb, 54 days postcoital. The basement membrane and a second, partially incomplete lamella can be seen. The surrounding cells are not particularly differentiated and exhibit a conspicuous rough endoplasmic reticulum.

(b) Another area of the lamina propria at the same stage of developmen showing elongated, rather differentiated cells, with less endoplasm reticulum and filaments in the periphery of their cytoplasm (Busto Obregón and Courot 1974).

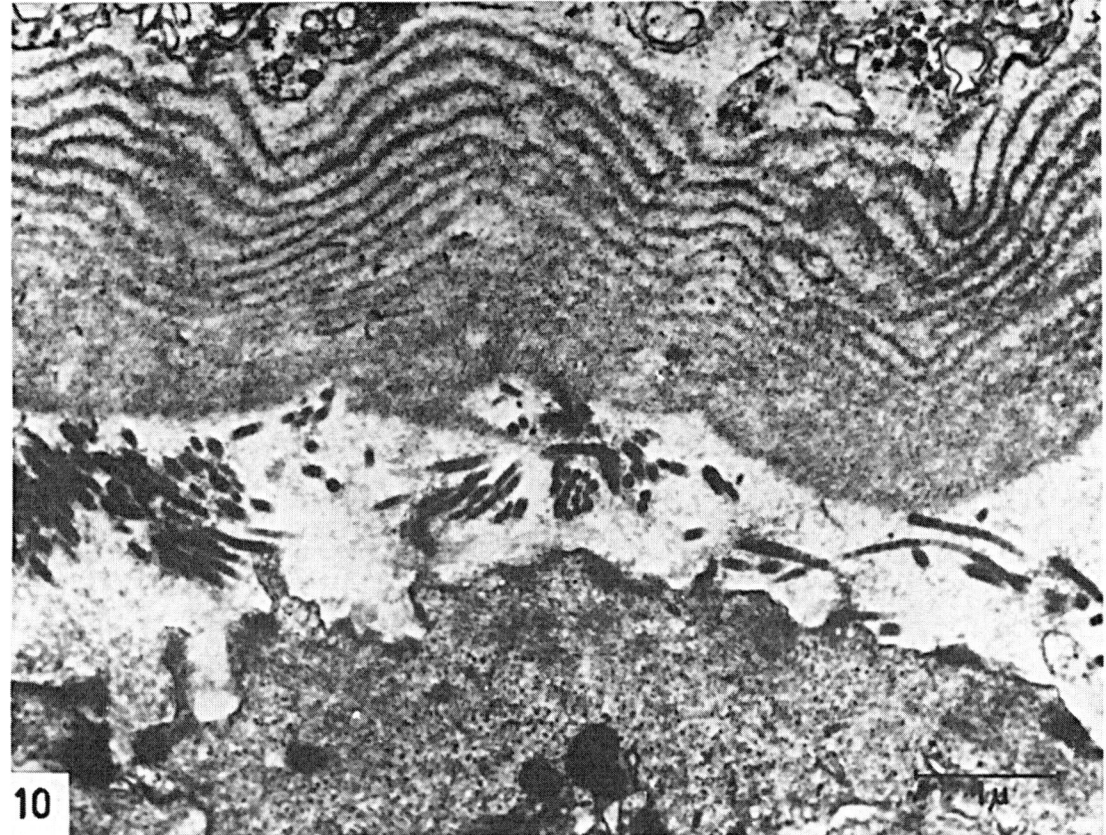

Figure 10. Lamina propria of adult ram. Note the multilamellar appearance of the noncellular component and the hazy aspect of the outer lamellae. The contractile cells have densities under the plasma membrane, where the filaments are anchored (Bustos-Obregón and Courot 1974).

REFERENCES

Attal J: Levels of testosterone, androstenedione, estrone and estradiol-17 B in the testis of fetal sheep. Endocrinol 85: 280-289, 1969.

Bock P, Breitnecker G, Lunglmayr G: Kontraktile Fibroblasten (Myofibroblasten) in der Lamina propria der Hodenkanälchen vom Menschen. Cell Tiss Res 133: 519-527, 1972.

Bouffard G: Injection des couleurs de benzidine aux animaux normaux. Ann Inst Pasteur 20: 539-546, 1906.

Bressler RS, Ross MH: Peritubular myoid cell differentiation. Biol Reprod 6: 148-159, 1972.

Burgos MH, Vitale-Calpe R, Aoki A: Fine structure of the testis and its functional significance. In: The testis. Johnson AD, Gomes WR, Vandemark NL (eds), New York, Academic Press, 1970, vol 1, 551-649.

Bustos-Obregón E: Description of the boundary tissue of human seminiferous tubules under normal and pathological conditions. Verh Anat Ges 68: 197-201, 1974.

Bustos-Obregón E: Ultrastructure and function of the lamina propria of mammalian seminiferous tubules. Andrologia 8: 179-185, 1976.

Bustos-Obregón E, Courot M: Ultrastructure of the lamina propria in the ovine seminiferous tubules: development and some endocrine considerations. Cell Tiss Res 150: 481-492, 1974.

Bustos-Obregón E, Holstein AF: On structural patterns of the lamina propria of human seminiferous tubules. Cell Tiss Res 141: 413-425, 1973.

Bustos-Obregón E, López ML: The lamina propria of cat seminiferous tubule. Rev Micr Electr 3: 26-27, 1976.

Clermont Y: Contractile elements in the limiting membrane of seminiferous tubules of the rat. Exp Cell Res 15: 438-440, 1958.

Cook P: A filamentous cytoskeleton in vertebrate smooth muscle fibers. J Cell Biol 68: 539-556, 1976.

Courot M: Endocrine control of the supporting and germ cells of the impuberal testis. J Reprod Fertil, suppl 2: 89-101, 1967.

De la Balze FA, Mancini RA, Arrillaga F, Andrada J, Vilar O, Gurtman AI, Davidson OW: Puberal maturation of the normal human testis: a histologic study. J Clin Endocr 20: 266-285, 1960.

Dubois M, Mauleon P: Mise en évidence par immunofluorescence des cellules à l'activité gonadotrope LH dans l'hypophyse du fœtus de brébis. CR Acad Sci Paris 269: 219-222, 1969.

Dym M: The fine structure of the monkey (*Macaca*) Sertoli cell and its role in maintaining the blood-testis barrier. Anat Rec 175: 639-656, 1973.

Dym M, Cavicchia JC: Further observations on the blood-testis barrier in monkeys. Biol Reprod 17: 390-403, 1977.

Eigel T: Histologische und autoradiographische Untersuchungen zur Kinetik der Wandzellen während der Evolution der II-Gonocyten. Dissertation, Düsseldorf, 1973.

Fawcett DW: Observations on the organization of the interstitial tissue of the testis and on the occluding cell junctions in the seminiferous epithelium. Adv Biosciences 10: 83-99, 1973.

Fawcett DW, Heidger PM, Leak LV: Lymph vascular system of the interstitial tissue of the testis as revealed by electron microscopy. J Reprod Fertil 19: 109-119, 1969.

Fawcett DW, Leak LV, Heidger PM: Electron microscopic observations on the structural components of the blood-testis barrier. J Reprod Fertil, suppl 10: 105-122, 1970.

Flechon JE, Bustos-Obregón E, Steger RW, Hafez ESE: Ultrastructure of testes and excurrent ducts in the bonnet monkey (*Macaca radiata*). J Med Primatology 5: 321-335, 1976.

Furuya S: Studies on testicular function 5: electron microscopic studies on the changes of the peritubular wall of the human seminiferous tubules in hypospermatogenesis. Jap J Urol 66: 809-828, 1975.

Furuya S, Jumamoto Y, Suguki T, Takauji M, Nagai T: Actin-like filaments in the peritubular cells of human testis: chemical extraction and binding with heavy meromyosin. Andrologia 9: 349-356, 1977.

Goldacre RJ, Sylvén N: On the access of blood-borne dyes to various tumour regions. Brit J Cancer 16: 306-322, 1962.

Hadžiselimović F, Seguchi H: Entwicklung der peritubularen Struktur des Tubulus seminiferus bei Kindern. Verh Anat Ges 69: 525-731, 1975.

Hovatta O: Contractility and structure of adult rat seminiferous tubules in organ culture. Cell Tiss Res 130: 171-179, 1972a.

Hovatta O: Effect of androgens and antiandrogens on the development of the myoid cells of the rat seminiferous tubules (organ culture). Cell Tiss Res 131: 299-308, 1972b.

Kormano M: Dye permeability and alkaline phosphatase activity of testicular capillaries in the postnatal rat. Histochemie 9: 327-338, 1967.

Kormano M, Hovatta O: Contractility and histochemistry of the myoid cell layer of the rat seminiferous tubules during postnatal development. Anat Embryol 137: 239-248, 1972.

Lacy D, Rotblat J: Study of normal and irradiated boundary tissue of the seminiferous tubules of the rat. Cell Res 21: 49-70, 1960.

Langford GA, Heller GC: Fine structure of muscle cells of the human testicular capsule: basis of testicular contractions. Science 179: 573, 1973.

McCord RC: Fine structure observations of peritubular cell layer in the hamster testis. Protoplasma 69: 283-289 (1970).

Mihatsch W: Über die Anwendung der Semidünnschnitt Technik als Routinemethode für die Untersuchung von Hodenbiopsie Material. Dissertation, Hamburg, 1973.

Neaves WB: The blood-testis barrier. In: The testis, Johnson AD, Gomes WR (eds), New York, Academic Press, 1977, vol 4, p 125-162.

Regaud C: Études sur la structure des tubes séminifères et sur la spermatogénèse chez les mammifères. Arch Anat Microsc Norphol 4: 101-156, 231-380, 1901.

Ribbert H: Die Abscheidung intravenös injizierten gelösten Karmins in den Geweben. Z Allgem Physiol 4: 201-214, 1914.

Roosen-Runge EC: Motions of the seminiferous tubules of rat and dog. Anat Rec 109: 413, 1951.

Ross MH: The fine structure and development of the peritubular contractile cell component in the seminiferous tubule of the mouse. Am J Anat 121: 523, 528, 1967.

Ross MH, Long JR: Contractile cells in human seminiferous tubules. Science 153: 1271-1273, 1966.

Setchell BP, Waites GMH: The blood-testis barrier. In: Handbook of Physiology, Hamilton DW, Greep RO (eds), Baltimore, Williams and Wilkins, 1975, vol 5, p 143-172.

Suvanto O, Kormano M: The relation between in vitro contractions of the rat seminiferous tubules and the cyclic stage of the seminiferous epithelium. J Reprod Fertil 21: 227-232, 1970.

Wissler RW: The arterial medial cell, smooth muscle or multifunctional mesenchyme? Circulation 36: 1-5, 1967.

7. THE BLOOD-TESTIS BARRIER

S. Furuya, Y. Kumamoto, M. Mori and S. Sugiyama

1. INTRODUCTION

The existence of the blood-testis barrier has been established morphologically and physiologically in some experimental animals such as guinea pigs, rats and mice. Since the seminiferous tubules were not stained by intravenously injected dyes, it was at first assumed that the blood-testis barrier probably located in the capillary wall of the testis, as with the blood-brain barrier (Kormano 1967). By cannulation into the rete testis of the ram, however, it has been demonstrated physiologically that there are some differences between components of testicular fluid and testicular lymph, and that the components of blood and testicular lymph are almost the same. Some substances tested (urea, ethanol, Na, K, Cl, creatinine, etc.) passed into the testicular fluid and testicular lymph, while others (inulin, para-amino-hippuric acid, albumin, etc.) passed readily into the testicular lymph but did not enter the testicular fluid. It has been concluded, therefore, that the blood-testis barrier is not in the capillary wall but in the peritubular wall (Setchell 1967, 1970). Electron-microscopic study, using the tracer method, has revealed that the penetration of the electron-dense tracer into the seminiferous tubules was prevented by the tight junction between the myoid cells and the Sertoli cell tight junction (Fawcett et al. 1970). At present it is considered that the myoid cell layer acts as a partial barrier while the specialized Sertoli junction constitutes a basic and essential blood-testis barrier.

This barrier effectively excludes certain substances from the seminiferous epithelium and creates a specific fluid environment inside the seminiferous tubules where the spermatogenesis is carried out. Moreover this barrier appears postnatally at the time when spermatogenesis is initiated. Thus it should be emphasized that the blood-testis barrier is closely associated with spermatogenesis.

A limited number of papers on the human blood-testis barrier have been reported (Furuya 1975; Nagano and Suzuki 1976a, 1976b, 1976c; Kumamoto and Furuya 1976; Bigliardi and Vegni-Talluri 1976; Furuya et al. 1978). Factors influencing the initiation and maintenance of the blood-testis barrier as well as the relationship between the blood-testis barrier and spermatogenesis and the secretion of gonadotropin have not been demonstrated. In order to clarify these factors and this relationship, in this chapter, we will consider the ultrastructure, development and morphological integrity of the blood-testis barrier in man.

2. MORPHOLOGY OF THE BLOOD-TESTIS BARRIER

2.1. Permeability of lanthanum tracer into seminiferous tubules

Substances transported from the bloodstream must first cross the capillary endothelium, penetrate the peritubular wall and then reach the seminiferous epithelium. The morphological characteristics of their pathway should be clarified by using the lanthanum tracer method.

The capillary endothelium in the testis has no apparent pores or fenestrations. It is surrounded by a complete continuous investment of basement membrane. These features resemble those of the brain and muscle. However, occluding junctions are absent in the endothelium of the testis, although they are always noted in those of the brain. In addition, there are comparatively few micropinocytotic vesicles on the surface of the endothelium in the testicular capillary. The thin margin of these endo-

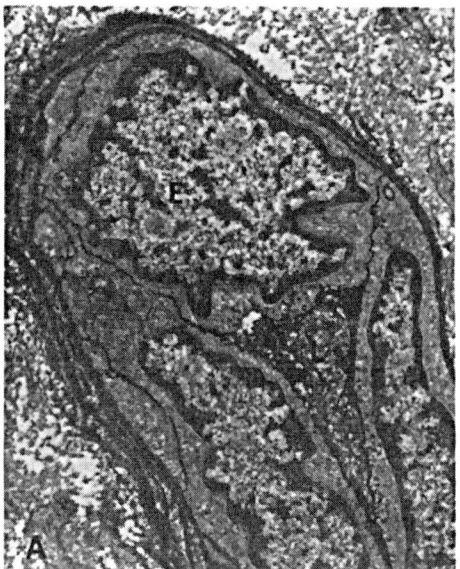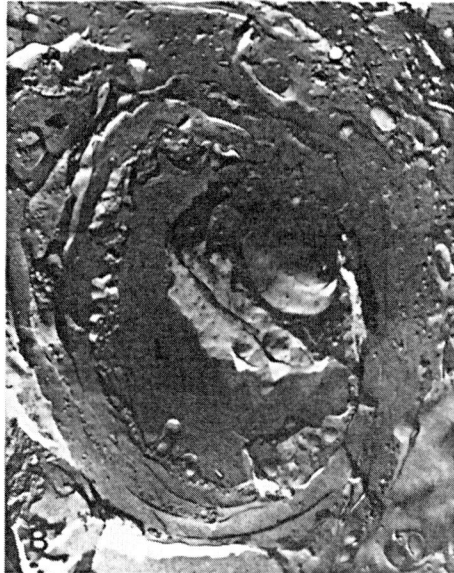

Figure 1. Electron micrographs of the testicular capillary in man. (A) The penetration of lanthanum into the intercellular spaces between the capillary endothelium (× 7,500). (B) Freeze-etched replica – note no specialized junctions (× 6,000). E: capillary endothelium; L: capillary lumen.

thelia often overlaps, but a 200 Å intercellular cleft is seen throughout most of this region of overlap. There are close appositions in limited areas (Fawcett et al. 1969). In the human testis, lanthanum penetrated freely into the intercellular clefts between the capillary endothelium with no specialized junctional complexes being observed (Figure 1).

The peritubular walls are generally composed of the basement membrane, myoid cell layer and collagen fiber layer. In the guinea pig, the tracer carbon and colloidal thorium could not penetrate the peritubular walls, while both ferritin and horse-radish peroxidase readily passed (Fawcett et al. 1970). In the rat, it has been noted that the penetration of lanthanum was prevented by inter-cellular tight junctions between the myoid cells. However, intercellular open junctions were seen occasionally and lanthanum did penetrate this myoid cell layer in 10-15% of the tubular cross-section examined (Dym and Fawcett 1970). In man, lanthanum penetrated this layer freely through the intercellular spaces between the myoid cells. These cells showed desmosome-like junctions in limited areas (Figure 2).

Inside the seminiferous tubules, lanthanum passed through the intercellular clefts between the seminiferous epithelium. However, the penetration of lanthanum was blocked at a short distance after

slight penetration within the Sertoli junctions. Lanthanum could rarely be found in the tubular lumen. Thus, the Sertoli junctions effectively pre-vented the penetration of lanthanum deeply into the seminiferous tubules (Figure 3).

2.2. *Ultrastructural characteristics of the Sertoli junction*

In previous studies, there has been a difference of opinion as to what type of junctional complexes the Sertoli cell would have. It has been referred to as 'narrow junction' (Nicander 1967) or 'close junction' (Flickinger and Fawcett 1967) and in one case a 'desmosome-like' structure has been described in the human testis (Bawa 1963). Using the en-block uranyl acetate staining method, it has been firstly demonstrated that the Sertoli junction in the rat is a tight junction (Dym and Fawcett 1970). Later, with application of the tracer technique and the freeze-fracture method, the same results have been clearly revealed in other animals and man (Dym 1973; Neaves 1973; Furuya 1975; Nagano and Suzuki 1976a, 1976b, 1976c; Gilula et al. 1976; Connell 1978).

The Sertoli junctions are characterized by three components: (1) multiple membrane fusions; (2) subsurface cisternae of endoplasmic reticulum

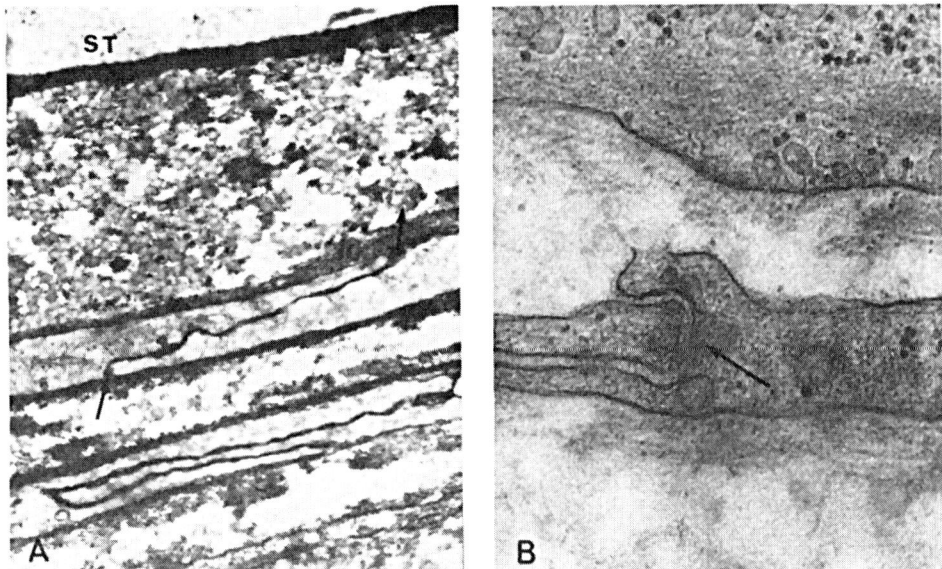

Figure 2. Electron micrographs showing the intercellular junctions between the peritubular myoid cells in man. (A) Lanthanum tracer penetrates into the peritubular walls (arrow) via the interstices between the myoid cells (×20,000). (B) The desmosome-like junction, arrowed (×95,000). ST: seminiferous tubule.

oriented in parallel with the Sertoli cell plasma membrane; and (3) bundles of microfilaments.

2.2.1. Membrane fusions. In this sections, the intercellular spaces between the Sertoli cells were approximately 50-150 Å, showing some close points here and there which may be indicative of membrane fusions (Figure 3). Pictures of lanthanum-filled Sertoli junctions showed their ultrastructural characteristics more clearly than those of thin sections. In longitudinal-section pictures of lanthanum-filled Sertoli junctions, membrane fusions were clearly recognized as tight junctions with a pentalaminar structure (Figure 4a). Oblique-section pictures and en-face section pictures showed a characteristic structure with an alternating arrangement of electron-dense bands and electron-lucent lines (Figure 4b). The former corresponded to the intercellular spaces filled with lanthanum. The latter corresponded to the membrane fusions, and were approximately 100 Å in width. These lines were parallel with each other in a linear fashion. At times they showed branching and blind-ending which made a bypass for communication between adjacent electron-dense bands (Figure 4c, d). This picture seemed to indicate a partial discontinuity of membrane fusion. For this reason, we could see a short-distance penetration of lanthanum within the Sertoli junctions. In a freeze-etched Sertoli junction, thirty

or more strands were observed (Figure 5). These strands were parallel with each other and formed anastomosing networks, like complicated compartments. The strands corresponded to the electron-lucent lines in the lanthanum tracer method. The majority of strands appeared to be continuous, but disinterconnection of strands which made possible communication between adjacent compartments was at times seen. These findings were the same as in the blind-ending of electron-lucent lines.

It has been shown that the permeability of tight junctions in various types of epithelium is correlated with the number of strands. 'Tight' epithelium exhibits more than five strands, whereas 'leaky' epithelium shows few strands (Claude and Goodenough 1973). The number of strands in Sertoli tight junctions in man is over thirty, which is considered as 'very tight' in grade. Moreover, the size and configuration of these junctions have a significant effect as a barrier.

2.2.2. Subsurface cisternae. The Sertoli junctions were bounded on each side by cisternae of the endoplasmic reticulum. These subsurface cisternae ran parallel to the junctions, located 500-1000 Å from the Sertoli cell plasma membrane. Ribosomes were noted on the cytoplasmic surface of the cisternae, but at times they were present on both surfaces. Continuity between these specialized cisternae and rough endoplasmic reticulum was frequently seen (Figure 6).

2.2.3. Microfilaments (HMM-binding filaments). Bundles of microfilaments were noted between the Sertoli cell plasma membrane and the associated subsurface cisternae. They were parallel to each other and to the cell membrane, and were about 50 Å in diameter. These filaments formed characteristic arrowhead complexes, when incubated with heavy meromyosin (Figure 7). The arrowhead complexes were inhibited when incubated with HMM plus

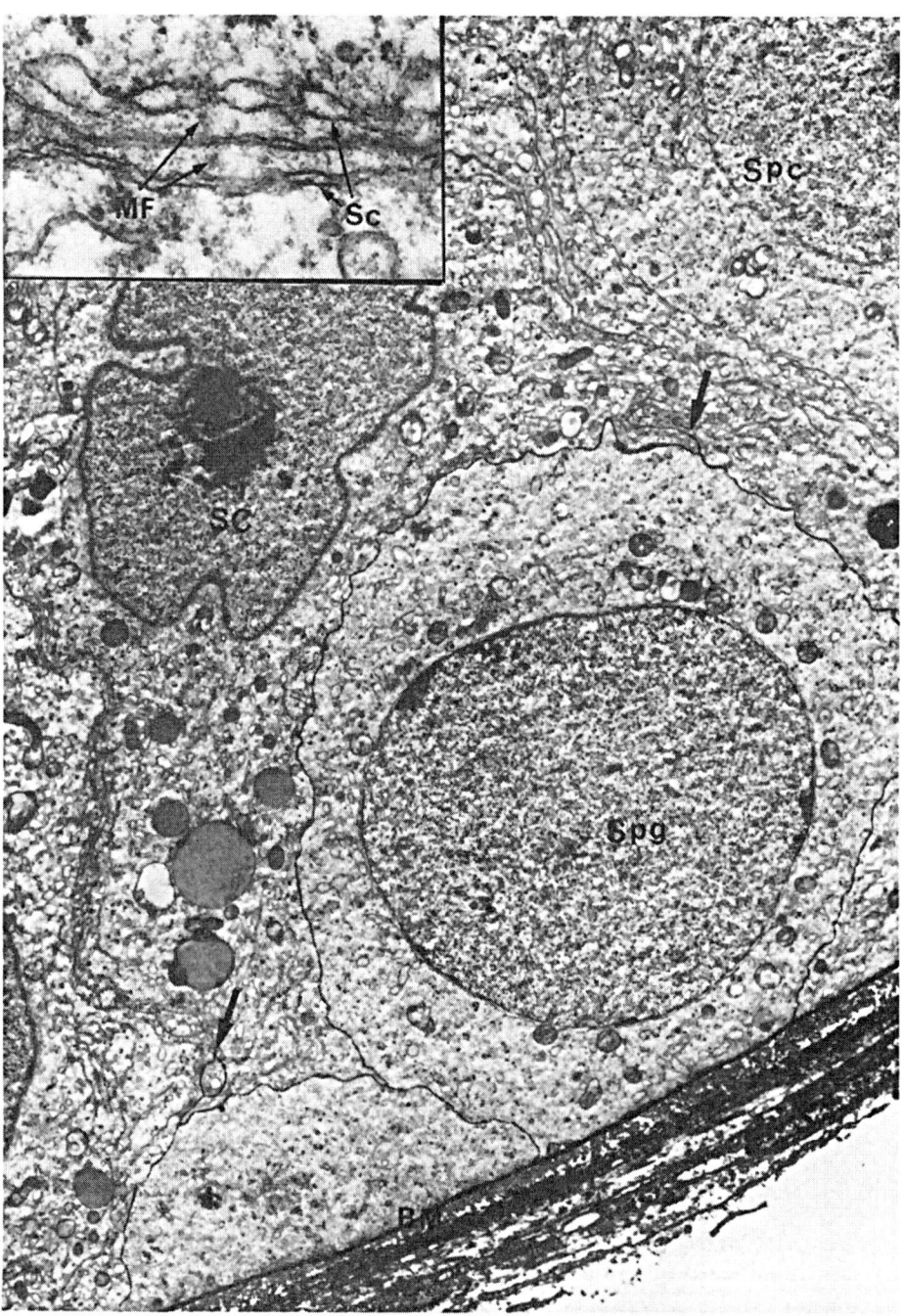

Figure 3. Electron micrograph showing the penetration of lanthanum into the seminiferous tubules of an adult normal testis. The penetration of lanthanum is blocked by the Sertoli junctions after a slight permeation (arrows) into the intercellular spaces between the Sertoli cells (×8,000). *Inset:* Thin section picture of the specialized Sertoli junctions (×47,000). BM: basement membrane; MF: microfilament; Sc: subsurface cisternae; SC: Sertoli cell; Spc: spermatocyte; Spg: spermatogonia.

ATP. The same result has been revealed in the Sertoli junctions of swine and mouse testes (Toyama 1976). These findings may indicate that these microfilaments are actin-like and that a contractile system exists in the Sertoli junctions. Therefore, it is suggested that the microfilaments may be involved in a 'zipper-up' function of the Sertoli junctions for movement of the developing germ cells upward from the basal compartment to the adluminal compartment (Dym and Fawcett 1970; Toyama 1976).

3. FUNCTIONS OF THE BLOOD-TESTIS BARRIER

It is considered that the main function of the blood-testis barrier is to establish and maintain a stable and

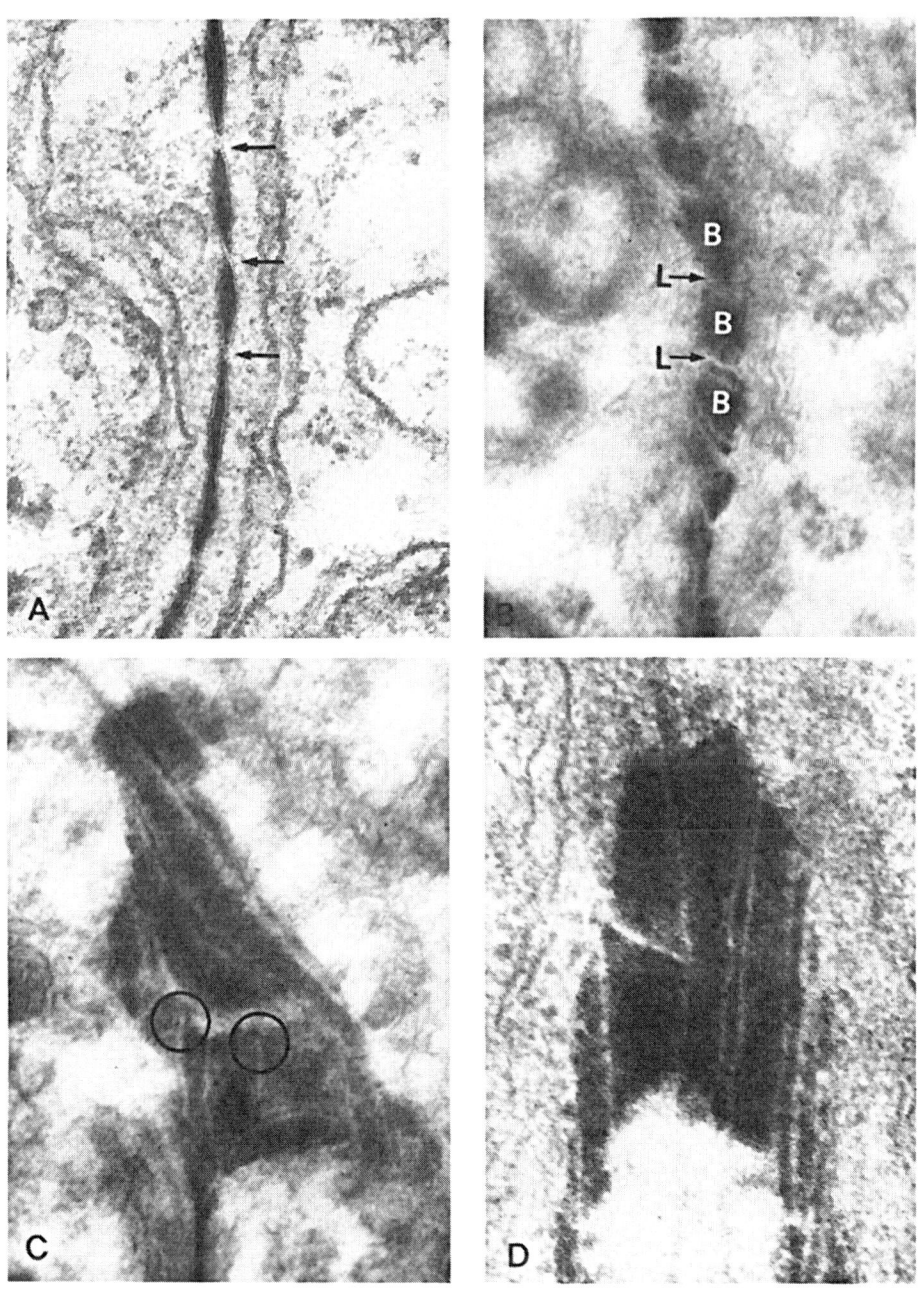

Figure 4. Electron micrographs of the lanthanum-filled Sertoli junctions. (A) Longitudinal section picture – arrows indicate the membrane fusions (×90,000). (B) Oblique section picture (×60,000) – note characteristic feature of an alternating arrangement of electron-lucent lines (L) and electron-dense bands (B). (C, D) En-face section pictures – the electron-lucent lines show blind-ending (circles) and branching (C: ×60,000; D: ×66,000).

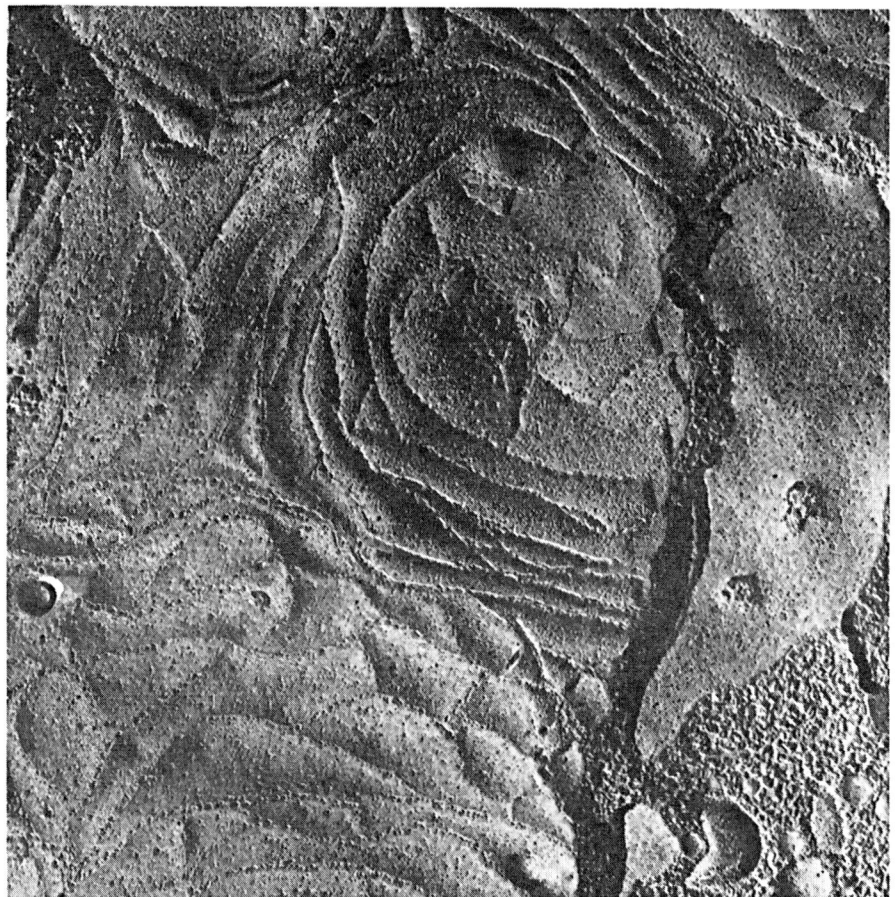

Figure 5. Freeze-etched replica of the Sertoli junctions (× 40,000).

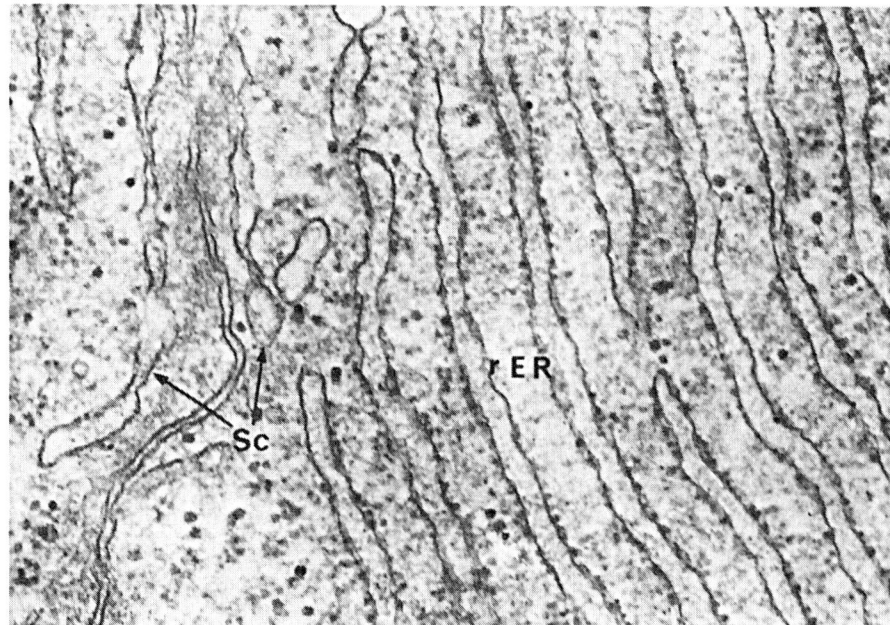

Figure 6. Electron micrograph (× 10,000) showing subsurface cisternae (Sc) associated with rough endoplasmic reticulum (rER).

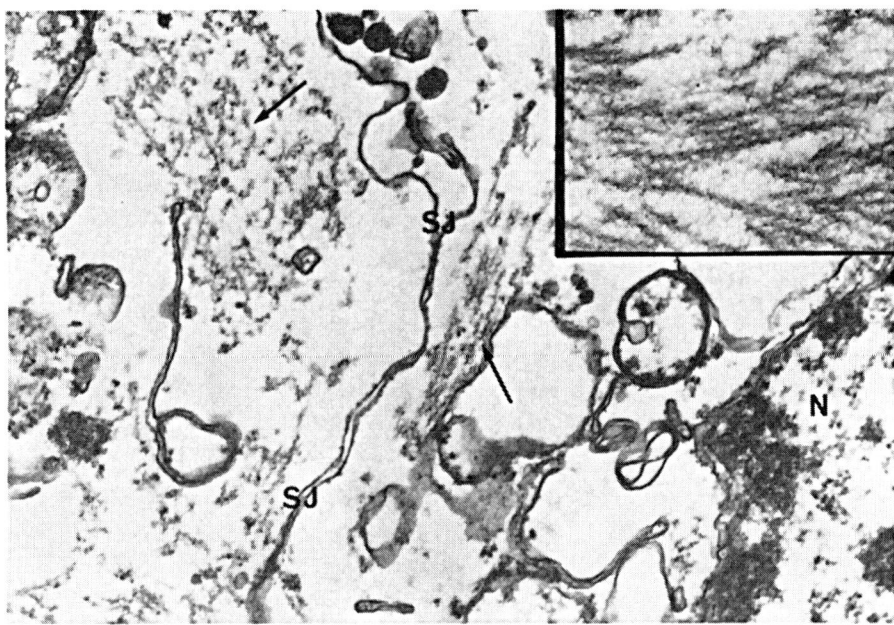

Figure 7. Electron micrographs (× 40,000) showing the microfilaments of the Sertoli junction treated with heavy meromyosin (arrows). *Inset:* High magnification of the HMM complexed filaments – note characteristic arrowhead complexes (× 80,000). N: nucleus of the Sertoli cell; SJ: Sertoli junction.

beneficial environment for spermatogenesis. The seminiferous tubules are divided into two physiological compartments by the Sertoli junctions. One is the basal compartment including spermatogonia and primary spermatocytes between the Sertoli junctions and basement membrane, and the other is the adluminal compartment including developing spermatocytes and spermatids – Figure 8 (Dym and Fawcett 1970). The basal compartment forms a environment where substances transported from blood plasma after penetrating the peritubular walls come directly in contact with the germ cells. On the other hand, in the adluminal compartment the substances are blocked by the Sertoli junctions and the germ cells are placed in an environment where they cannot come in contact with the substances except through the cytoplasm of the Sertoli cells. The composition of the testicular fluid in the adluminal compartment is different from that of blood plasma or testicular lymph. A greater potassium content, some aminoacids in high concentration, and proteins in low concentration, with the exception of β-macroglobulin and specific protein, have been found in the seminiferous fluid (Setchell and Waites 1975). It is suggested that the testicular fluid has an important effect on spermatogenesis. On the other hand, the fluid transports the testicular spermatozoa from the germinal epithelium to the caput epidi-

dymis and supplies the spermatozoa with various substances for survival. The peculiar composition of the testicular fluid is probably caused by secretion of the Sertoli cells and the regulation of the entry of various substances by the blood-testis barrier. Thus, it is assumed that meiosis and sperm maturation are carried out in the specific environment which is created by the Sertoli cells and the blood-testis barrier.

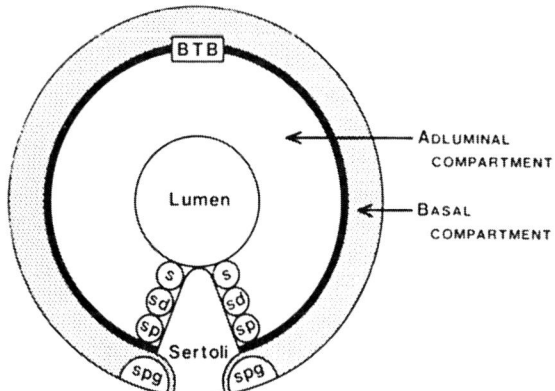

Figure 8. The blood-testis barrier and compartments in the seminiferous tubules. Mitosis of the young germ cells is carried out in the adluminal compartment which is created by the blood-testis barrier. The main function of the blood-testis barrier is considered to establish and to maintain a stable and beneficial environment for spermatogenesis- BTB: blood-testis barrier; s: spermatozoa; sd: spermatids; sp: spermatocytes; spg: spermatogonia.

There are specific substances such as androgen-binding protein (ABP) and inhibin in the testicular fluid. ABP has been suggested to form the high local concentration of androgen required for spermatogenesis and to facilitate the transport of androgen (Steinberger and Steinberger 1977). Inhibin has been postulated as the basis of a feedback mechanism to pituitary on the rate of spermatogenesis. Thus, the blood-testis barrier may play a role in retaining some specific substances of endocrinological significance formed inside the tubules (Setchell and Waites 1975).

As another specific role, the blood-testis barrier has an effect on the immunological isolation of the developing germ cells (Neaves 1973). The developing spermatocytes, spermatids and spermatozoa which appear at puberty have an auto-antigen. It has been well demonstrated that immunization with testicular homogenate or extract, or spermatozoa in Freund's adjuvant make an autoimmune reaction in the guinea pig testis which leads to aspermatogenesis. However, under natural conditions this immunological response does not occur. There is no detectable γ-globulin or IgG in the seminiferous tubules. In addition, no intratubular fluorescence has been observed after intravenous injections of fluorescence-conjugated γ-globulin and albumin, yet the interstitial space and peritubular wall have fluoresced very clearly (Tung et al. 1970; Johnson 1972). Thus it may be said that the blood-testis barrier acts as an immunologically protective mechanism which prevents the sperm-specific antibody from entering into the adluminal compartment and the sperm-specific antigen from leaking from the seminiferous tubules.

It has been shown that the blood-testis barrier retards or blocks the penetration of some chemicals. It has also been suggested that the blood-testis barrier prevents the permeation of toxins and mutagens, and that it protects the developing germ cells against these noxious substances (Dixon and Lee 1973).

4. POSTNATAL DEVELOPMENT OF THE BLOODTESTIS BARRIER

4.1. Time of appearance of the blood-testis barrier

The postnatal development of the Sertoli junctions of rats and mice has been clearly elucidated by the freeze-fracture method (Gilula et al. 1976; Nagano and Suzuki 1976b). In the newborn, gap junctions consisting of an aggregation of the intramembranous particles are frequently found. The initial formation of tight junctions is also seen in limited areas. As development progresses, those gap junctions become less numerous and ultimately disappear, while the tight junctions appear to increase in size and in number. Around sixteen days of age or thereabouts, many parallel rows of intramembranous particles appear to be circumferentially oriented on the Sertoli cell surface. Moreover, it has been revealed by the tracer method that the blood-testis barrier appears to be established between sixteen and nineteen days of age (Vitale et al. 1973; Tindall et al. 1975). In the seminiferous tubules of this period, spermatogenesis has progressed to pachytene spermatocytes and tubular canalization is completed. Thus, it may be stated that the blood-testis barrier is not present at birth, but develops shortly before and after onset of spermatogenesis (Fawcett et al. 1976).

In the prepubertal testis of man (3-8 years old), the tracer lanthanum permeated freely through the interstices between the immature Sertoli cells, reaching even the centre portion of the seminiferous tubules (Figure 9a). It was difficult to find specialized junctions between these cells, but interdigitation-like complexes were frequently seen (Figure 9b, c). Subsurface cisternae were noted in the testes of seven and eight-year-old boys (Figure 9d). In the pubertal testis (11-13 years old), specialized junctional complexes, composed of membrane fusions, subsurface cisternae, and bundles of microfilaments, were observed between the mature Sertoli cells. These tight junctions blocked the deep penetration of lanthanum into the seminiferous tubules (Figure 10a). Longitudinal and en-face section pictures of lanthanum-filled Sertoli junctions clearly showed the membrane fusions, resembling those in the normal control (Figure 10b, c). In one of these cases (11 years old), the spermatocytes did not appear in the seminiferous tubules, but the spermatogonia increased in number. In another cases (12-13 years old), spermatogenesis had been initiated and lumen formation had been accomplished. Thus, it is suggested the human blood-testis barrier is established shortly before and after the spermatogonia proliferate to give rise to the primary spermatocytes (Furuya et al. 1978).

4.2. Relationship between maturation of Sertoli cells and the blood-testis barrier

4.2.1. Morphological characteristics of immature and mature Sertoli cells. It has been revealed in the rat that there are two morphological indexes of Sertoli cell maturation: (1) specialized tight junctions between adjacent Sertoli cells (blood-testis barrier); and (2) tripartite structures of nucleolus (Flickinger 1967).

In the human testis, prepubertal immature Sertoli cells were cuboidal or columnar in shape, resting on

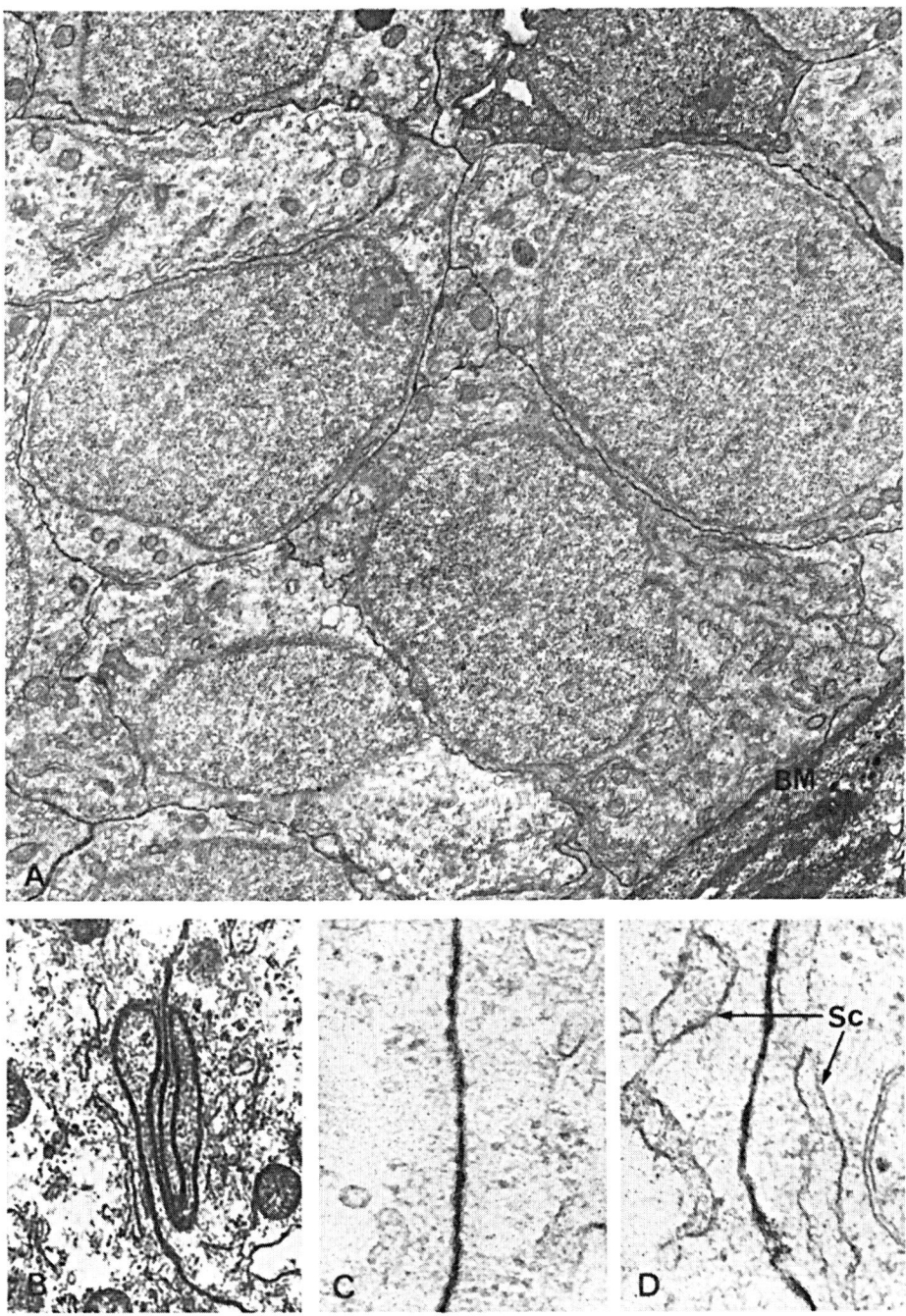

Figure 9. Electron micrographs showing the distribution of lanthanum in the prepubertal testis (A) and the lanthanum-filled intercellular junctions between the immature Sertoli cells (B-D). (A) The blood-testis barrier is not formed (× 6,000). (B) Interdigitation-like junction (× 80,000). (C) No specialized junctional complexes (× 75,000). (D) Subsurface cisternae (Sc) are observed in the testes of seven and eight-year-olds (× 75,000).

the basement membrane. They were compactly arranged in the seminiferous tubules. Mitochondria were round or oval, sometimes rodlike in shape. A few tubular cristae were seen. Smooth and rough endoplasmic reticula were noted in moderate abundance. The Golgi complexes were clearly seen, but not so well-developed. Lipid droplets and lysosomes were sometimes present; polyribosomes were also seen. The nucleus was oval-shaped, the nuclear envelope having a smooth outline, but

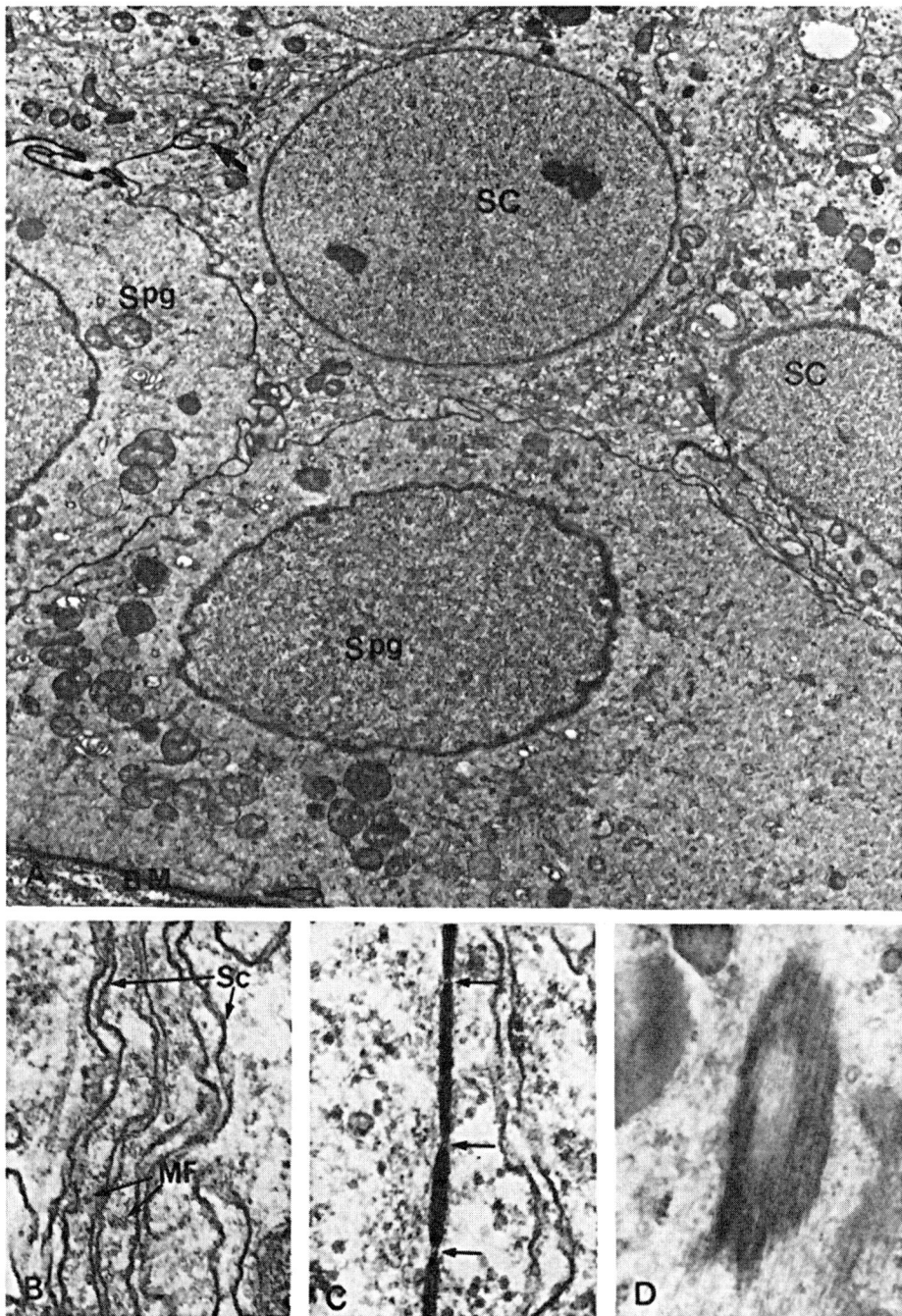

Figure 10. Electron micrographs showing the penetration of lanthanum into the seminiferous tubules (A), specialized Sertoli junctions (B, C) and Sertoli cell crystalloid (D) in the pubertal testis. (A) The Sertoli junctions block the deep penetration of lanthanum – arrows (×6,500); BM: basement membrane; SC: Sertoli cell; Spg: spermatogonia. (B, C) The Sertoli junctions are composed of membrane fusions (arrows), subsurface cisternae (Sc) and microfilaments (MF) – both ×70,000. (D) Note typical crystalloid of Charcot-Böttcher (×35,000).

sometimes showing a small irregular indentation. The nucleus contained karyosomes and peripheral clumps of heterochromatin (Figure 11a). One or two nucleoli were noted, frequently located near the nuclear envelope. They displayed various forms: (1) round dense body (Figure 11b) and (2) reticular formation of anastomosing strands (nucleolonema) associated with or without round pars amorpha (Figure 11c). On the other hand, pubertal mature Sertoli cells extended radially from the basement membrane to the tubular lumina. In the cytoplasm, there was a striking increase of smooth endoplasmic reticulum and the Golgi complexes were well-developed. Fine cytoplasmic filaments, microtubules, lipid droplets and lysosomes were ordinarily noted. The Sertoli cell crystalloids, the so-called

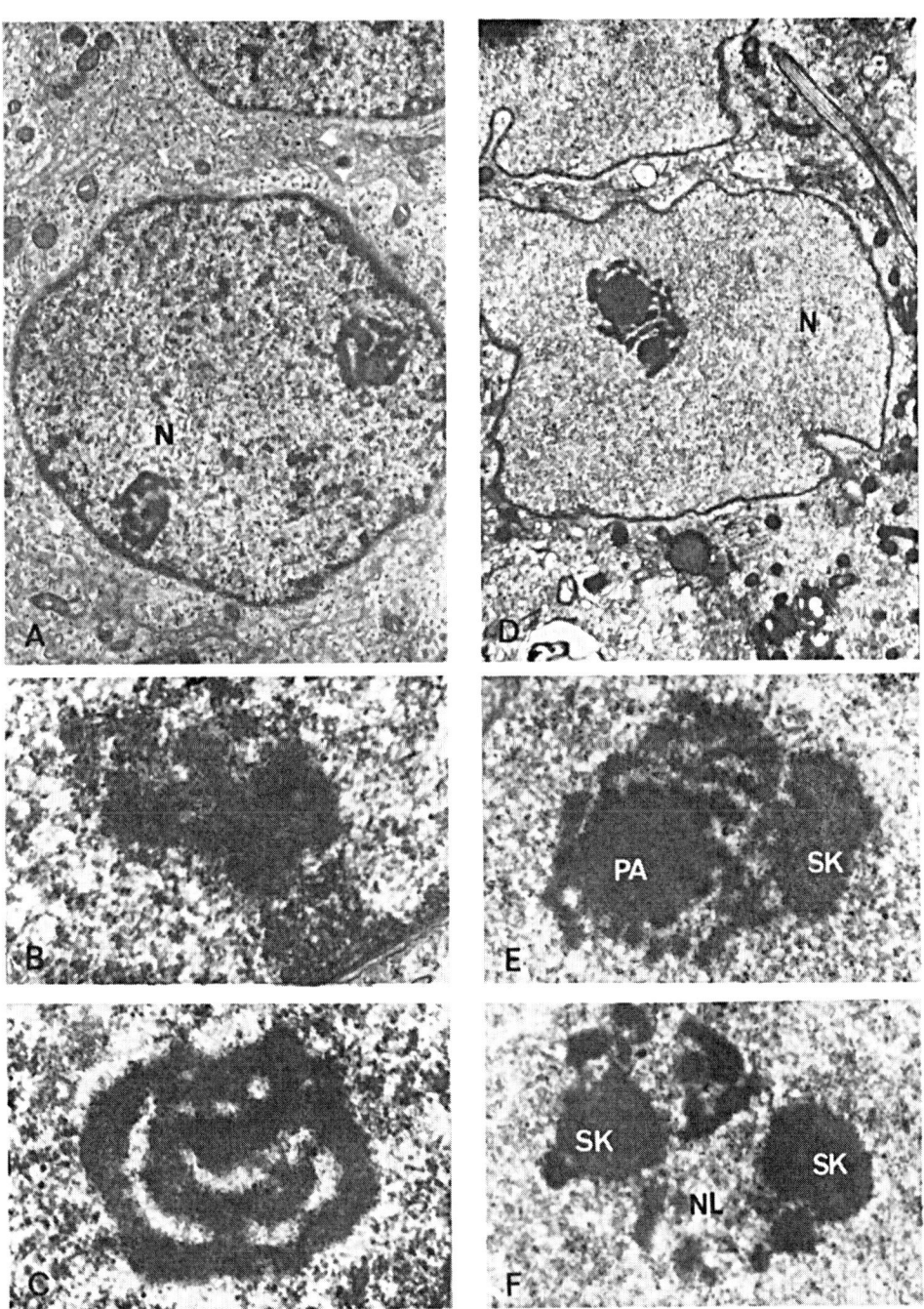

Figure 11. Electron micrographs showing the nucleus and nucleolus of immature Sertoli cells (A-C) and mature Sertoli cells (D-F). Note the tripartite structure of the nucleus in (F). A: ×7,800; B: ×27,000; C: ×28,000; D: ×4,800; E: ×17,000; F: ×17,000. N: nucleus; NL: nucleolonema; PA: pars amorpha; SK: satellite karyosome.

Charcot-Böttcher crystalloid, were found in the testis of an eleven-year-old boy (Figure 10d). The nucleus was irregularly shaped with deep infoldings of the nuclear envelope and had relatively homogenous nucleoplasm (Figure 11d). The nucleolus showed a tripartite structure. It consisted of a typical nucleolonema associated with large round pars amorpha and lateral satellite karyosomes (Figure 11e, f). Thus, we observed the differences in the configuration and cytoplasmic organelles between the immature and mature Sertoli cells of man. Their morphological differences are summarized in Table 1.

Table 1. Comparative morphological characteristics of cell shape and cytoplasmic organelles in immature and mature Sertoli cells.

	Immature Sertoli cells	*Mature Sertoli cells*
shape	cuboidal or columnar	radially elongated
nucleus	oval	irregularly infolded
nucleolus	dense body or nucleolonema	tripartite structure
endoplasmic reticulum	moderate	abundant
lipid droplet	few	regularly present
filament and microtubule	moderate	abundant
crystalloid	absent	present
junctional complex	interdigitation	specialized tight junction (blood-testis barrier)

4.2.2. Sertoli cell proliferation. It has been reported that the number of immature Sertoli cells in the rat increases progressively until eighteen days of age and that the mitosis of these cells ceases at fifteen days of age (Clermont and Perey 1957; Hilscher and Makoski 1968). An autoradiographic study revealed that the incorporation of ^{3}H-thymidine in the Sertoli cells decreased progressively after birth, and became negligible at fifteen days of age (Steinberger and Steinberger 1971). Our result, utilizing a flash-labelling method with ^{3}H-thymidine in the rat, also supported this finding (Figure 12).

Only very little mitosis was seen in the prepubertal human testis. Under light microscopy, however, it was difficult to distinguish whether the mitotic cells were the Sertoli cells or the germ cells. Ultrastructurally the mitotic picture of the immature Sertoli cells was recognized (Figure 13). In addition, it was noted that the number of Sertoli cells per cross-section of tubules decreased after puberty (Figure 14).

Thus, it would appear that the Sertoli cells divide and proliferate before appearance of the blood-testis barrier. After a period of proliferation, the Sertoli cells become mature and form the blood-testis barrier.

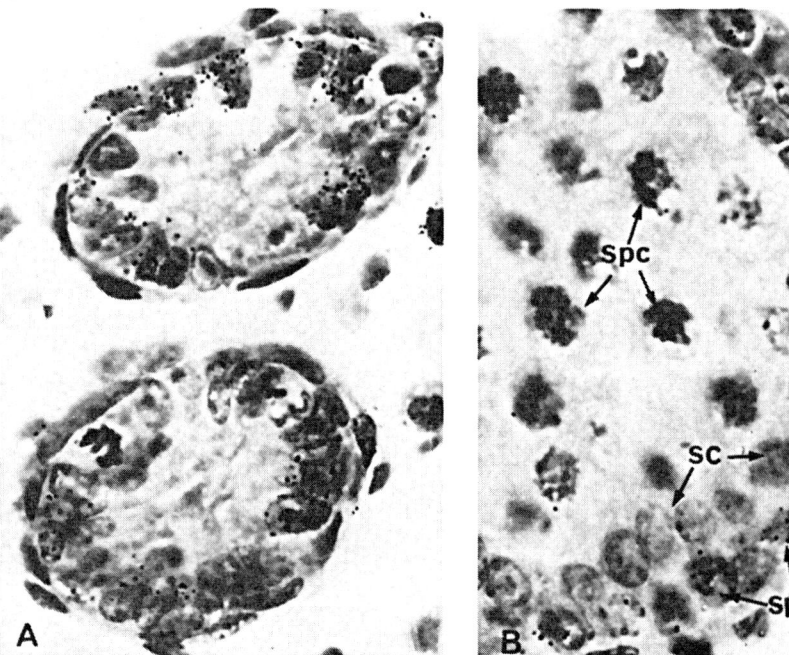

Figure 12. Radioautographs showing the incorporation of ^{3}H-thymidine in the testes of wister rats. (A) Seven days of age – note the incorporation of ^{3}H-thymidine into the immature Sertoli cell nucleus ($\times$840). (B) Eighteen days of age – ^{3}H-thymidine is not incorporated into the mature Sertoli cells, but is incorporated into the nucleus of spermatogonia. SC: Sertoli cell; Spc: spermatocyte; Spg: spermatogonia ($\times$840).

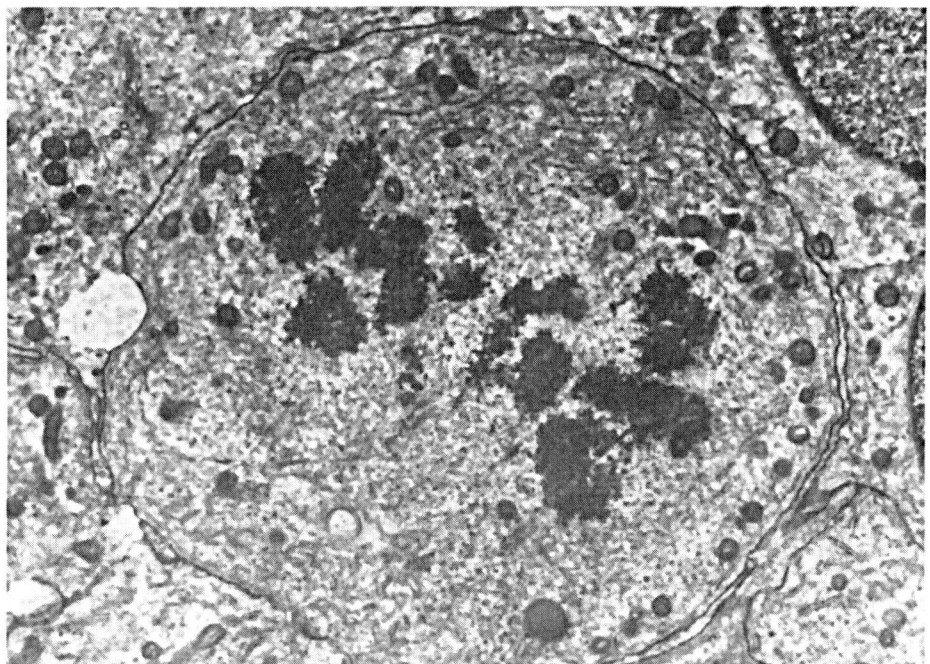

Figure 13. Electron micrograph showing the early metaphase in mitosis of the immature human Sertoli cell (× 7,500).

4.3. *Factors influencing development of the blood-testis barrier*

4.3.1. Gonadotropins. In the rat testis, the blood-testis barrier is formed between sixteen and nineteen days after birth (Vitale et al. 1973; Tindall et al. 1975), at which time a peak in the concentration of LH, FSH and testosterone is noted (Miyachi et al. 1973). This finding suggested that the formation of the blood-testis barrier might appear to be under hormone control. However, the suppression of gonadotropin secretion by daily injections of estrogen or clomiphene in the rat after birth resulted in a delay in the appearance of the blood-testis barrier. The formation of tight junctions between the Sertoli cells was delayed approximately by seven days and was accomplished 26 days after birth (Vitale et al. 1973). Thus, the development of the blood-testis barrier does not appear to be directly dependent upon gonadotropins. On the contrary, in experimental conditions where the testes taken from newborn mice were implanted into the testes of normal and hypophysectomized mice, the Sertoli cells in implants in normal hosts exhibited a normal developmental pattern, whereas those in implants in hypophysectomized hosts retained the feature observed in the newborn control. In the former, the

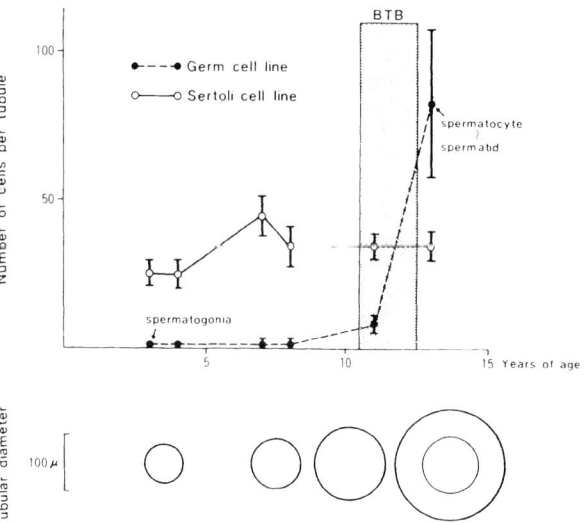

Figure 14. Diagram of changes in a number of Sertoli and germ cells per cross-section of tubules and the tubular diameter in the human testis during postnatal development. The Sertoli cells increase in number during the prepubertal period. The blood-testis barrier (BTB) appears at 11-13 years of age when spermatogenesis is initiated and lumen formation is completed.

specialized junctions between the Sertoli cells were noted in ultra-thin section preparations, but in the latter, these were not seen (Bressler 1976). Moreover, it has been reported that the transformation of the immature Sertoli cells in prepubertal testis into mature-type Sertoli cells was prevented by hypophysectomy in the lamb (Courot 1967), and that only immature Sertoli cells were found in patients of hypogonadotropic eunuchoidism ranging 17 to 37 years of age, whereas after treatment with chorionic and pituitary gonadotropin, the Sertoli cells exhibited the characteristic features of mature Sertoli cells (De Kretser and Burger 1972). These findings suggest that the development of the blood-testis barrier has a close relation to gonadotropin. Although it is difficult to interpret the above contradictory findings, the possibility of difference in materials and experimental methods cannot be ruled out.

In patients with hypogonadotropic eunuchoidism aged between 16 and 22 years old, the seminiferous tubules were filled mainly with immature Sertoli cells and a few spermatogonia were seen. The ultrastructural characteristics of cell shape and the intracytoplasmic organelles of these immature Sertoli cells were quite similar to those in the prepubertal testis. Lumen formation had not occurred as yet. The lanthanum passed through the intercellular spaces between these immature Sertoli cells and reached the centre portion of the seminiferous tubules (Figure 15a, b). Thus, the barrier structure which blocks the penetration of lanthanum was not observed. After hCG treatment, the testis increased in size and spermatogenesis was initiated. Spermatocytes and spermatids were seen, but the number of these cells was moderately few. Tubular canalization occurred. In ultra-thin section preparations and lanthanum-filled preparations, the morphological characteristics of the Sertoli cells as well as Sertoli junctions were comparable to those in normal control. These junctions excluded deep penetration of lanthanum into the seminiferous tubules. The lanthanum was found to be distributed into the basal compartment (Figure 15c, d). Thus, it is suggested that the initiation and development of the blood-testis barrier in man is dependent upon gonadotropins, at least in part.

4.3.2. Germ cells. It has been demonstrated that the formation of the blood-testis barrier is associated with the appearance of the spermatocytes in the rat testis (Vitale et al. 1973) and an increased number of spermatogonia in the human testis (Furuya et al. 1978). Thus, the development of the blood-testis barrier may be associated with the differentiation of the germ cells.

In the case of male offspring whose mother rat was irradiated during pregnancy, the germ cells could not develop and the Sertoli-cell-only testis was formed. However, the blood-testis barrier appeared even in these testes at thirty days after birth (Tindall et al. 1975). In addition, normal development of the Sertoli junctions was demonstrated in the Sertoli-cell-only testis of the rat whose mother was given Buzulfan during pregnancy (Gilula et al. 1976).

Congenital germ-cell-free mice, whose seminiferous tubules were devoid of germ cells throughout life, were obtained by a cross between two inbred strains (C57BL-W^v/+ and WN-W^n/+). At four to six weeks after birth, the seminiferous tubules consisted only of Sertoli cells, arranged in one layer in contact with the basement membrane. Tubular lumina appeared. Large and oval mitochondria were highly visible in the cytoplasm of the Sertoli cells (Figure 16a). After slight penetration of lanthanum into the interstices between the Sertoli cells, the Sertoli junctions blocked its penetration (Figure 16b). In the observations of ultra-thin sections and lanthanum-filled sections, these Sertoli junctions consisted of membrane fusions, subsurface cisternae and microfilaments, and showed the same characteristics as those in the normal control (Figure 16c, d). The same finding has been reported by using the freeze-fracture method (Nagano et al. 1977).

The syndrome called Sertoli-cell-only syndrome (germ cell aplasia) is characterized by seminiferous tubules containing only Sertoli cells. The only presenting complaint is infertility. Azoospermia, slightly small testis with normal consistence, elevated FSH titres, no gynecomastia and no abnormality in sex chromosomal configuration constitute the clinical features. It has been postulated that the congenital absence of germ cells is the basis for this syndrome, but no direct evidence for this exists. The seminiferous tubules showed a moderate decrease in size and no peritubular hyalinization. Ultrastructurally the Sertoli cells had normal structure characterized by an irregularly shaped nucleus with deep infolding, typical nucleoli, abundant smooth ER and crystalloids of Charcot-Böttcher. However, the infoldings of basement membrane into the cytoplasm of Sertoli cells were plainly observed. The Sertoli junctions prevented lanthanum from penetrating inside the seminiferous tubules (Figure 16a). Lanthanum could not be found in the lumina.

These Sertoli junctions consisted of membrane fusions, subsurface cisternae and bundles of microfilaments, and were identical with those in the normal control (Figure 17b, c).

Thus, the Sertoli cells and Sertoli junctions developed normally in spite of the absence of germ cells. It is therefore suggested that the formation of the blood-testis barrier is independent of the existence of germ cells.

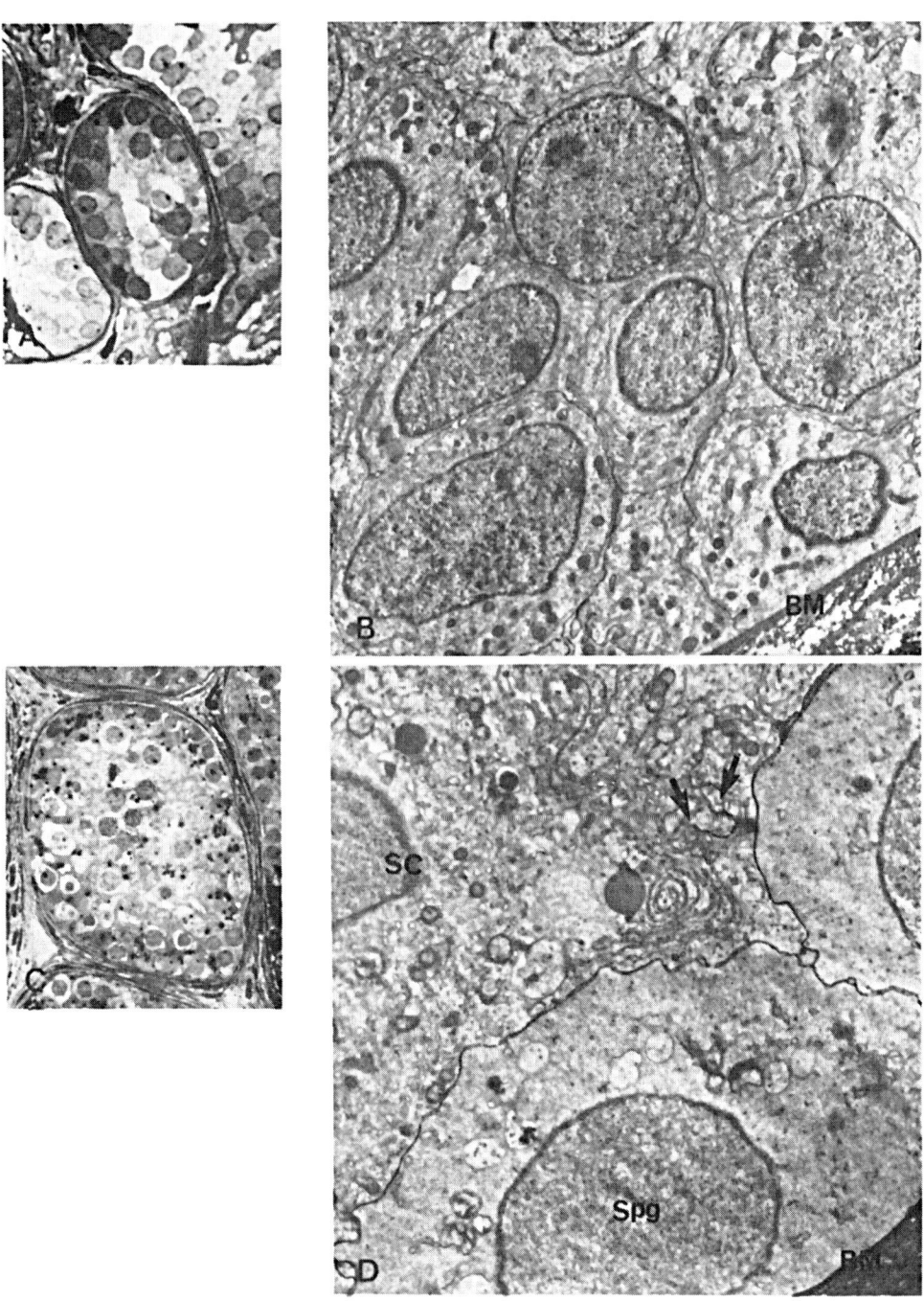

Figure 15. Light micrographs (A, C) and electron micrographs (B, D) showing morphological changes of the seminiferous tubules in patients with hypogonadotropic eunuchoidism before and after hCG treatment. (A, B) Before hCG treatment: note immature Sertoli cells which do not form the blood-testis barrier (A: ×240; B: ×3,800). (C, D) After hCG treatment: spermatogenesis has been initiated and has progressed; the blood-testis barrier (arrows) has been established (C: ×240; D: ×5,500). BM: basement membrane; SC: Sertoli cell; Spg: spermatogonia.

5. MORPHOLOGICAL INTEGRITY OF THE BLOOD-TESTIS BARRIER

5.1. Hypospermatogenic testis

By using the lanthanum tracer method, the ultra-structure of the Sertoli junctions was observed in hypospermatogenic testes which were obtained from infertile patients (Furuya 1975). In these testes the seminiferous tubules showed a moderately

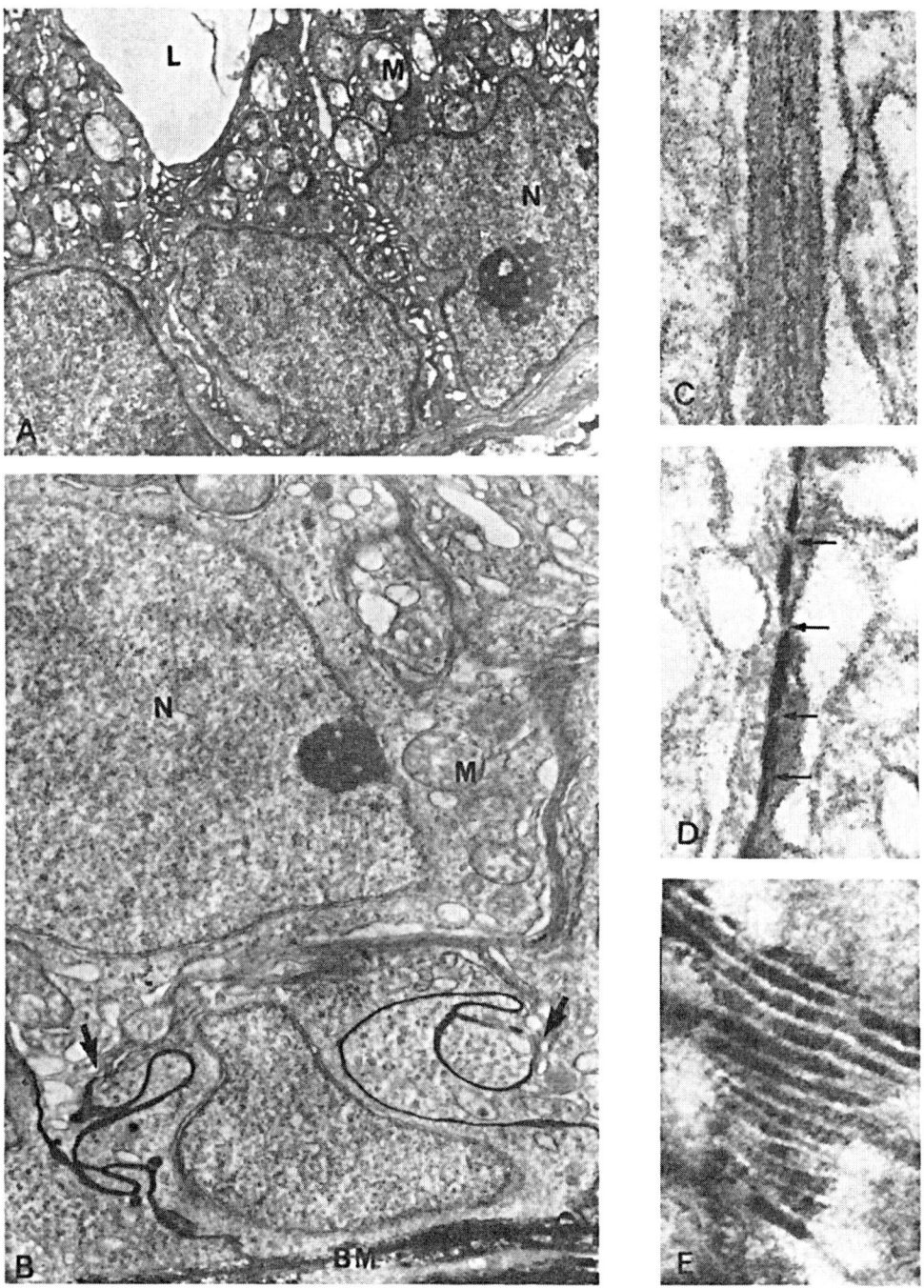

Figure 16. Electron micrographs showing the Sertoli cells and Sertoli junctions in congenital germ-cell-free mice of four weeks of age. (A) Thin section picture of the seminiferous tubule (×5,500). (B) The penetration of lanthanum is blocked (arrows) by the Sertoli junctions (×16,000). (C) Thin section picture of the Sertoli junction (×80,000). (D) Longitudinal section picture of the lanthanum-filled Sertoli junction – note arrowed membrane fusions (×80,000). (E) En-face section picture of the lanthanum-filled Sertoli junction (×80,000). BM: basement membrane; L: tubular lumen; M: mitochondria; N: nucleus.

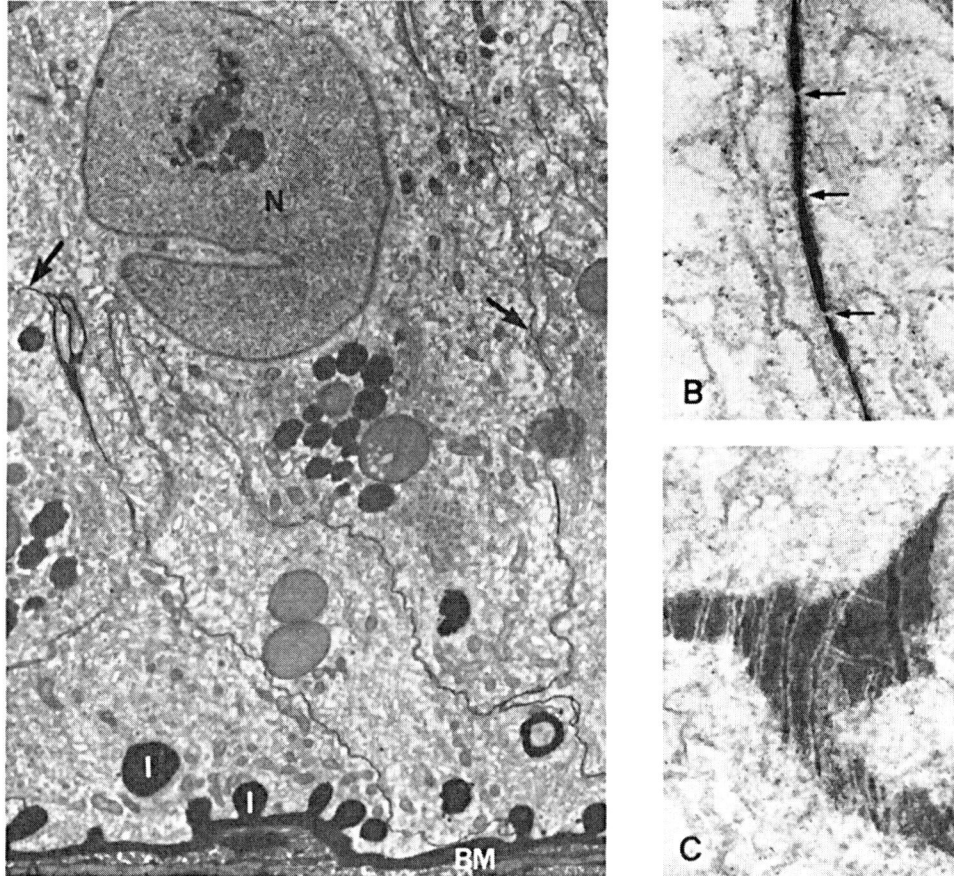

Figure 17. Electron micrographs showing the seminiferous tubules of Sertoli-cell-only syndrome treated with lanthanum tracer. (A) Complete penetration of lanthanum is blocked by the Sertoli junctions (arrows) at some points (× 5,000). (B) Longitudinal section picture of the lanthanum-filled Sertoli junction - arrows indicate membrane fusions (× 80,000). (C) En-face section picture of the lanthanum-filled Sertoli juncton (× 50,000). BM: basement membrane; I: infolding of the basement membrane; N: nucleus.

decreased number of spermatocytes and spermatids. After a slight penetration of lanthanum into the interstices between the Sertoli cells, the specialized Sertoli junctions blocked deep penetration of lanthanum (Figure 18). Ultrastructurally these Sertoli junctions showed specialized tight junctions comparable to those in normal control. The same result has been reported in the testes of infertile oligospermia and azoospermia patients by applying freeze-fracture method and lanthanum tracer technique (Bigliardi and Vegni-Talluri 1977). Therefore, these findings suggest that the Sertoli junctions morphologically appear to be intact in the hypospermatogenic testis of the man.

5.2. Hypophysectomy

It has been revealed that the acriflavin staining pattern in the seminiferous tubules of the hypo-

physectomized adult rat, after being injected subcutaneously, did not differ from that in sham-operated controls (Johnson 1970). Ultrastructurally, the penetration of lanthanum into the adluminal compartment was prevented by the Sertoli junctions in the testes of the hypophysectomized rats (Hagenäs et al. 1978). Therefore, it is suggested that the maintenance of the blood-testis barrier is not dependent upon gonadotropic hormones.

In hypophysectomized patients, the seminiferous tubules showed severe hypospermatogenesis. Only a few spermatogonia and Sertoli cells were noted. The peritubular walls were severely thickened and tubular diameter was decreased. Lanthanum penetrated into the interstices between the Sertoli cells, but complete penetration of lanthanum was prevented by the Sertoli junctions at some points (Figure 19a). Lanthanum was not found at the centre parts of the seminiferous tubules. In ultra-

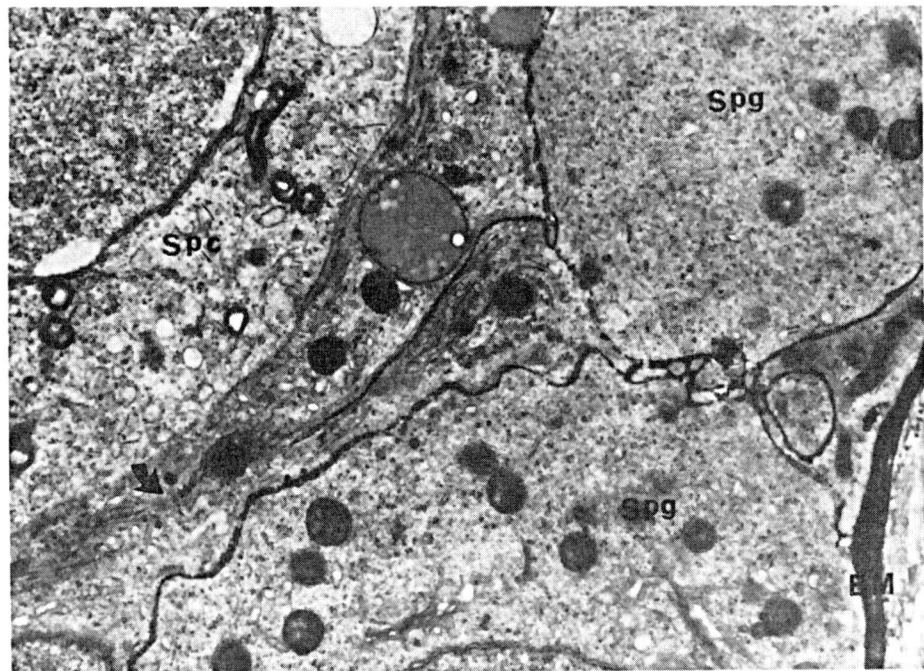

Figure 18. Electron micrograph (×9,500) showing the penetration of lanthanum in the hypospermatogenic testis of an infertile patient. The Sertoli junction excludes the deep penetration of lanthanum (arrow). BM: basement membrane; Spc: spermatocyte; Spg: spermatogonia.

thin section preparations and lanthanum-filled preparations, ultrastructural morphology of the Sertoli junctions was quite similar to that in the normal control (Figure 19b, c). It appears that the Sertoli junctions are not damaged by suppression of gonadotropin secretion in the human testis.

5.3. *Other conditions*

5.3.1. *Cryptorchidism.* It is well-known that experimental cryptorchidism prevents spermatogenesis. Ultrastructurally, using the lanthanum tracer method over twelve days, no breakdown of the Sertoli junctions was observed in the rat cryptorchid testis (Hagenäs 1976).

5.3.2. *Vasectomy.* Electron-microscopic study has revealed no change in the rat testis after vasectomy (Flickinger 1972). Moreover, it has been reported that the Sertoli junctions maintained normal ultrastructural characteristics after vasectomy in the rat, and that the permeability of these junctions to lanthanum was not altered (Neaves 1973).

5.3.3. *Ligation of efferent ductuli.* It has been shown that ligation of the efferent ductuli in the rat is followed by an increase in the diameter of the

seminiferous tubules and in the testicular weight, and eventually resulted in testicular atrophy (Smith 1962). It has also been reported that lanthanum penetrated into the Sertoli junctions and entered the adluminal compartment 24 hours after efferent ductuli ligation in the rat (Neaves 1973). However, another report has revealed that lanthanum could not penetrate beyond the Sertoli junctions 12 hours after efferent ductuli ligation in the mouse (Ross 1977). In ultra-thin sections, it was also noted that the Sertoli junctions were not changed and the components of these junctions, membrane fusions, subsurface cisternae and microfilaments, persisted for 24 hours – four weeks after efferent ductuli ligation in the rat (Furuya et al. 1977). Thus it would appear that the morphological integrity of the Sertoli junctions was maintained after efferent ductuli ligation.

5.3.4. *Immune orchitis.* The breaking of the blood-testis barrier has been reported in the testis of allergic aspermatogenesis produced in guinea pigs by iso-immunization with homologous sperm, homogenized testis or testicular antigens in complete Freund's adjuvant. In such cases, acriflavin and γ-globulin entered readily in the seminiferous tubules beyond the barrier (Johnson 1970a).

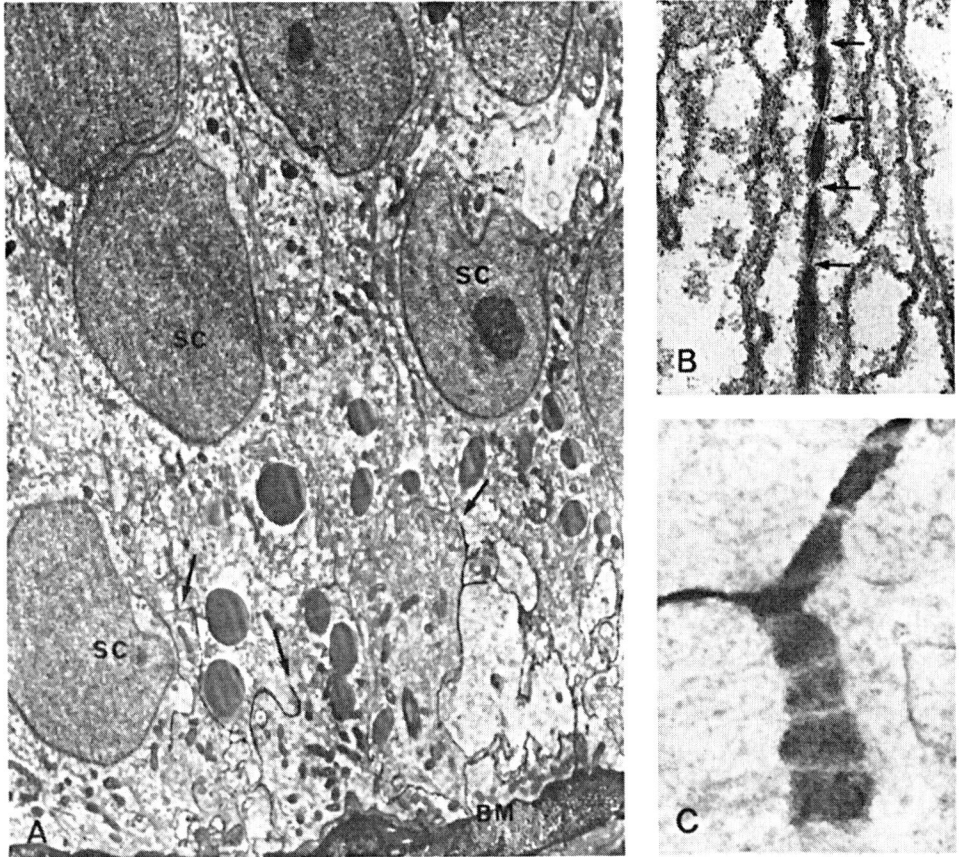

Figure 19. Electron micrographs showing the penetration of lanthanum (A) and lanthanum-filled Sertoli junction (B. C) in the damaged testis of a patient with hypophysectomy. (A) Arrows indicate the blockage of lanthanum penetration into the seminiferous tubules. BM: basement membrane: SC: Sertoli cell (× 4.000). (B) Longitudinal section picture – note arrowed membrane fusions (× 80.000). (C) Oblique section picture (× 60.000).

Regarding the manner in which the antibody gains access to the spermatogenic antigen, three hypothetical concepts have been considered: first, the antibody is taken up by the Sertoli cells and spermatogonia, and is next transferred to the target cells (developing germ cells) – intravenously injected horseradish peroxidase was found in the cytoplasm of the Sertoli cells and spermatogonia type B, while it failed to pass beyond the Sertoli junctions (Willson et al. 1973); second, the antibody can readily enter the rete testis, and is refluxed back to the seminiferous lumen – indeed it has been revealed that the immunological reaction was found in the rete testis and that injected antibody produced a reaction in the rete testis (Tung et al. 1970; Johnson 1970b, 1972); third, the Sertoli junctions have sporadic breaking points where the antibody penetrates (Castro and Seiguer 1974). It has been reported in allergic orchitis of guinea pigs that the Sertoli junctions

became fragmented, probably resulting in leakage (Nagano and Suzuki 1976a) and that mononuclear cells infiltrated into the seminiferous tubules (Tung et al. 1970).

5.3.5. Hypertonic solutions. It has been revealed that the Sertoli tight junctions differ from other epithelial tight junctions in their stability and resistance to the effects of hypertonic solutions. After perfusion with hypertonic solutions (lithium chloride, sucrose and urea), the Sertoli junctions showed no alteration, while the spermatogonia were almost invariably detached from the basement membrane and remarkably shrunken. The spermatocytes and spermatids occupying the adluminal compartment were not affected over a short time interval. Thus, the Sertoli junctions are highly impermeable and resistant to osmotic damage (Gilula et al. 1976).

5.3.6. Epinephrine-induced testicular damage. Testicular degeneration, after injections of epinephrine and papaverine in the Syrian hamster, was induced by ischemia produced by vasoconstriction. Even in these degenerating tubules, penetration of horse-radish peroxidase and lanthanum traces was prevented by the Sertoli junctions (Gravis et al. 1977).

6. CONCLUDING REMARKS

The blood-testis barrier is a morphological and physiological entity in the testis. This barrier may play a role in establishing and maintaining a specific and beneficial fluid environment for spermatogenesis.

We observed, by using the lanthanum tracer method, that the Sertoli junctions acted as a basic blood-testis barrier in man. These Sertoli junctions displayed specialized tight junctions, characterized by three components: (1) membrane fusions; (2) subsurface cisternae of endoplasmic reticulum oriented in parallel with the Sertoli cell plasma membrane; and (3) bundles of microfilaments located between the Sertoli cell plasma membrane and the associated cisternae. Membrane fusions were clearly recognized as electron-lucent lines in lanthanum-filled preparations and anastomosing strands in freeze-etched preparations. The micro-filaments are suggested to be actin-like, because they are bound with heavy meromyosin and form arrowhead complexes. The functions of the subsurface cisternae and microfilaments, however, remain to be clarified.

Specialized tight junctions between the Sertoli cells were noted in the testes of 11-13-year-old boys. In these testes, spermatogenesis was initiated and lumen formation occurred. These specialized junctions were created by mature Sertoli cells, characterized by an irregularly shaped nucleus with deep infoldings, tripartite complexes of nucleolus, abundant smooth ER and crystalloid of Charcot-Böttcher. We suggest that the human blood-testis barrier is established shortly before and after the spermatogonia proliferate to give rise to the primary spermatocytes.

We studied ultrastructurally factors influencing the development and maintenance of the blood-testis barrier (Table 2). The specialized Sertoli junctions were formed after hCG treatment in patients with hypogonadotropic eunuchoidism. It

Table 2. Factors influencing development and maintenance of the blood-testis barrier in man.

Blood-testis barrier	Factors	Relationship
Development	gonadotropins	dependent
	germ cells	independent
Maintenance	hypospermatogenesis	independent
	hypophysectomy	independent

was noted that the Sertoli junctions normally developed in congenital germ-cell-free mice, and that the Sertoli junctions in the Sertoli-cell-only syndrome were identical with those in the normal control. These findings suggest that the initiation and development of the blood-testis barrier is dependent upon gonadotropins, but is not dependent upon the existence of germ cells. On the other hand, the Sertoli junctions ultrastructurally appeared to be intact in the hypospermatogenic testis of infertile patients and in damaged testis of patients with hypophysectomy. Therefore, it is suggested that the etiology of infertility is not directly attributable to the morphological change of the blood-testis barrier, and that the maintenance of the blood-testis barrier is independent of the suppression of gonadotropins.

ACKNOWLEDGEMENTS

This study was supported by grants of the Japanese Ministry of Education. The authors would like to thank Prof. T. Nagano for helpful advice; Prof. K. Matsumoto for generous supply of the congenital germ-cell-free mice; and Mr. S. Mutoh, Miss K. Shiraki and Miss M. Asao for their assistance.

REFERENCES

Bawa SR: Fine structure of the Sertoli cell in the human testis. J Ultrastruct Res 9: 459, 1963.
Bigliardi E, Vegni-Talluri M: Gap junctions between Sertoli cells in the infertile human testis. Fertil Steril 28: 755, 1977.
Bressler RS: Dependence of Sertoli cell maturation on the pituitary gland in the mouse. Am J Anat 147: 447, 1976.
Castro AE, Seiguer AC: The permeability of the blood-testis barrier to lanthanum during the immune-induced aspermatogenesis and following vasectomy in the guinea pig. Virchows Arch Cell Path 16: 297, 1974.
Claude P, Goudenough D: Fracture faces of zonulae occludentes from 'tight' and 'leaky' epithelia. J Cell Biol 58: 390, 1973.

Clermont Y. Perey B: Quantitative study of the cell population of the seminiferous tubules in immature rats. Am J Anat 100: 241. 1957.

Connell CJ: A freeze-fracture and lanthanum tracer study of the complex junction between Sertoli cells of the canine testis. J Cell Biol 76: 57. 1978.

Courot M: Endocrine control of the supporting and germ cells of the impuberal testis. J Reprod Fertil, suppl 2: 89. 1967.

De Kretser DM. Burger HG: Ultrastructural studies of the human Sertoli cell in normal men and males with hypogonadotropic hypogonadism before and after gonadotropic treatment. In: Gonadotropins. Saxena BB. Beling CG. Grandy MH (eds). New York: John Wiley and Sons. 1972. p 640.

Dixon RL. Lee IP: Possible role of the blood-testicular barrier in dominant lethal testing. Environ Health Perspect 6: 59. 1973.

Dym M: The fine structure of the monkey (Macaca) Sertoli cell and its role in maintaining the blood-testis barrier. Anat Rec 175: 639. 1973.

Dym M. Fawcett DW: The blood-testis barrier in the rat and the physiological compartmentation of the seminiferous epithelium. Biol Reprod 3: 308. 1970.

Fawcett DW. Gilula NB. Aoki A: Recent observations on the organization of the seminiferous epithelium. Gumma Symp Endocr 13: 49. 1976.

Fawcett DW. Heidger PM. Leak LV: Lymph vascular system of the interstitial tissue of the testis as revealed by electron microscopy. J Reprod Fertil 19: 109. 1969.

Fawcett DW. Leak LV. Heidger PM: Electron microscopic observations on the structural components of the blood-testis barrier. J Reprod Fertil, suppl 10: 105. 1970.

Flickinger CJ: The postnatal development of the Sertoli cells of the mouse. Cell Tiss Res 78: 92. 1967.

Flickinger CJ: Ultrastructure of the rat testis after vasectomy. Anat Rec 174: 477. 1972.

Flickinger CJ. Fawcett DW: The junctional specializations of Sertoli cells in the seminiferous epithelium. Anat Rec 158: 207. 1967.

Furuya S: Electron microscopic studies (lanthanum tracer and freeze-etching method) on the blood-testis barrier in human testis. Jap J Urol 66: 829. 1975.

Furuya S. Kumamoto Y. Sugiyama S: Fine structure and development of Sertoli junctions in human testis. Arch Androl 1: 211. 1978.

Furuya S. Miyake M. Shiraki K. Kumamoto Y: Spermatogenesis and Sertoli junction after efferent ductuli ligation in the rat: abstract. Jap Cong Fertil Steril 22: 120. 1977.

Gilula NB. Fawcett DW. Aoki A: The Sertoli cell occluding junctions and gap junctions in mature and developing mammalian testis. Dev Biol 50: 142. 1976.

Gravis CJ. Chen I. Yates RD: Stability of the intra-epithelial component of the blood-testis barrier in epinephrine-induced testicular degeneration in Syrian hamsters. Am J Anat 148: 19. 1977.

Hagenäs L. Ploën L. Ekwall H: Blood-testis barrier: evidence for intact inter-Sertoli cell junctions after hypophysectomy in the adult rat. J. Endocr 76: 87. 1978.

Hagenäs L. Ploën L. Ritzen EM. Ekwall H: Blood-testis barrier: maintained function of inter-Sertoli cell junctions in experimental cryptorchidism in the rat. as judged by a simple lanthanum-immersion technique. Andrologia 9: 250. 1977.

Hilscher W. Makoski HB: Histologische und autoradiographische Untersuchungen zur Präspermatogenese und Spermatogenese der Ratte. Cell Tiss Res 86: 327. 1968.

Johnson MH: Changes in blood-testis barrier of the guinea pig in relation to histological damage following iso-immunization with testis. J Reprod Fertil 22: 119. 1970a.

Johnson MH: The pituitary and the blood-testis barrier. J Reprod Fertil 22: 181. 1970b.

Johnson MH: The distribution of immunoglobulin and spermatozoal autoantigen in the genital tract of the male guinea pig: its relationship to autoallergic orchitis. Fertil Steril 23: 383. 1972.

Kormano M: Dye permeability and alkaline phosphatase activity of testicular capillaries in the postnatal rat. Histochemie 9: 327. 1967.

Kumamoto Y. Furuya S: Morphological study of the blood-testis barrier in human testis. Gumma Symp Endocr 13: 69. 1976.

Miyachi Y. Nieschlag E. Lipsett MB: The secretion of gonadotropins and testosterone by the neonatal male rat. Endocrinol 92: 1. 1973.

Nagano T. Suzuki F: Freeze-fracture observations on the intercellular junctions of Sertoli cells and Leydig cells in the human testis. Cell Tiss Res 166: 37. 1976a.

Nagano T. Suzuki F: The postnatal development of the junctional complexes of the mouse Sertoli cells as revealed by freeze-fracture. Anat Rec 185: 403. 1976b.

Nagano T. Suzuki F: Freeze-fracture observations on the junctional complexes of Sertoli cells in the seminiferous tubule. Gumma Symp Endocr 13: 61. 1976c.

Nagano T. Suzuki F. Kitamura Y. Matsumoto K: Sertoli cell junctions in the germ-cell-free testis of the congenic mouse. Lab Invest 36: 8. 1977.

Neaves W: Permeability of Sertoli cell tight junctions to lanthanum after ligation of ductus deferens and ductuli efferentes. J Cell Biol 59: 559. 1973.

Nicander L: An electron microscopical study of cell contacts in the seminiferous tubules of some mammals. Cell Tiss Res 83: 375. 1967.

Ross MH: Sertoli-Sertoli junctions and Sertoli-spermatid junctions after efferent ductule ligation and lanthanum treatment. Am J Anat 148: 49. 1977.

Setchell BP: The blood-testicular fluid barrier in sheep. J Physiol (London) 189: 63. 1967.

Setchell BP: Testicular fluid. In: The testis. Johnson AD. Gomes WR. Vandenmark NL (eds). New York. Academic Press. 1970, vol 1. p 101.

Setchell BP. Waites GM: The blood-testis barrier. In: Handbook of physiology, sec 7: Endocrinology; vol 5: Male reproductive system. Greep RO. Astwood EB (eds). Baltimore. Williams and Wilkins. 1975. p 143.

Steinberger A. Steinberger E: Replication pattern of Sertoli cells in maturing rat testis in vivo and in organ culture. Biol Reprod 4: 84. 1971.

Steinberger A. Steinberger E: The Sertoli cells. In: The testis. Johnson AD. Gomes WR (eds). New York: Academic Press. 1977, vol 4, p 371.

Tindall DJ. Vitale R. Means AR: Androgen-binding protein as a biochemical marker of formation of the blood-testis barrier. Endocrinol 97: 636. 1975.

Toyama Y: Actin-like filaments in the Sertoli cell junctional specializations in the swine and mouse testis. Anat Rec 186: 477. 1976.

Tung KST. Unanue ER. Dixon FJ: The immunopathology of experimental allergic orchitis. Am J Pathol 60: 313. 1970.

Vitale R. Fawcett DW. Dym M: The normal development of the blood-testis barrier and the effect of clomiphene and estrogen treatment. Anat Rec 176: 333. 1973.

Willson JT. Jones NA. Katsch S. Smith SW: Penetration of the testicular-tubular barrier by horseradish peroxidase induced by adjuvant. Anat Rec 176: 85. 1973.

8. NEURO-ENDOCRINE CONTROL OF SPERMATOGENESIS

C. GIROD and J.C. CZYBA

The development and the function of the testicular germ line on both the prepubertal and the adult testis are subject to a hypothalamo-hypophyseal regulation, which has been the subject of several recent reviews (Franchimont et al. 1975, Gupta et al. 1975; Jeffcoate 1975; Steinberger 1975, Courot 1976; Forest et al. 1976; Hansson et al. 1976).

1. HYPOPHYSIS AND SEMINIFEROUS TUBULES

1.1. Prepuberty

Before puberty the testis undergoes a process of morphological evolution resulting in the formation of the germ line in contact with the Sertoli cells.

1.1.1. Prepubertal seminiferous tubules. In man, the evolution of the organization of the seminiferous tubules starts during the intrauterine period and continues until puberty.

1.1.1.1. In the fetus. In the fetus the seminiferous tubules, which should more correctly be called seminiferous cords, are of small *diameter* (50-60 μm), and have a *solid appearance* (absence of lumen). They are made up of three basic elements:

– a *limiting membrane* (basal lamina or membrana propria), thin and little differentiated, made up only of a doubled basal membrane with a few fibroblastic cells without myoid characteristics;
– the *supporting cells* which will become the Sertoli cells, and which consist of two distinct populations: the first appear early (between the 42nd and the 49th days) and consist of light-coloured cells, the second appear two weeks later and consist of darker cells; these two populations each exercise a distinctive physiological control over the primitive germinal

cells, and they are given the names 'meiosis-preventing (MP) Sertoli cells' and 'meiosis-inducing (MI) Sertoli cells' (Wartenberg 1978);
– the *primitive germinal cells*, called pro-spermatogonia, appear, under electron microscopy, to consist of three different types: multiplying (M), transitional$_1$ (T_1), and transitional$_2$ (T_2) pro-spermatogonia (Wartenberg 1976).

1.1.1.2. In the neonate. In the newborn the seminiferous cords have only slightly increased in *diameter* (60-70 μm) and retain a *solid appearance* (absence of lumen) but, within certain tubes, cellular debris, corresponding to degenerated spermatogonia, may be observed. The *lamina propria* remains little differentiated.

1.1.1.3. In the child. From birth to the age of 10-11 years, the seminiferous cords increase only slightly in *diameter*, but they elongate and become convoluted. They retain their *solid appearance*. Degenerescence of the central cells can be seen more frequently than in the neonate. The *membrana propria* is still made up of a basal membrane surrounded by a layer of fibrous conjunctive tissue. The *spermatogonia* have a typical appearance: large cells situated close to the membrana propria of the seminiferous cords; their voluminous nuclei contain a large nucleolus; mitoses can be observed. In children over eight years old, binucleated and hypertrophied spermatogonia may be observed.

1.1.1.4. At puberty. The seminiferous tubules attain a considerable *diameter* at puberty: average diameter at ten years is 72 μm, at twelve years it is 85 μm, and at fifteen years it is 100-150 μm (the mean diameter in adults is from 150-300 μm). A lumen opens within the tubes.

The *membrana propria* differentiates, and the five layers which typify the seminiferous tubule of the adult man develop. In particular the myoid cells, situated in the middle of the membrana propria, acquire the characteristics of contractile cells and enter into mutual contact by differentiation of the membranes of the zonula adhaerens type, suggesting a role in the blood-testis barrier.

The *spermatogonia* show a high mitotic activity. Signs of cellular differentiation can be observed with the appearance of spermatogonia Ad, Ap, and B (Clermont's terminology). These spermatogonia develop into spermatocytes, but spermatogenesis proceeds only slowly.

At the same time the MI Sertoli cells differentiate into mature Sertoli cells and hence nuclear division among the supporting cells becomes infrequent; the fundamental difference is the appearance of 'junctional specializations' (terminology of Flickinger and Fawcett 1967) or 'ectoplasmic specializations' (Russell 1977) of the plasma membrane which contribute to the blood-testis barrier. In the human pubertal testis, 'the blood-testis barrier is established shortly before or after the spermatogonia proliferate to give rise to the primary spermatocytes' (Furuya et al. 1978).

1.1.2. Effects of experimental prepubertal hypophysectomy.

The ablation of the hypophysis in prepubertal animals results in several testicular alterations (reviewed in Courot and Ortavant 1972; and Hochereau de Reviers and Courot 1978):

– reduction in the weight of the testes, together with a reduction in the length and diameter of the tubules;
– a lack of development and differentiation, and a reduction in the number of the supporting cells;
– retention of the pro-spermatogonia in undifferentiated state.

During puberty the following weeks or months, no modification in the organization of the seminiferous tubules can be observed.

Rhesus monkey fetuses were hypophysectomized at 111 to 116 days of gestation (Gulyas et al. 1977); at birth the weight of the testes was significantly low, as was the number of spermatogonia per testis, however the diameter of the seminiferous cords was unchanged.

1.1.3. Administration of gonadotropins before puberty.

The administration of FSH or LH to subjects hypophysectomized before puberty results in various modifications which are most pronounced when the gonadotropins are administered shortly after hypophysectomy. Only minor modifications are observed when the gonadotropins are injected several weeks after the operation.

1.1.3.1. Macroscopic characteristics. The modifications depend upon the nature of the gonadotropin (and also its origin, e.g., bovine, ovine, and so on). In general it can be stated that:

– FSH results in a slight but significant increase in testicular weight, although this remains inferior to that of controls;
– LH increases the testicular weight beyond that of controls;
– the association of FSH and LH at the same dose administered separately produces a synergistic action and the weight increase of the testes can become considerable.

1.1.3.2. Microscopic characteristics. Examination of sections of testes from prepubertal hypophysectomized subjects treated with FSH reveals the following modifications:

– two general modifications may be noted: first, the *diameter* of the tubules, much reduced after hypophysectomy, is only slightly increased by FSH; treatment with LH results in a greater increase in diameter and in the appearance of a lumen; the combination of FSH and LH induces a still greater increase in diameter; secondly, the *length* of the tubules is greatly increased by FSH but only slightly by LH; a combination of the two gonadotropins again results in a still greater increase in length;
– cytologically, FSH results in the stimulation of spermatogenesis (meiosis can be observed), but has only little effect on the differentiation of the supporting cells; LH stimulates mitotic activity of the supporting cells and partially favours their membrane differentiation. The combination of FSH and LH results in the simultaneous development and differentiation of all of the cellular elements of the tubules, particularly those of the membranes of the Sertoli cells which contribute to the formation of the blood-testis barrier.

1.1.4. Some factors influencing the testicular development in prepubertal hypophysectomized subjects. In nonhypophysectomized prepubertal subjects the direct action of FSH can be demonstrated by the radioimmunological measurement of gonadotropins after hemi-castration: when 25-day-old rats are hemi-castrated the remaining testicle increases significantly in weight over the next five days; at this time the amount of FSH present is significantly increased although that of intratesticular testosterone remains unaltered (Moger 1977). Similar results have been observed in rats operated on at five days old (Cunningham et al. 1978).

It is, however, certain that the prepubertal testis is sensitive to androgens. A direct influence of androgens on the prepubertal testis can be demonstrated under certain experimental conditions (intratesticular injection or implantation of microcrystals of testosterone), in animal pathology (Tfm mice), or in human pathology (unilateral Leydigian tumours of children) – see review in Bressler (1978). Testosterone includes:

– the maturation and differentiation of the elements of the membrana propria (its thickening and the differentiation of myoid elements);
– the appearance of spermatogenesis (very localized, in regions in contact with the hormone crystals in the case of implantation);
– the precocious appearance of lumen in seminiferous tubules.

The influence of testosterone can be confirmed by the administration of anti-androgens (cyproterone or cyproterone acetate). In the prepubertal rat the administration of anti-androgen 'prevents stem cell mitosis or differentiation, resulting in a depletion of the yield of spermatogonial divisions, either directly or by a modification of Sertoli cell metabolism' (Viguier-Martinez and Hochereau de Reviers 1977). Injections of antiserum to highly purified FSH produce clear modifications of testicular weight and of the diameter of the seminiferous cords in immature rats (Raj and Dym 1976).

1.2. Adult

Complete testicular organization is achieved at a variable time after puberty (depending upon the species considered).

1.2.1. The adult seminiferous tubule. In man the seminiferous tubule of the adult is composed of several elements (Vilar 1973; Steinberger and Steinberger 1975; Bustos-Obregón et al. 1975; Fawcett 1976; Neaves 1977; Dym and Cavicchia 1978):

– the *membrana propria*, which is some 3-5 μm thick, and has a heterogeneity of structure under electron microscopy (Böck 1978; Hermo and Lalli 1978);
– the *germinal line*, an assembly of cells which develop from the stem cells into the male gamete, through a series of cellular divisions and differentiations; the kinetics of these transformations follows a precise chronology (Clermont 1972; Hilscher and Hilscher 1976); electron-microscopical studies have shown that, in rats, the presence of intercellular bridges complicates the description of the evolution of the seminal epithelium; in man the mechanism of this evolution may be less complex 'but it seems likely that the same principles apply' (Fawcett 1976);
– the *Sertoli cells* extend from the membrana propria to the lumen of the tubule; their lateral prolongations make contact with the cells of the seminal epithelium; at their apical pole, next to the lumen of the tubule, they enter into close contact with the spermatids undergoing spermiogenesis; their organelles are distributed unevenly; at the basal pole, next to the membrana propria, are found a system of smooth endoplasmic reticulum, many mitochondria, lipid droplets occasionally surrounded by cisternae of rough endoplasmic reticulum, glycogen granules, thin filaments, lysosomes, annulate lamellae, and crystals of Charcot-Böttcher (in man only); at the apical pole are found some rod-shaped mitochondria, microtubules and microfilaments; the distribution of the organelles led Schulze (1974) to describe five normal morphological types in man; the nucleus appears, especially on electron microscopy, to be irregular, indented, and provided with a large nucleolus; the nucleus is generally separated from the organelles by fine intracytoplasmic filaments; the Golgi apparatus is situated near to the nucleus; finally, the Sertoli cells are characterized by several types of membrane differentiations: some are found at zones of contact with cells of the germinal line at different stages of differentiation, and others at zones of contact between two Sertoli cells (Fawcett 1975; Ross 1976; Russell 1977); the topography of the membrane

specializations of the Sertoli cells allows the distinction between two regions of the seminal epithelium: the *basal compartment* – peripheral distribution and membrane differentiations between adjacent Sertoli cells – and the *adluminal compartment* – more internal with respect to the lumen of the tubule and membrane differentiations on Sertoli cells in contact with cells of the germinal line (Dym and Fawcett

1970); another region of the seminal epithelium may be distinguished: this is the *intermediate compartment* (Russell 1978) and corresponds to the zone where one finds spermatocytes in the leptotene stage.

The components of testicular tubules at the various stages of life are summarized in Table 1.

Table 1. The components of testicular tubules at various stages of life.

Stage	Seminal elements	Supporting cells	Interstitial cells
Fetus	Pro-spermatogonia (M-, T_1 and T_2 - P. sp)	Meiosis-preventing Sertoli cells Meiosis-inducing Sertoli cells	Present between 3rd and 7th months
Child	Spermatogonia	Meiosis-inducing Sertoli cells	Dedifferentiation of the fetal cells
Onset of puberty	Differentiation and multiplication of spermatogonia (Ad, Ap, B sperm) Spermatocytes	Mature Sertoli cells	Differentiation of the interstitial gland
After puberty	Seminal epithelium: – spermatogenesis – spermiogenesis	Differentiation of the functional specializations; constitution of 3 compartments: – basal intermediate – adluminal	Active interstitial cells

1.2.2. Effects of experimental adult hypophysectomy. Removal of the hypophysis of a postpubertal animal results in several testicular modifications (see review in Steinberger and Steinberger 1972):

– a reduction in the weight of the testes, which is most marked when the weight of the testes was elevated at the moment of the hypophysectomy;
– a marked regression of the seminal epithelium with: (1) degeneration of cells which have progressed beyond the pachytene stage; (2) reduction of the transformation of Ap spermatogonia into B spermatogonia; and (3) alterations in the spermatocytes entering into meiotic prophase;
– no reduction in the overall number of Sertoli cells, but alterations of their morphology (especially cytomembranary systems) and their metabolic function – reduction in several enzyme activities, and of the synthesis of androgen-binding protein (ABP).

These testicular modifications after adult hypophysectomy are thus different from those seen in the subject treated before puberty; they allow us to conclude that certain stages of the development of

the seminal epithelium are absolutely dependent on the hypophyseal hormones, while for other stages these hormones exert a modulating influence. It should, however, be emphasized that there are species differences, and while the above description corresponds to the effects of hypophysectomy in rats, in man the totality of the seminal epithelium is sensitive to the effects of hypophysectomy.

1.2.3. Administration of gonadotropins to hypophysectomized pubescents and adults. The administration of FSH or LH results in modifications which differ somewhat in subjects hypophysectomized at the moment of puberty and in those operated after the completion of puberty.

1.2.3.1. Macroscopic characteristics. The modifications produced depend, as in the prepubertal subject, on the nature and the origin of the gonadotropin used:

– if the hypophysectomy is performed at the start of the process of puberty, FSH increases the weight of the testes beyond the values observed in nonhypophysectomized controls; LH increases testicular weight over that of hypophysectomized controls but does not re-establish a normal weight for nonoperated animals; the combination of FSH with LH has a synergic effect;

– if the hypophysectomy is performed on the adult subject, FSH does not increase testicular weight; LH results in an increase similar to that observed with prepubescent subjects; the combination of FSH and LH gives a result slightly more marked than that seen with LH alone.

1.2.3.2. Microscopic characteristics. As in the case of the prepubertal subject, the administration of FSH or LH to subjects hypophysectomized at or after completion of puberty causes generalized modifications:

– regarding the *general* characters of the seminal tubules, the following results are noted: the *diameter* of the tubules, which is only slightly reduced after hypophysectomy, is restored under the same conditions, predominantly by LH and especially by the combination of FSH and LH; the *length* of the adult seminiferous tubules is much less modified by hypophysectomy and treatment with FSH and/or LH than is that of the prepubertal tubules;

– regarding their *cytological* characteristics, FSH administered to subjects hypophysectomized just before puberty stimulates spermatogenesis (or at least some meiosis); in subjects hypophysectomized after puberty FSH has only a limited activity on the seminal epithelium (maintenance of stem spermatogonia and some spermatogonia division); LH stimulates the reappearance of meiosis of the spermatocytes; the combination of FSH and LH restores spermatogenesis and spermiogenesis to a nearly 'normal' condition.

These observations allow the conclusion that the maintenance of the structural and functional integrity of the seminiferous tubules requires the simultaneous and synergic action of gonadotropic hormones. However, since the restoration of the experimentally hypophysectomized animal is never complete using these two gonadotropins, it can be supposed that the physiological development of the seminiferous tubules requires the action of other pituitary hormones, notably prolactin and somato-

tropic hormone, as well as that of peripheral hormones, especially the androgens.

1.3. Relation between the seminiferous epithelium and FSH

In man, there is a close relationship between the phase of development (or of nondevelopment, e.g., Sertoli-cell-only syndrome, severe germ cell depletion, or idiopathic disorders of spermatogenesis) of the seminal line and the plasmatic or urinary level of FSH (see reviews in Hansson et al. 1975; Baker et al. 1976). These correlations can also be related to the parallel modifications to the Sertoli cells (Chemes et al. 1977). Briefly, it is observed that there is:

– a high level of FSH in men whose seminiferous tubules are depleted of spermatids,
– a correlation between number of spermatogonia and level of FSH,
– a link between the presence of lesions of the Sertoli cells (often only visible on electron microscopy) and rises in FSH levels.

These observations suggest that the exocrine testis exerts an influence upon the antehypophyseal gonadotropic activity.

1.4. Prolactin and spermatogenesis

While it is certain that FSH and LH exert an influence on spermatogenesis, the action of prolactin on the exocrine testis is somewhat controversial (review in Bartke 1976).

Two recent experimental observations may be considered here:

– in lambs treated with CB-154 (2-bromo-α-ergocryptine) at the moment of puberty, a histological study of the testes showed that 'the establishment of spermatogenesis was not delayed by the treatment' (Ravault et al. 1977);
– in rats hypophysectomized 28 days previously, treatment with prolactin (100 μg/100 g bodyweight) does not modify the appearance of the seminiferous tubules; the combination of FSH with prolactin produces the same results as treatment with FSH alone (Sivelle et al. 1978).

It is possible that prolactin exerts some indirect influence 'due to augmenting the effect of endogenous or exogenous LH on testicular steroidogenesis rather than to potentiating the effects of androgens on the seminiferous epithelium' (Bartke et al. 1978). Prolactin acts indirectly upon spermatogenesis by its influence on the testicular LH receptors (Zipf et al. 1978). In the male, prolactin has a direct action on the hypothalamo-hypophyseal system: 'prolactin may sensitize the hypothalamus and/or pituitary gland to the negative feedback of gonadal steroids' (McNeilly et al. 1978).

1.5. Mechanism of action of the gonadotropins

1.5.1. General mechanisms. The antehypophyseal gonadotropins act on the seminiferous tubules by two general mechanisms (review in Means et al. 1976; Means 1977):

– an action on adenyl cyclase and on cAMP; FSH increases the formation of cAMP in the seminiferous tubules of the prepubertal subject, but not in the adult; LH, on the other hand, increases cAMP production in both prepubertal and adult tubules;
– an action on the production of nucleic acids; FSH stimulates the incorporation of ^{3}H-thymidine into spermatogonia and leptotene spermatocytes in prepubescent subjects, whereas LH stimulates a similar incorporation in adults; in addition FSH stimulates the synthesis of RNA in the seminiferous epithelium, and consequently the synthesis of protein in those cells; LH exerts a comparable action on protein synthesis in the seminiferous epithelium.

1.5.2. Role of Sertoli cells. The role of Sertoli cells in endocrine control of spermatogenetic function has been the object of much research described in recent reviews (Fawcett 1975; Means et al. 1976, 1978; Means 1977; Chemes et al. 1977; Dym 1977; Steinberger and Steinberger 1977; Fritz et al. 1978; Hansson et al. 1978; Hochereau de Reviers and Courot 1978; Kotite et al. 1978). The Sertoli cells perform several other general functions which we will mention briefly.

1.5.2.1. General functions. These general functions influence the normal development of spermatogenesis and spermiogenesis.

– *Supporting role.* The Sertoli cells ensure the maintenance of contacts between the cells of the seminal epithelium (Figure 1). The displacement of

newly-differentiated cells from the periphery to the lumen of the tubule could imply active movement of the Sertolian cytoplasm, in which filaments of contractile proteins (actin-like and myosin-like proteins) have been demonstrated, and perhaps also certain simultaneous and temporary modifications of the tight junctions allowing the translation of cells of the seminal line from the basal to the adluminal compartment. At apical pole, the Sertoli cells are in contact with the spermatids undergoing spermiogenesis; next to these cells, which are deeply inserted into the Sertolian cytoplasm (often to the perinuclear region) at the beginning of spermiogenesis, the Sertoli cells possess membrane modifications and the surrounding cytoplasm is rich in mitochondria; these structures certainly play a role in the maturation of the spermatids and in spermiation. It is, however, not known what control processes influence this differentiation and the mechanisms of spermiation, and, particularly, whether the control is hormonal.

– *Nutritional role.* Given the absence of capillaries within the seminiferous tubules, it may be supposed that the Sertoli cells which extend to the membrana propria, which is in contact with blood and lymphatic capillaries, ensure the transport of the necessary materials for the various biosynthetic activities of the cells in the seminal epithelium.

– *Secretory role.* The lumen of the seminiferous tubules contains a liquid which can be sampled by micro-puncture. This is not a plasmatic filtrate, but is produced by the Sertoli cells and persists even when the germinal line is experimentally destroyed. In these conditions (on use of antimitotics for example) the production of the tubular liquid is even greater than that of controls, and is reduced only after the complete reappearance of spermatogenesis. Among the products synthesized by the Sertoli cells, special mention should be given to the 'ABP' (androgen-binding protein), so called because it binds to the androgens produced by the Leydig cells. It has also proved possible to culture Sertoli cells in vitro, and these cultured cells retain their secretory ability and their capacity to produce ABP.

– *Role in the blood-testis barrier.* The chemical composition of the tubular fluid, especially with respect to proteins, is different to that of blood or of testicular lymph: the protein content of testicular fluid is much lower than that of intravascular liquids. This fluid is thus not a simple filtrate, and

Lumen of seminiferous tubule

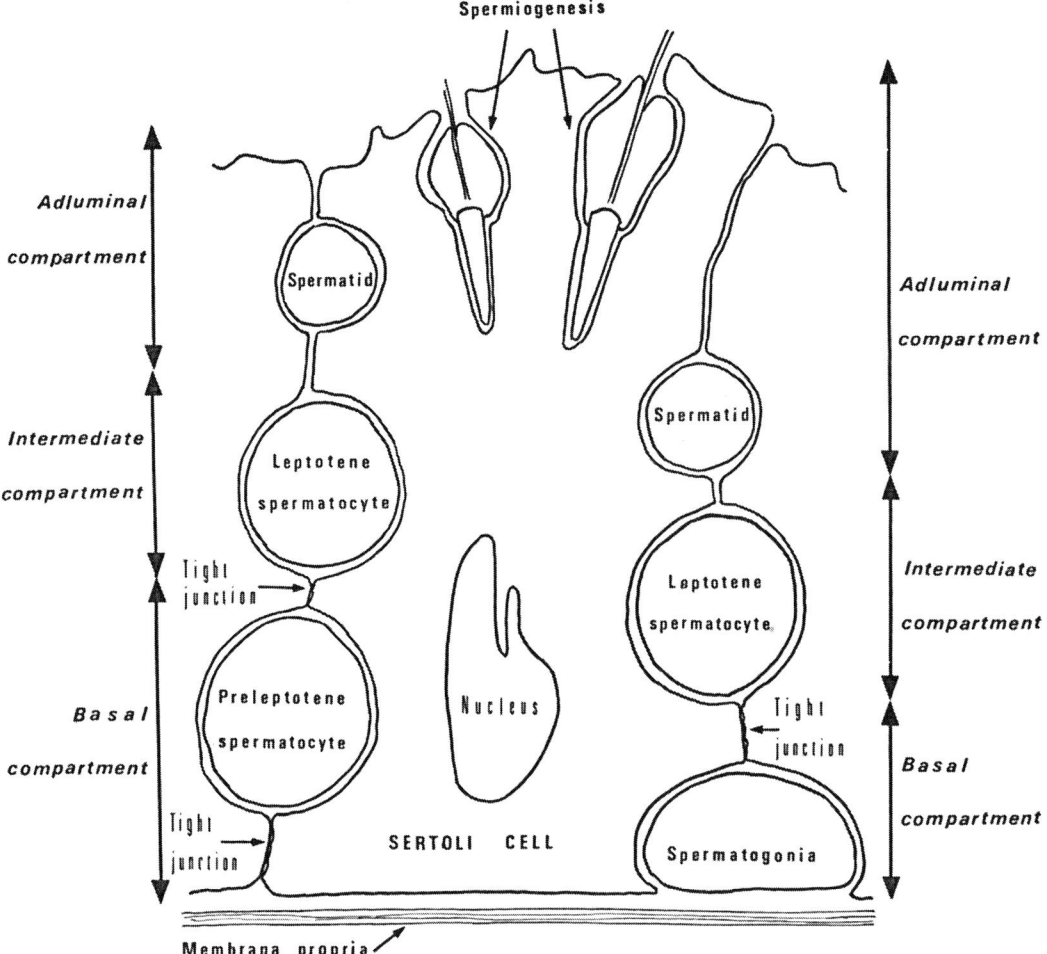

Figure 1. The interrelations between Sertoli cells and germinal cells, and the subdivision of seminiferous epithelium into three compartments.

the Sertoli cells play a role in the blood-testis barrier. This blood-testis barrier can be localized to the tight junctions by the use of markers specific for the intracellular spaces (lanthanum nitrate in particular). The composition of the fluid within the adluminal compartment, where meiosis is completed and spermiogenesis occurs, suggests that the Sertoli cells provide an environment indispensable for the occurrence of these phenomena, as well as an isolation of this territory from exogenous toxic factors possibly present in the bloodstream. This blood-testis barrier at the level of the Sertoli cells also protects the seminal epithelium from any possible antibody activity as it is impermeable to γ-globulins.

– *Phagocytic role.* During the normal development of the seminal line, a certain number of cells, including spermatogonia and type-I spermatocytes, degenerate. This degeneration can be followed by labelling the seminal line cells at an early stage with ^{3}H-thymidine and autoradiography: 24 hours after injection of label, silver grains can be seen over nuclear debris associated with lysosomes within the cytoplasm of the Sertoli cells.

– *Role in steroidogenic activity.* The Sertoli cells can transform pregnenolone and progesterone into testosterone, and testosterone into 17β-estradiol; they must therefore contain the enzymes necessary for these transformations, although they do not contain the enzymes required for the cleavage of the cholesterol side chain; it is noteworthy that their cytoplasm is rich in endoplasmic reticulum, like that of cells which secrete steroids.

1.5.2.2. Sertoli cells and the endocrine control of spermatogenesis. Sertoli cells contribute to the endocrine control of spermatogenesis by several mechanisms; this control requires a synergic action of FSH and androgens.

– *Sertoli cells as the primary target cells for the action of FSH*. Sertoli cells are susceptible to the action of FSH. This is indicated by several types of observations:

- in the prepubertal hypophysectomized subject, injections of FSH provoke a *hypertrophy* of the Sertoli cells with increase in production of tubular fluid;
- in adults whose germinal line cells have been destroyed by X-rays, FSH induces the synthesis of *new messenger-RNA* and *proteins* in Sertoli cells;
- in vitro, Sertoli cells can bind highly purified preparations of ^{125}I-labelled FSH;
- cultures of Sertoli cells are stimulated by FSH; two types of reactions can be observed: (1) *morphological* reactions with cytoplasmic and nuclear hypertrophy, with numerous cytoplasmic extensions: if the treated Sertoli cells are replaced in a medium lacking FSH they regain a morphology similar to that of untreated cells; (2) *metabolic* reactions, some of which appear rapidly such as the stimulation of adenyl cyclase and the metabolic consequences of modifications in the cyclic nucleotides, or the activation of an AMP-dependent protein kinase (these phenomena are responsible for a rapid protein synthesis), others appear more slowly, such as the aromatization of testosterone to 17β-estradiol;
- *membrane receptors for FSH* have been identified on Sertoli cells, which are the only testicular cells to have such receptors: peritubular cells have no specific affinity for FSH; it is estimated that each Sertoli cell possesses some 10,000 of these receptors; in adults these receptors are not modified by hypophysectomy which also causes no change in

the number of Sertoli cells; these receptors are present in the testicular tubules of rats irradiated at the eighteenth day of embryonic life, these tubules being uniquely composed of Sertoli cells as the irradiation completely destroys the gonocytes (Sertoli-cell-enriched testes); some 'control' could be imposed upon the binding of FSH to the receptors by the action of one or more 'inhibitory factors' whose nature is at present unknown, but which are probably produced in the seminiferous tubule;

- under the influence of the reactions induced by FSH, the Sertoli cells produce *diffusible substances*, whose nature is still controversial, which circulate in the intercellular spaces of the adluminal compartment to reach the germinal cells and stimulate both their proliferation and differentiation.

– *Sertoli cells and androgens*. The role of Sertoli cells in the regulation of spermatogenesis is closely linked to the androgens, as FSH alone is capable of maintaining spermatogenesis; in addition, the action of FSH is not only potentiated by androgens but is also inhibited by anti-androgens. The action of androgens on Sertoli cells is proved by the study of seminiferous tubules after treatment with anti-gonadotropin (anti-LH) serum which provokes a rapid (five days in adult rats) and considerable reduction in the plasmatic testosterone levels, and in the weight of the seminal vesicles; there is an increase in the number of lipid droplets in the basal cytoplasm of the Sertoli cells, and spermatids undergoing spermatogenesis are retained and degenerate within the Sertoli cells; degenerative lesions of the germinal cells (spermatocytes and spermatids) are also observed. Two special aspects of the relation between Sertoli cells and androgens should be emphasized: the synthesis by Sertoli cells of androgen-binding protein (ABP), and the presence of androgen receptors on Sertoli cells:

- *androgen-binding protein* is produced in the seminiferous tubules and is present in the tubular fluid; ABP is a glycoprotein of molecular weight around 65,000-68,000 composed of 70-80% aminoacids and 20-30% carbohydrates; production of ABP ceases after hypophysectomy, but the administration of FSH to the hypophysectomized subject restores its production; however, since LH also stimulates the biosynthesis of ABP at the same time as an increase in production of testosterone, it is considered that the biosynthesis of ABP depends upon both FSH and testosterone; it would appear, however, that testosterone is the principal regulating factor in adults (FSH has a greater action in immature subjects); in addition, different in vivo and in vitro experiments indicate that testosterone stabilizes ABP towards the activity of proteolytic tissues factors;

• *another androphilic protein*, different from ABP, can be isolated from Sertoli cells; it has a sedimentation coefficient of 6-8 S, is unstable to heat, and has a slow complex dissociation rate; these characteristics resemble those of intracellular androgen (and steroid) receptors; these can be considered to be Sertoli cell *androgen receptors* and are present in the cytoplasm and the nuclei of these cells; progesterone and dihydrotestosterone (as well as cyproterone acetate) compete to various degrees with testosterone for the binding sites; estradiol and cortisol do not compete; it should, however, be emphasized that similar androgen receptors are also present in cells of the germinal line.

The hormonal relationships between the Sertoli cell and other components of the testicular parenchyma are illustrated schematically in Figure 2.

1.6. Central control of hypophyseal gonadotropins

Antehypophyseal gonadotropic function is under hypothalamic control. The hypothalamus produces a decapeptide called Gn-RH (gonado-tropin-releasing hormone); this peptide, which is synthesized in neurones situated in various regions of the hypothalamus (principally in the medio-basal and the anterior hypothalamus), reaches the anterior lobe of the hypophysis by the hypothalamo-hypophyseal portal vessels. A single hypothalamic hormone controls pituitary secretion of FSH and LH (ICSH), both these hormones being the product of a single type of antehypophyseal cell. The role of Gn-RH in the control of spermatogenesis is proved by experiments measuring the involution of the germinal line after hypothalamo-hypophyseal disconnection or after administration of anti-Gn-RH antibodies. Conversely, in animals bearing pituitary grafts under the renal capsule (and whose tubules contain only spermatogonia and spermatocytes-I), treatment with Gn-RH induces a complete restora-

tion of spermatogenesis; similarly, in oligospermic men, injections of Gn-RH have sometimes resulted in an increase in the number of gametes in the sperm. Treatment with Gn-RH agonists such as (D-Ala^6, Des-Gly-NH$_2$^{10})-LHRH ethylamide causes a reduction in testicular FSH and LH receptors; in such cases lesions of the Sertoli cells and degeneration of the seminal line are observed; such observations should incite caution in the use of synthetic agonists of Gn-RH in long-term treatment of dysfunction of spermatogenesis.

The predominant influence of Gn-RH on the production and/or cessation of production of FSH or LH is influenced by several factors: the specific action of the hypothalamic peptide on the receptors of the pituitary cells, the overall endocrine status and age of the subject, involvement with retroactive phenomena mediated by the sexual steroids, and by another testicular factor, inhibin (see below).

Activating or inhibitory influences are constantly acting on the hypothalamic centres. These receive multiple inputs from, on the one hand, all the encephalic regions, and, on the other hand, the extra-hypothalamic routes for Gn-RH which carry this peptide into regions other than the median eminence where the nerve-blood junction, which allows the passage of the hormone from the hypothalamus to the hypophysis, normally occurs; numerous inter-relations thus exist between the hypothalamus and other regions of the encephalon.

It can therefore be considered that multiple factors may be expected to influence the process of spermatogenesis.

2. TESTICULAR INHIBIN

2.1. Original observations

The existence of hypophyso-gonadal interactions implies not only the idea of a hypophysary influence upon the testis, but also a feedback mechanism. In fact, the supposed feedback by the tubular secretions remained for a long time purely hypothetical.

Studies of the cytological modifications in the anterior pituitary of irradiated animals whose germinal epithelium was destroyed led to the postulation of a secretion from the epithelium of the seminiferous tubules. Suppression of this secretion would induce the appearance of 'castration cells' in

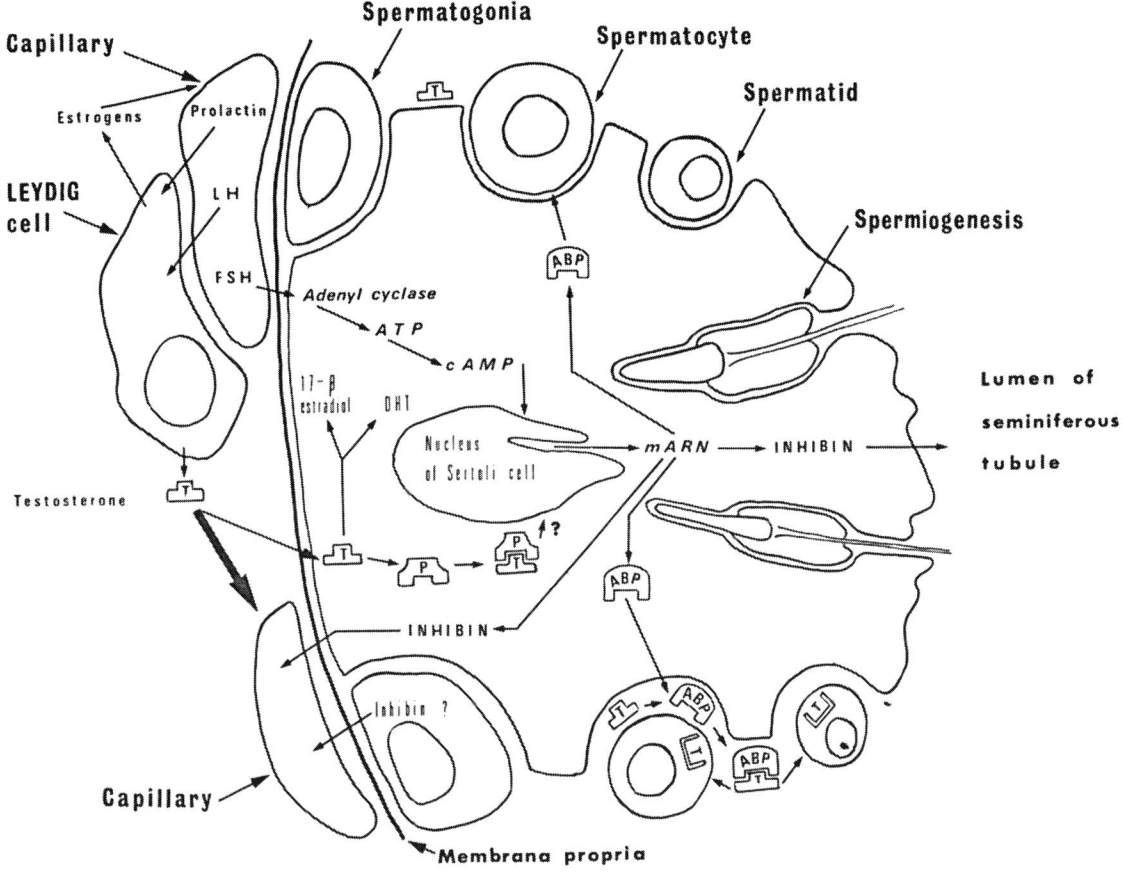

Figure 2. The hormonal correlations between Sertoli cells and other components of the testicular parenchyma.

the pituitary gland. The observation of similar modifications of the hypophysis in parabiotic rats support the hypothesis of the production of a tubular factor: this factor, which was initially considered hydrosoluble and to differ from the steroids, was named *inhibin* by MacCullagh (1932). The absence of inhibin was considered to be responsible for the increase in the level of FSH in subjects with damaged epithelium.

However, from the first, the inhibin theory was contested as no cell could be identified in the seminal epithelium as being responsible for the secretion of the factor. There was proposed an alternative hypothesis to explain the increase of FSH after destruction of the seminal line, the 'utilization hypothesis', which stated that under normal conditions FSH was 'utilized' or degraded by the seminal epithelium, and therefore that when the epithelium was destroyed the lack of intratubular 'utilization' led to the increase in circulating FSH. This theory was based on no valid

findings, and recent studies totally refute any such interpretation.

2.2. *Present status of the hypothesis*

At present there are a good number of arguments which support the existence of a factor which may properly be called inhibin because it inhibits the secretion of FSH. The name 'FSH-inhibiting factor' has also been used, but as this name resembles the nomenclature of the hypothalamic 'factors' very closely, it would be preferable to retain the name inhibin. Although the physiological reality of inhibin can be considered to be demonstrated, certain unknowns remain, especially concerning the nature and number of factor(s) concerned (cf. reviews in Baker et al. 1976; Franchimont et al. 1977, 1978; Prasad and Rajalakshmi 1977; Setchell et al. 1977; Eddie et al. 1978).

2.2.1. Demonstration of the existence of 'inhibin'. Injection of testicular extracts, from which the steroids have been removed, into adult animals causes a modification in the secretion of antehypophyseal gonadotropins; there is either a selective suppression of FSH (e.g. in sheep), or a major reduction of FSH accompanied by a diminution in LH (e.g. in rats).

The addition of such extracts to cultures of antehypophyseal cells or to incubated pituitary halves results in the reduction of the secretion of FSH by the pituitaries. The co-culture of pituitary cells with Sertoli cells or addition to a pituitary cells culture of the medium in which Sertoli cells have been grown, causes a reduction in the basal level of secretion of FSH, and suppresses the production of FSH following the addition of Gn-RH to the culture. However, when pituitary cells from rats are treated with extracts of rat seminal tubules under these conditions the production of LH is also slightly diminished.

Measurement of the steroids present in the culture medium shows that this suppression or reduction of secretion of FSH is not mediated by testosterone or estradiol. Neither is this response due to the 'ageing' of the cells in vitro with a consequent incapacity to produce pituitary hormones as these same cells produce TSH when stimulated with TRH.

It should be emphasized that, under experimental conditions, different responses to extracts containing 'inhibin' are observed according to the injection route employed; when given intra-peritoneally they induce a reduction of liberation of FSH only after injection of Gn-RH while, when given intravenously, a reduction in liberation of both FSH and LH is observed after administration of Gn-RH.

2.2.2. Nature of 'inhibin'. The exact chemical nature of 'inhibin' is not yet known. It would appear to be *a protein or a peptide* as the activity of preparations with the properties of inhibin is destroyed by heat and by proteolytic enzymes, but is unaltered by steroid solvents; the molecule differs from that of ABP.

Separation of testicular extracts by Sephadex filtration yields two active fractions, one with a molecular weight of 15-25,000 daltons, and the other of 70-80,000 daltons. It is at present not known whether these are monomeric and a polymeric form of the same molecule, or whether the molecule can be firmly bound to another protein. In vitro under certain experimental conditions, both fractions have the same activity, but more usually the active fraction is the smaller protein.

The capacity to reduce the level of FSH secretion is also found in the 'inhibin' extracted from seminal fluid; precipitation of the proteins by ethanol followed by molecular filtration on Sephadex G-100 gives two fractions of which only one, called Ac-II (Franchimont et al. 1975), possesses the property of specific suppression of FSH without alteration of the level of LH. Administration of anti-Ac-II antibody to rats causes the suppression of endogenous secretion of the 'inhibin' and an increase in circulating FSH levels. Using different methods of protein separation on liquid obtained by aspiration from the rete testis of sheep, several fractions contain inhibin-like activity; this might be due either to the association of inhibin with different proteins or to the existence of several forms of inhibin.

2.2.3. Origin of 'inhibin'. Inhibin is undoubtably produced in the seminiferous tubules, but what type of cell is responsible for its synthesis?

– From *observations on human testes* with more or less extensive lesions in their seminal epithelium, the secretion of the inhibin appeared to be associated with the spermatids or perhaps the spermatogonia as there was a correlation between the number of these cells present and the level of circulating FSH. However, owing to the disparities between different series and the considerable individual variations observed, no certain conclusions could be drawn.

– From *experimental observations* on the testes of animals treated by heat, X-rays (especially during the prenatal period, giving rise to Sertoli-cell-enriched testes) or antimitotics, it would appear that the synthesis of inhibin can be principally localized to the Sertoli cells, whence the alternative name of 'Sertoli cell factor'.

At present, therefore, it would appear that inhibin derives from the seminiferous tubules; the principal producers would appears to be the Sertoli cells, but the synthesis of this factor by other cells of the seminal epithelium cannot be excluded.

2.2.4. Physiological properties of 'inhibin'. Inhibin is synthesized in the seminal epithelium and appears in the tubular fluid, in the rete testis fluid, and in the seminal fluid; an inhibin-like activity has been observed in spermatozoa.

Testicular inhibin could reach the general circulation either directly via the vessels in the interstitial spaces of the testis, or through the vessels beside the lining of the rete testis whose epithelium possesses reabsorbin properties, or even by the epididymal vessels. The inhibin would then pass into the general circulation through the spermatic veins. The means by which inhibin passes into the circulation might depend upon the type of cell which synthesizes it: passage into the interstitial vessels if the synthesis took place in the spermatogonia, or passage into the vessels of Highmore's body or the epididymis if synthesis occurred in cells in the adluminal compartment of the tubule. The reabsorption of the inhibin present in the testicular fluid is certainly incomplete, and the spermatozoa actively absorb the remaining fraction.

By passage through the systemic circulation the inhibin reaches the pituitary. It is generally supposed that it exerts an influence upon the ante-hypophyseal cells by blocking the control of secretion of FSH mediated by Gn-RH, but some experimental findings (intraventricular injections of preparations with inhibin-like activity from spermatozoa) suggest that it also has some direct action on the hypothalamic synthesis of Gn-RH.

Inhibin might also act on the synthesis of FSH: in vitro, in organotypic hypophyseal cultures, inhibin produced by Sertoli cell culture 'can selectively reduce the incorporation of ^{3}H-leucine into immunoprecipitable FSH without decreasing the incorporation into LH' (Chowdhury et al. 1978).

Under experimental conditions, the effects of an injection of inhibin, or, more accurately, of testicular extracts from sheep or of substance(s), proteinaceous in nature, from the seminal plasma of bulls or of men, are limited in time: the fall in the level of FSH is observed some three to six hours after the injection and is maintained for some 24 to 36 hours only.

These effects of inhibin on the direct or indirect production of FSH are well established, but under physiological conditions FSH is above all necessary for the development of the testis during the pre-pubertal phase. This raises questions concerning the significance of inhibin in adults in whom the influence of FSH on the seminiferous tubule is less marked. This requires further research, as does the

existence of inhibin-like activity in females, and the influence of extracts of testis or of seminal plasma with inhibin-like activity on hypophyso-ovarian functions.

3. ACTION OF OTHER FACTORS

The normal development of spermatogenesis requires the participation of factors other than the hypothalamo - hypophyseal hormones. The influence of the *pineal gland* should be mentioned (review in Johnson and Reiter 1978; Vaughan et al. 1978); but since the relations between the epiphysis and the exocrine testis are of the nature of an epiphyso-pituitary antagonism, this represents only another link in the chain of neuro-endocrine relations.

Two other groups of physiological factors exert an important influence on the development of spermatogenesis: *vascular* factors and *nervous* factors (review in Bell 1972; Baumgarten et al. 1975). We shall not consider the influence of physical factors (e.g. temperature, radiation) or pharmacological factors.

3.1. Vascular factors

The vascular integrity of the testis is an essential factor. For example, in man a testicular torsion with arrest of circulation causes lesions of the seminiferous tubules after 8-10 hours, and a true tubular necrosis after 15-24 hours.

Some pharmacological vaso-constrictors (especially serotonin) cause seminal lesions by their action on the testicular vascularization. The action of an endocrine factor influencing visceral vascularization, including that of the gonads, hypophyseal corticotropic hormone, should also be noted.

3.2. Nervous factors

3.2.1. *The extra-hypothalamic central nervous system.* The extra-hypothalamic central nervous system is involved in the control of spermatogenesis either indirectly through its connections with the hypothalamus, or directly through the innervation of the testis itself. It is, for example, known that spermatogenesis is altered in paraplegia, in spinocerebellar heredo-ataxia, in Steinert's disease, and in the Laurence-Moon-Bardet-Biedl syndrome. This link between the germinal epithelium and the central nervous system, especially clear in pathological conditions, permits the definition of a corresponding group of pathologies: the neuro-germinal degenerative diseases.

3.2.2. The vegetative nervous system. The vegetative nervous system, through the vasomotor or proprioceptive innervation, appears to influence the regulation of spermatogenesis. Lesions of the prostato-vesiculo-deferential ganglion cause a regression of the seminal epithelium despite the presence of a normal secretion of gonadotropic hormones.

4. SUMMARY AND GENERAL CONCLUSIONS

Experimental and clinical observations allow us at present to affirm the existence of a neuro-endocrine loop which controls the spermatogenetic function of the testis. The principal stages can be summarized as follows (see also Figure 3):

– *The hypothalamus* produces a decapeptide, so-called Gn-RH; this production of Gn-RH is influenced by several modulating factors, either an intra-hypothalamic control through the direct action of Gn-RH on the neurones which synthesize it through the participation of their retrograde collateral axons (ultra-short feedback), or a control via afferent fibers of extra-hypothalamic origin which carry various neuro-transmitters (mono-amines and perhaps peptides of the endorphin or enkephalin types).
– *The Gn-RH peptide* reaches the pituitary gonadotropic cells through 'neuro-vascular synapses' in the median eminence and the hypothalamo-hypophyseal portal vascularization; the passage of the hypothalamic peptide in the infundibular loops of the median eminence depends upon local controlling factors, notably monoamines.
– *The pituitary gonadotropic cells* produce FSH and LH (ICSH); the production of both factors is certainly localized within the same cell; the preferential production of one or other hormone depends upon factors regulating the membrane receptors for Gn-RH.
– *The gonadotropins* reach the testes by the bloodstream; several types of testicular cells possess

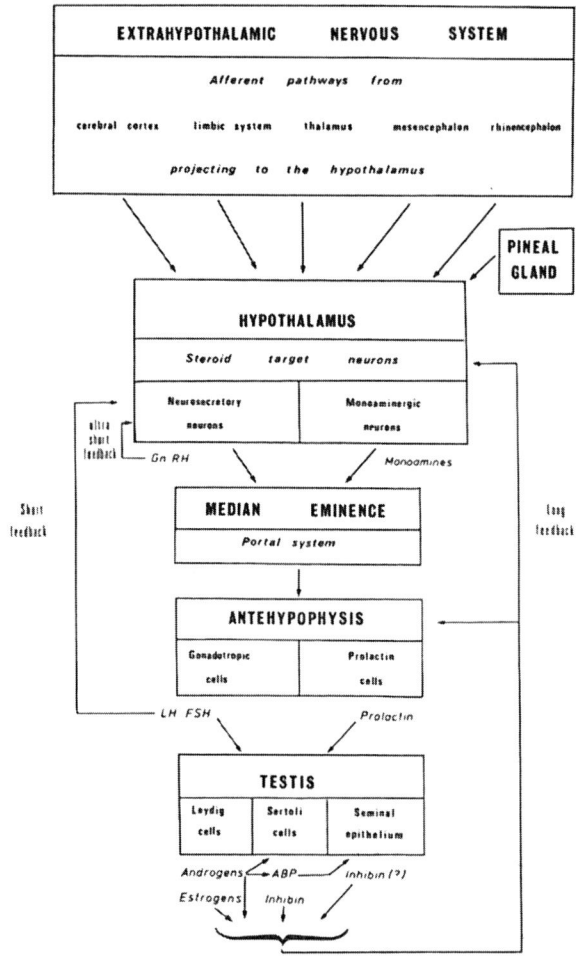

Figure 3. An overview of different factors implicated in the regulation of the testis activities.

membrane receptors for gonadotropic hormones; it is also likely that, through the 'ascending' flow, some part of the gonadotropins reaches the hypothalamus directly, producing a 'short feedback'.
– *In the testis*, the gonadotropins provoke either a stimulation of the Leydig cells (by LH-ICSH) or of the Sertoli cells (by FSH):
• under the influence of ABP, androgens are transported into contact with the cells in the seminal epithelium; proteins produced in the Sertoli cells also reach this epithelium; the reaction of the seminal epithelium is rapid;
• inhibin, which passes into the general circulation, exerts a 'long feedback' effect on the hypothalamo-hypophyseal centres.

The totality of present-day observations leads us to emphasize the close relationship which exists between the exocrine and the endocrine testis. For example, testosterone and its metabolites reduced in the 5α position are necessary for the induction and continuation of meiosis as well as for the phenomena of spermiogenesis. However, testosterone and its metabolites also exert a feedback on the control centres. In addition the testis also produces estrogens, notably estradiol, and estradiol exerts a negative feedback effect on the secretion of FSH and LH.

It is, therefore, possible to conclude that a neuro-endocrine control of spermatogenetic function really exists, but, because of the intimate interrelation with the endocrine testicular activity, it is preferable to emphasize the global nature of the control of testicular function, a parallel and interdependent control of the exocrine and endocrine activities of the testis.

REFERENCES

Baker HWG, Burger HG, De Kretser DM, Hudson B, O'Connor S, Wang C, Mirovics A, Court J, Dunlop M, Rennie GC: Changes in the pituitary-testicular system with age. Clin Endocrinol 5: 349-372, 1976.

Bartke A: Pituitary-testis relationships: role of prolactin in the regulation of testicular function: sperm action. Progr Reprod Biol 1: 136-152, 1976.

Bartke A, Hafiez AA, Bex FJ, Dalterio S: Hormonal interactions in regulation of androgen secretion. Biol Reprod 18: 44-54, 1978.

Baumgarten HG, Owman C, Sjöberg NO: Neural mechanisms in male fertility. In: Control of male fertility, Sciarra JJ, Markland C, Speidel JJ (eds), New York, Harper and Row, 1975, p 26-40.

Bell C: Autonomic nervous control of reproduction: circulatory and other factors. Pharmacol Rev 24: 657-736, 1972.

Böck P: Histochemical demonstration of disulfide-groups in the lamina propria of human seminiferous tubules. Anat Embryol 153: 157-166, 1978.

Bressler RS: Hormonal control of postnatal maturation of the seminiferous cord. Ann Biol Anim Bioch Biophys 18: 535-540, 1978.

Bustos-Obregón E, Courot M, Fléchon JE, Hochereau de Reviers M-T, Holstein AF: Morphological appraisal of gametogenesis. spermatogenetic process in mammals with particular reference to man. Andrologia 7: 141-163, 1975.

Chemes HE, Dym M, Fawcett DW, Javadpour N, Sherins RJ: Patho-physiological observations of Sertoli cells in patients with germinal aplasia or severe germ cell depletion: ultrastructural findings and hormone levels. Biol Reprod 17: 108-123, 1977.

Chowdhury M, Steinberger A, Steinberger E: Inhibition of de novo synthesis of FSH by the Sertoli cell factor (SCF). Endocrinol 103: 644-647, 1978.

Clermont Y: Kinetics of spermatogenesis in mammals: seminiferous epithelium cycle and spermatogonial renewal. Physiol Rev 52: 198-236, 1972.

Courot M: Hormonal regulation of male reproduction (with reference to infertility in man). Andrologia 8: 187-193, 1976.

Courot M, Ortavant R: Contrôle gonadotrope de la spermatogénèse chez les mammifères. In: Fécondité et stérilité du mâle: acquisitions récentes, Thibault C (ed), Paris, Masson, 1972, p 1-18.

Cunningham GR, Tindall DJ, Huckins C, Means AR: Mechanisms for the testicular hypertrophy which follows hemicastration. Endocrinol 102: 16-23, 1978.

Dym M: The role of the Sertoli cell in spermatogenesis. In: Male reproductive system, Yates RD, Gordon M (eds), New York, Masson, 1977, p 155-169.

Dym M, Cavicchia JC: Functional morphology of the testis. Biol Reprod 18: 1-15, 1978.

Dym M, Fawcett DW: The blood-testis barrier in the rat and the physiological compartmentation of the seminiferous epithelium. Biol Reprod 3: 308-326, 1970.

Dym M, Fawcett DW: Further observations on the number of spermatogonia, spermatocytes and spermatids joined by intercellular bridges in mammalian spermatogenesis. Biol Reprod 4: 195-215, 1971.

Eddie LW, Baker HWG, Dulmanis A, Higginson RE, Hudson B: Inhibin from cultures of rat seminiferous tubules. J Endocr 78: 217-224, 1978.

Fawcett DW: Ultrastructure and function of the Sertoli cell. In: Handbook of physiology, sec 7: Endocrinology; vol 5: Male reproductive system, Greep RO, Astwood EB (eds), Baltimore, Williams and Wilkins, 1975, p 21-55.

Fawcett DW: The male reproductive system. In: Reproduction and human welfare: a challenge to research, Greep RO, Koblinsky MA, Jaffe FS (eds), Cambridge, Massachusetts, MIT Press, 1976, p 165-277.

Forest MG, De Peretti E, Bertrand J: Hypothalamic-pituitary-gonadal relationships in man from birth to puberty. Clin Endocrinol 5: 551-569, 1976.

Franchimont P, Chari S, Demoulin A: Hypothalamus-pituitary-testis interaction. J Reprod Fertil 44: 335-350, 1975.

Franchimont P, Chari S, Hazee-Hagelstein MT, Debruche ML, Duraiswami S: Evidence for the existence of inhibin. In: The testis in normal and infertile men, Troen P, Nankin HR (eds), New York, Raven, 1977, p 253-270.

Franchimont P, Demoulin A, Verstaelen-Proyard J, Hazee-Hagelstein MT, Walton JS, Waites GMH: Nature and mechanisms of action of inhibin: perspective in regulation of male fertility. Int J Androl, suppl 2, part 1: 69-80, 1978.

Fritz IB, Louis BG, Tung PS, Dorrington J: Action of hormones on Sertoli cells during maturation. Ann Biol Anim Bioch Biophys 18: 555-563, 1978.

Furuya S, Kumamoto Y, Sugiyama S: Fine structure and development of Sertoli junctions in human testis. Arch Androl 1: 211-219, 1978.

Gulyas BJ, Tullner WW, Hodgen GD: Fetal and maternal hypophysectomy in rhesus monkeys (*Macaca mulatta*): effects on the development of testes and other endocrine organs. Biol Reprod 17: 650-660, 1977.

Gupta D, Rager K, Zech K, Voelter W: Hypothalamic-pituitary-testicular feedback mechanism during mammalian sexual maturation. In: Hypothalamic hormones: structure, synthesis and biological activity, Gupta D, Voelter W (eds), Weinheim, Verlag Chemie, 1975, p 179-206.

Hansson V, Calandra R, Purvis K, Ritzén M, French FS: Hormonal regulation of spermatogenesis. Vitam Horm 34: 187-214, 1976.

Hansson V, Purvis K, Ritzén EM, French FS: Hormonal regulation of Sertoli cell function in the rat. Ann Biol Anim Bioch Biophys 18: 565-572, 1978.

Hansson V, Weddington Sc, McLean WS, Smith AA, Nayfeh SN, French FS, Ritzén EM: Regulation of seminiferous tubular function by FSH and androgen. J Reprod Fertil 44: 363-375, 1975.

Hermo L, Lalli M: Monocytes and mast cells in the limiting membrane of human seminiferous tubules. Biol Reprod 19: 92-100, 1978.

Hilscher W, Hilscher B: Kinetics of the male gametogenesis. Andrologia 8: 105-116, 1976.

Hochereau de Reviers M-T, Courot M: Sertoli cells and development of seminiferous epithelium. Ann Biol Anim Bioch Biophys 18: 573-583, 1978.

Jeffcoate SL: The control of testicular function in the adult. Clin Endocr Metab 4: 521-543, 1975.

Johnson LY, Reiter RJ: The pineal gland and its effects on mammalian reproduction. In: The pineal and reproduction, Reiter RJ (ed), Basel, Karger, 1978, p 116-156.

Kotite NL, Nayfeh SN, French FS: FSH and androgen regulation of Sertoli cell function in the immature rat. Biol Reprod 18: 65-73, 1978.

McNeilly AS, Sharpe RM, Davidson DW, Fraser HM: Inhibition of gonadotropin secretion by induced hyperprolactinaemia in the male rat. J Endocr 79: 59-68, 1978.

Means AR: Mechanisms of action of follicle-stimulating hormone (FSH). In: The testis, Johnson AD, Gomes WR (eds), New York, Academic Press, 1977, vol 4, p 163-188.

Means AR, Dedman JR, Tindall DJ, Welsh MJ: Hormonal regulation of Sertoli cells. Int J Androl, suppl 2, part 2: 403-423, 1978.

Means AR, Fakunding JL, Huckins C, Tindall DJ, Vitale R: Follicle-stimulating hormone, the Sertoli cell, and spermatogenesis. Recent Progr Hormone Res 32: 477-522, 1976.

Moger WH: Endocrine responses of the prepubertal male rat to hemiorchidectomy. Biol Reprod 17: 661-667, 1977.

Neaves WB: The blood-testis barrier. In: The testis, Johnson AD, Gomes WT (eds), New York, Academic Press, 1977, vol 4, p 125-162.

Prasad MRN, Rajalakshmi M: Recent advances in the control of male reproductive functions. In: Reproductive physiology II, Greep RO (ed), Baltimore, University Park Press, 1977, p 153-199.

Raj MHG, Dym M: The effects of selective withdrawal of FSH or LH on spermatogenesis in the immature rat. Biol Reprod 14: 489-494, 1976.

Ravault JP, Courot M, Garnier D, Pelletier J, Terqui M: Effect of 2-bromo-α-ergocryptine (CB 154) on plasma prolactin, LH and testosterone levels, accessory reproductive glands and spermatogenesis in lambs during puberty. Biol Reprod 17: 192-197, 1977.

Ross MH: The Sertoli cell junctional specialization during spermiogenesis and at spermiation. Anat Rec 186: 79-103, 1976.

Russell L: Observations on rat Sertoli ectoplasmic ('junctional') specializations in their association with germ cells of the rat testis. Tiss Cell 9: 475-498, 1977.

Russell LD: The blood-testis barrier and its formation relative to spermatocyte maturation in the adult rat: a lanthanum tracer study. Anat Rec 190: 99-111, 1978.

Schulze C: On the morphology of the human Sertoli cell. Cell Tiss Res 153: 339-355, 1974.

Setchell BP, Davies RV, Main SJ: Inhibin. In: The testis, Johnson AD, Gomes WR (eds), New York, Academic Press, 1977, vol 4, p 189-238.

Sivelle PC, McNeilly AS, Collins PM: A comparison of the effectiveness of FSH, LH and prolactin in the reinitiation of testicular function of hypophysectomized and estrogen-treated rats. Biol Reprod 17: 878-885, 1978.

Steinberger A, Steinberger E: The Sertoli cells. In: The testis, Johnson AD, Gomes WR (eds), New York, Academic Press, 1977, vol 4, p 371-399.

Steinberger E: Hormonal regulation of the seminiferous tubule function. In: Hormonal regulation of spermatogenesis, French FS, Hansson V, Ritzen EM, Nayfeh SN (eds), New York, Plenum, 1975, p 337-352.

Steinberger E, Steinberger A: Testis: basic and clinical aspects. In: Reproductive biology, Balin H, Glasser S (eds), Amsterdam, Excerpta Medica, 1972, p 144-267.

Steinberger E, Steinberger A: Spermatogenic function of the testis. In: Handbook of physiology, sec 7: Endocrinology vol 5: Male reproductive system, Greep RO, Astwood EB (eds), Baltimore, Williams and Wilkins, 1975, p 1-19.

Vaughan GM, Meyer GG, Reiter RJ: Evidence for a pineal-gonad relationship in the human. In: The pineal and reproduction, Reiter RJ (ed), Basel, Karger, 1978, p 191-223.

Viguier-Martinez MC, Hochereau de Reviers M-T: Comparative action of cyproterone and cyproterone actetate on pituitary and plasma gonadotropins levels on male genital tract and spermatogenesis of prepubertal rats. Ann Biol Anim Bioch Biophys 17: 1069-1076, 1977.

Vilar O: Spermatogenesis. In: Human reproduction, Hafez ESE, Evans TN (eds), New York, Harper and Row, 1973, p 12-37.

Wartenberg H: Comparative cytomorphologic aspects of the male germ cells, especially of the 'gonia'. Andrologia 8: 117-130, 1976.

Wartenberg H: Human testicular development and the role of the mesonephros in the origin of a dual Sertoli cell system. Andrologia 10: 1-21, 1978.

Zipf WB, Payne AH, Kelch RP: Prolactin, growth hormone, and luteinizing hormone in the maintenance of testicular luteinizing hormone receptors. Endocrinol 103: 595-600, 1978.

9. BIOGENESIS OF ANDROGENS AND ESTROGENS BY THE NORMAL TESTIS

B.K. TSANG and G.A. KINSON

1. THE TESTIS AS A SOURCE OF MALE SEX HORMONE

The description of interstitial cells by Leydig in 1857 and the epithelium of the seminiferous tubules by Sertoli in 1865 laid the foundation for the present concepts of testicular function (Steinberger and Steinberger 1975). By 1903, Bouin and Ancel had linked the interstitium of the testis with male endocrine function. The finding of large quantities of androgenic material in interstitial tumours of the mouse testis convinced most that the Leydig cells were indeed the source of male hormone (Hooker and Pfeiffer 1942). The theory of one hormone for each sex evolved and testosterone was to be the masculinizing hormone secreted by the testis whilst estrogenic principles were believed to be confined to the ovaries. As is so often the case in research, the theory of one hormone-one sex was being challenged even during its development.

1.1. Testicular cell types involved in androgen biosynthesis

The mammalian testis is generally divided into three major functional components; the capsule, seminiferous tubules, and interstitial tissue. The capsule serves not only as an envelope for the interstitial and tubular contents of the testis, but plays an important physiological role in testicular ductal motion by virtue of its contractile properties (Davis et al. 1970). The characteristics of the seminiferous tubules and their contents is the focus of the later portion of this chapter. The interstitial tissue forms an irregular network in the spaces between the seminiferous tubules. The interstitial tissue of the human testis occupies about 34% of the testicular volume and also contains blood vessels, lymphatic ducts, nerves and various connective tissue elements such as fibro-

blasts, macrophages, mast cells, collagen and elastic fibers (Figure 1). Leydig cells are basically similar throughout the mammalian kingdom and those of the human testis are of average dimensions compared to other species. Human Leydig cells are about 15 μm in diameter occupying 12% of the testicular volume while, in the rat, Leydig cells are approximately 10 μm in diameter accounting for only 2% of testicular volume. Boar testis presents an example of the other extreme where they measure 30 μm in diameter and constitute about 37% of the testicular volume (Christensen 1975).

Leydig cells lie in clusters around the blood vessels which in turn lie in irregular peritubular sinusoids. The capillaries of the testis appear to be oriented parallel to the seminiferous tubules, the latter being avascular. Leydig cells undergo two periods of growth in most mammals, during fetal development and again at puberty. Mesenchymal cells have begun differentiating into Leydig cells in the eight-week-old human embryo. At fourteen weeks, more than half of the testicular volume is occupied by masses of Leydig cells which closely resemble those of the adult testis. Optimal differentiation of interstitial tissue is maintained from the fourteenth to the eighteenth week of fetal life and is then followed by a gradual and progressive involution of the fetal Leydig cells. Numbers of Leydig cells are greatly reduced by seven months and, within a few months of birth, the interstitial tissue of the human testis becomes essentially devoid of Leydig cells. This state of affairs persists until puberty at about thirteen years of age at which time redifferentiation of Leydig cells takes place, presumably from fibroblast-like cells.

The substructure of Leydig cells presents many common features throughout the mammalia and, again, the human cell is around the average when compared with those of other species. The polygonal cell with a diameter of 15-20 μm is bounded by a

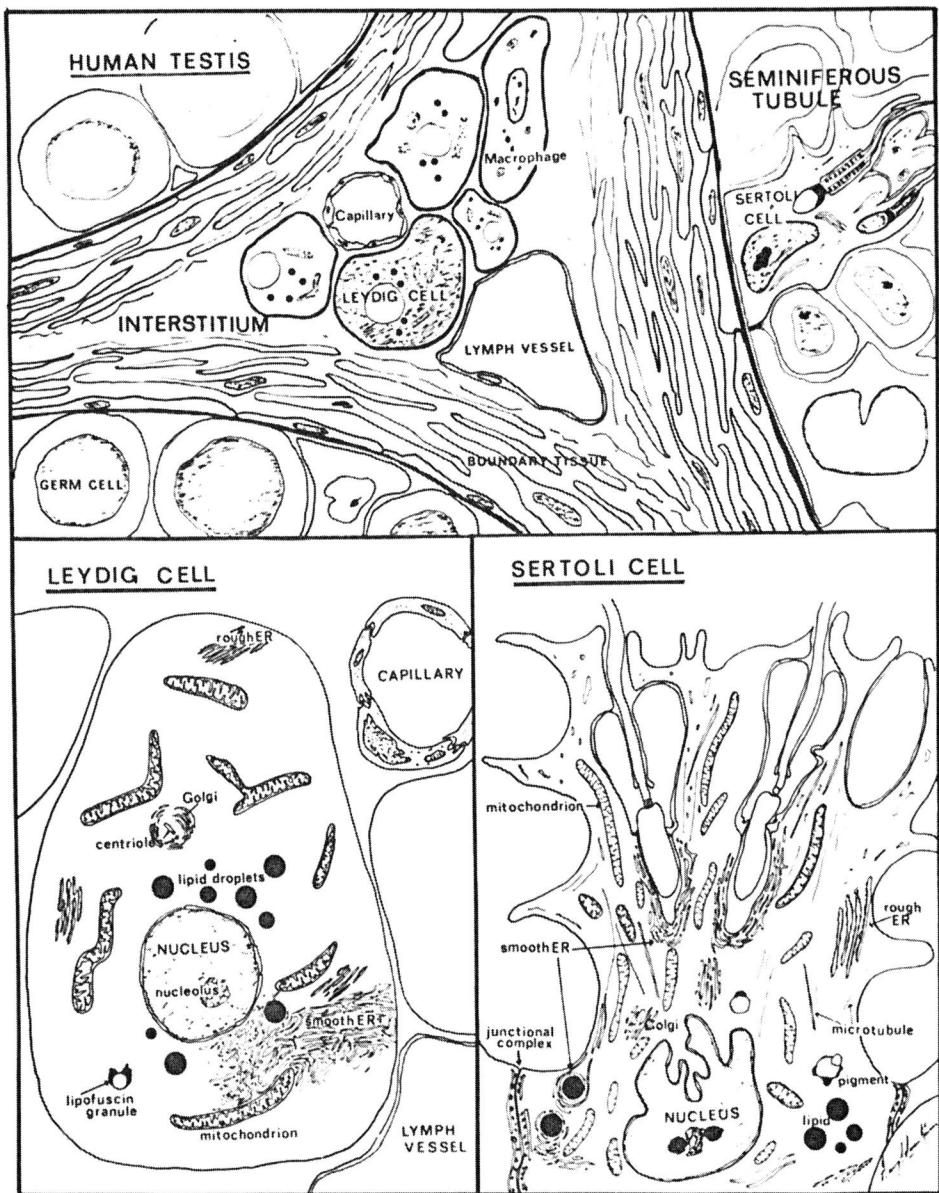

Figure 1. The interstitial tissue of the human testis in relation to the seminiferous tubules and the fine structures of the Leydig and Sertoli cells (redrawn from Christensen 1975 and Fawcett 1975).

typical plasma membrane possessing abundant microvilli (Christensen 1975). A smooth endoplasmic reticulum is, perhaps, the most striking cytoplasmic organelle which forms an extensive interconnecting network of membrane tubules throughout the cytoplasm. Scattered patches of rough endoplasmic reticulum interconnect with the smooth version. Moderate numbers of average-sized mitochondria contain cristae of characteristic lamellar form, yet many are tubular. Golgi elements composed of four to six flattened sacs with small vesicles at their periphery are usually at one pole of the nucleus although extensions of the complex can be seen elsewhere in the cytoplasm. The Golgi region contains two centrioles arranged perpendicular to one another. The cytoplasm also contains Reinke crystals, lipid droplets, microtubules and microfilaments. There are many primary lysosomes, digestive vacuoles (secondary lysosomes) and residual bodies (late secondary lysosomes), many of the latter containing lipofuscin pigment granules. The large nucleus is round or oval with one or two prominent nucleoli, and has a thin rim of heterochromatin interrupted only at pores through the nuclear envelope.

1.1.1. Synthesis of androgens by Leydig cells. Although initially difficult to demonstrate in the human testis (Maeir 1965), the histochemical localization of the steroidogenic enzyme 3β-hydroxysteroid dehydrogenase predominantly in the Leydig cells of mammalian testes (Baillie et al. 1966) was of tantamount significance. The separation of seminiferous tubules from interstitial tissue of the rat testis (Christensen and Mason 1965) led to the discovery that interstitial tissue transformed radiolabelled substrate into androgens far more effectively than did tubular preparations.

The main precursor for testosterone biosynthesis in several species is fatty acids, although glucose may also be a substrate. The fatty acids enter the cell from the plasma and are degraded to acetyl CoA via B-oxidation by an enzyme system within the mitochrondria. Acetyl CoA, destined for sterol biosynthesis, leaves the mitochondria for the formation of 3-hydroxy-3-methyl glutaryl-CoA and subsequent reduction to mevalonic acid. The successive production of farnesyl pyrophosphate involves soluble enzymes whereas the steps of cholesterol biosynthesis beyond farnesyl pyrophosphate are catalyzed by enzymes that are tightly bound to the smooth endoplasmic reticulum. The abundance of smooth endoplasmic reticulum probably reflects the ability of a steroid-secreting cell to produce its own cholesterol, rather than taking it up from the plasma. In contrast to the adrenal gland, the testis displays limited ability to take up cholesterol from circulating blood (Parvinen et al. 1970), most of the cholesterol being formed in situ in this organ. After synthesis, cholesterol is promptly esterified and accumulated in lipid droplets which are common in the Leydig cells cytoplasm of humans and other species. The lipid droplets contain mainly cholesterol esters and neutral fats and stored cholesterol esters can be hydrolyzed by cytoplasmic esterase to provide free cholesterol for steroid biosynthesis.

The cholesterol destined for testosterone biosynthesis, whether from de-novo synthesis, ester hydrolysis or from the plasma, first enters the mitochondria for cleavage of its side chain. The side-chain cleavage system, involving 20- and 22-hydroxylases and a 20,22-lyase, is presumably located on the mitochondrial inner cristae. This has been demonstrated in adrenocortical cells but not in Leydig cells. The two hydroxylases each involve an electron transport chain and are cytochrome-P-450-dependent, are abundant in mitochondria of boar testis and present in trace amounts in those of the human.

Following side-chain cleavage of cholesterol, the resulting 5-pregnenolone must pass through the mitochondrial membrane into the cytoplasm to engage the enzymes necessary for its conversion to testosterone. These are tightly bound to the endoplasmic reticulum, mainly the smooth variety. Androstenedione and testosterone are the major secretory products of the male gonad in all species investigated. Three different pathways are known to exist: the progesterone or delta-4 pathway, the dehydroepiandrosterone or delta-5 pathway, and the sulfate pathway. To what extent species differences exist in the use or preference of these pathways is presently unclear. 5-Androstenediol is a secretory product of the human testis (Laatikainen et al. 1971) and both 5-androstenediol-3β-yl sulfate and testosterone-17β sulfate are secreted by the human testis (Laatikainen et al. 1969; Saez et al. 1967). Administration of human chorionic gonadotropin to male subjects is associated with increased secretion of 5-pregnenolone and 5-androstenediol 3β-yl sulfates in spermatic venous blood (Laatikainen et al. 1971). Gonadal formation of testosterone-17β-yl sulfate presumably requires the intermediate formation of the disulfate of 5-androstenediol, but the latter has not yet been isolated from testicular tissue. Nevertheless, the delta-5 and sulfate pathways appear to be the major routes to the formation of testosterone in the human testis, although low levels of delta-4 intermediates have also been detected (Lipsett 1971).

Little is known regarding transport of steroids within the different testicular substructures as well as from the testis to the general circulation. Several proposals (Christensen 1975) have been put forward involving simple diffusion of cytoplasmic testosterone to the cell surface aided by a specific intracellular carrier protein. Testosterone may also remain in the membranes of the smooth endoplasmic reticulum and be transferred to the cell surface by movements of the endoplasmic reticulum itself. Transport within the cavity of the smooth endoplasmic reticulum might be facilitated by a specific carrier protein synthesized possibly on the polysomes of the rough endoplasmic reticulum.

1.2. Regulation of testicular androgen biosynthesis

The biosynthesis of androgenic steroids by the mammalian testis depends upon the secretions of the anterior pituitary and interstitial cell-stimulating hormone (ICSH) is essential for normal function of the Leydig cells. Testicular steroidogenesis is regulated by a complex of adenohypophyseal hormones. FSH and prolactin (PRL) are important constituents of this complex and, in certain animal species, other pituitary hormones play some role in this testicular function.

1.2.1. Role of pituitary hormones.
ICSH stimulates testosterone production and secretion by the mammalian testis of every species studied to date (Figure 2). Furthermore, ICSH stimulates testosterone output in in-vitro systems including perfused testis, incubations of testicular slices, minces, homogenates and, more recently, suspensions of purified Leydig cells. The acute Leydig cell response to ICSH depends largely upon activation of the mitochondrial enzymes controlling cholesterol side-chain cleavage (Marsh 1976) but the chronic effects of the gonadotropin on testicular steroidogenesis would appear to involve the synthesis of new protein and increase in activity of several of the enzyme systems beyond 5-pregnenolone leading to testosterone (Bartke et al. 1978). ICSH also activates cholesterol esterase thus liberating free cholesterol from the intracellular stores of lipid droplets. It plays a part in the uptake of cholesterol by the mitochondria and the exit of newly-formed 5-pregnenolone into the cytoplasm.

The nucleotide 3′,5′-AMP promotes increased production and secretion of testicular steroids, and its steroidogenic action is as fast as that of ICSH (Eik-Nes 1967). Gonadotropin stimulates testicular adenyl cyclase; the major location of the latter is the plasma membrane, although the testicular nucleus and mitochondria also contain the enzyme.

In experimental animals, FSH seems to augment the action of ICSH on plasma testosterone levels and on growth of the androgen-dependent accessory sex glands. FSH can significantly increase testosterone secretion by the perfused rabbit testis which was already exposed to excessive amounts of ICSH. In such a situation, the action of FSH could not have been due to contamination with ICSH (Johnson and Ewing 1971). In efforts to elucidate the mechanism of FSH action on testicular steroidogenesis, attention turned to the study of the effects of FSH on testicular binding of ICSH. FSH appears to be capable of inducing ICSH receptors and thus modulating the steroidogenic response to ICSH. Yet FSH specifically binds to the Sertoli cells of the seminiferous tubules and its binding to Leydig cells has never been convincingly demonstrated. In man, there is only fragmentary evidence to suggest that the response to human chorionic gonadotropin (HCG) is greater when FSH levels are higher.

Prolactin (PRL) potentiates the action of ICSH on the restoration of spermatogenesis and PRL may augment the effect of endogenous or exogenous ICSH on testicular steroidogenesis (Bartke 1971). Other animal data tend to support this contention. Effects of PRL on testis function can involve direct actions on the isolated interstitium (Charreau et al. 1977). Testicular concentrations of esterified cholesterol increase after PRL treatment, possibly to maintain pools of precursor for steroidogenesis and, thus, explain the increased ability of the testis to respond to ICSH (Bartke et al. 1973). Prolactin can be important to the testis during sexual maturation in the rat (Bartke et al. 1978). Very high levels of PRL, however, inhibit testicular function and are associated with hypogonadism and impotence in men (Thorner et al. 1977). Growth hormone (GH) potentiates the action of gonadotropins on spermatogenesis; the effects of this pituitary hormone may be of particular importance during puberty (Swerdoff and Odell 1977). Administration of adrenocorticotrophin (ACTH) reportedly both stimulates and inhibits plasma testosterone and testicular steroidogenesis.

1.2.2. Role of estrogens.
The presence of estradiol receptors in the Leydig cells of the rat testis (Mulder et al. 1976) and the ability of large doses of synthetic and natural estrogens to exert direct effects on testicular steroidogenesis (Samuels et al. 1964; Bartke et al. 1977b) indicates that estrogens may play a significant role in controlling interstitial androgenesis. Furthermore, the inhibitory actions of estrogens on androgen biosynthesis in vivo and in vitro by human testis have been clearly established (Yanaihara and Troen 1972; Oshima et al. 1974). Human testicular capacity to metabolize proges-

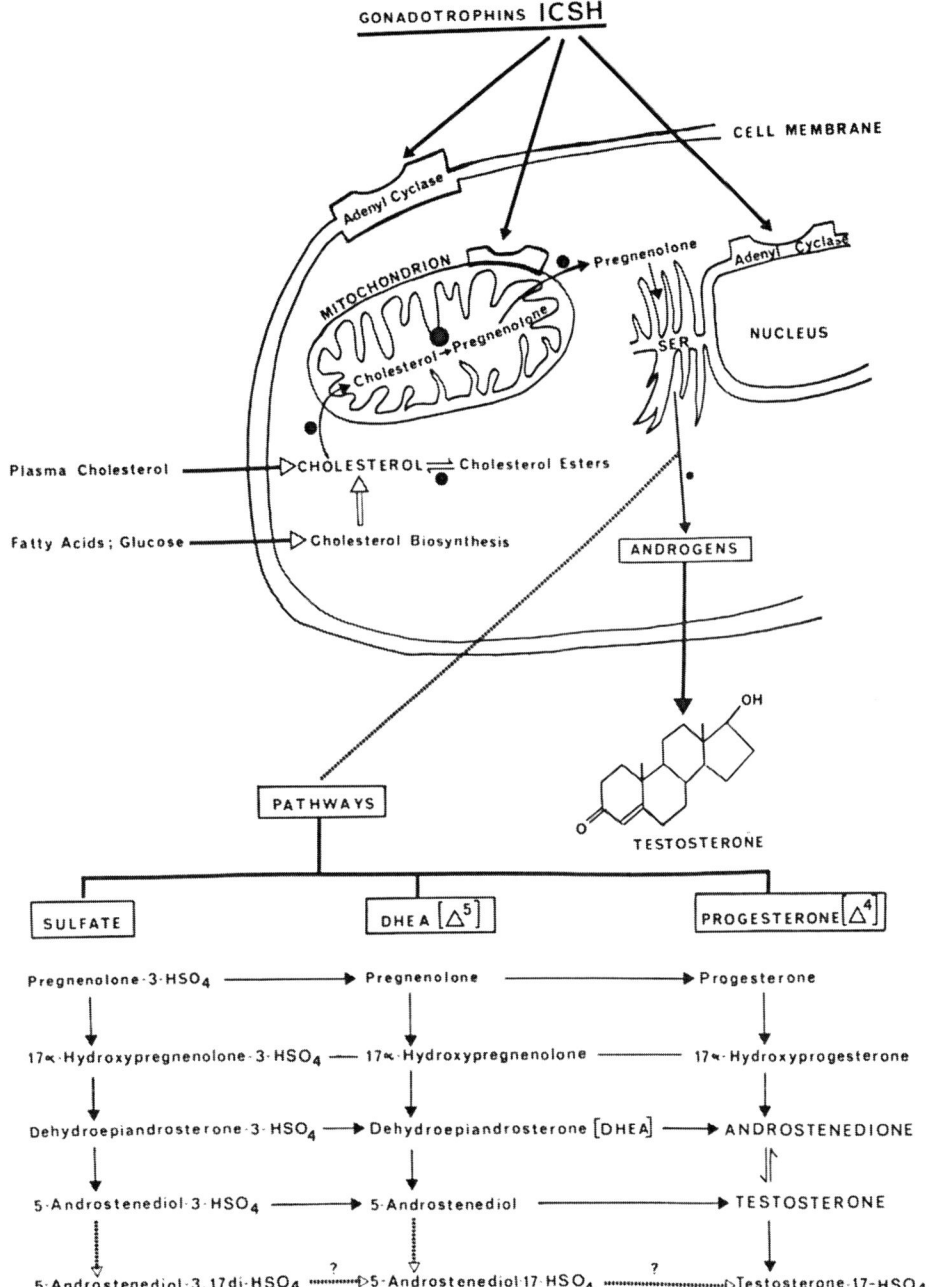

Figure 2. The role of ICSH in the regulation of Leydig cell androgenesis. The organelles involved are shown; the sites of gonadotropin influence are indicated by spots. Biosynthetic pathways between 5-pregnenolone and testosterone utilize enzyme systems located on the smooth endoplasmic reticulum (SER).

terone in vitro is severely curtailed after estrogen therapy (Rodriguez-Rigau et al. 1977) and is associated with a general depression of enzymatic activities related to androgen biosynthesis. Whether these long-term effects of high levels to estrogen were the result of hypothalamic-pituitary depression of gonadotropin output or a direct action on testicular androgenesis was not elucidated. If Sertoli cell estrogen (see below) is accessible to the Leydig cells, this may constitute an extension of the testicular two-cell concept whereby the Sertoli cells control their own ability to produce estrogens by directly influencing Leydig cell production of androgenic substrates for aromatization (Dorrington et al. 1978).

1.3. Ontogeny of the male gonads

The human fetal testis at an early age of development (fourteen weeks) possesses the essential enzymes for cholesterol formation and the subsequent synthesis of testosterone (Serra et al. 1970). Gonadotropins are present in the human fetus at ninety days and detectable quantities of FSH are to be found in the embryonic pituitary at seventy days (Kaplan et al. 1969).

Plasma levels of 4-androstenedione are higher than those of testosterone from birth to age eleven years in normal boys (Frasier et al. 1969). A dramatic change in the androstenedione-testosterone ratio of systemic blood accompanies puberty (Frasier and Horton 1966) and the late prepubertal testis responds to HCG administration with a marked increase in plasma testosterone (Saez and Bertrand 1968). Human testicular activity is optimal between 25 and 30 years when the testes produce around 7 mg testosterone per 24 hours. Decline in hormone production occurs in old age and is not a continuous process from adulthood to senescence: it begins at 55 to 60 years of age (Albeaux-Fernet et al. 1978). In ageing males, the 'andropause' does not exhibit a sudden onset and after age 50 years, males may be separated into two populations: one group showing elevated ICSH and FSH titres and the other with values of gonadotropins lower than those of younger men. The male andropause thus appears to involve primary testicular failure or failure secondary to pituitary gonadotropin declines. Plasma testosterone levels after 55 years of age are in the low range of normal and between 70 and 90 years the average level is significantly below normal. These changes do not always parallel the decrease in sexual activity which accompanies advancing age. Leydig cell response to HCG stimulation is impaired and there is change in the estrogen-androgen ratio; plasma estrogen is significantly elevated in the elderly male.

2. OCCURRENCE OF ESTROGENS IN THE MALE, AND THE TESTIS AS A SOURCE OF ESTROGEN

Estrogenic hormones were originally isolated from ovarian and placental tissues and were believed to occur only in the female. Although the occurrence of estrogens in male urine has been reported in several

species (Velle 1966), the precise origin and regulation of the secretion of these sex steroids is still somewhat unclear.

Estrogenic activity in testicular tissue was first shown in 1921 by Fellner, who described the effects of bovine testis extracts on uterus and mammary tissues of the rabbit. The histological effects were quite comparable with those obtained after injections of ovarian or placental extracts. Crude alcoholic preparations of horse testis displayed estrogenic potency which was due to the presence of estradiol and estrone (Beall 1940). Significant amounts of estrogen activity were subsequently demonstrated in testis extracts of the human (Goldzieher and Roberts 1952), hog (Haines et al. 1948) and fetal lambs (Attal 1969). Such findings dispelled the old concept that estrogens were confined to the female.

By measuring differences in concentration between peripheral and testicular venous plasma, the testes of several mammalia have been shown to secrete estradiol-17β in vivo. Numerous studies have revealed the presence of plasma estradiol gradients within the human, monkey, dog and rat testis (Table 1) and that testicular secretion may contribute 15-25% of the total estrogen bioproduction (Kelch et al. 1972; Scholler et al. 1973; De Jong et al. 1973).

2.1. Pathways of testicular estrogen biosynthesis

The main routes of testicular biosynthesis of steroids resemble those of other steroidogenic tissues such as the ovary, placenta and adrenal cortex, particularly with reference to the formation of common intermediates such as cholesterol and 5-pregnenolone. The conversion of pregnenolone to androstenedione and testosterone involves the enzymes 3β-hydroxysteroid dehydrogenase, 17α-hydroxylase and $C_{17,20}$-lyase via the delta-4 and delta-5 pathways. These tissues are capable of synthesizing estrogens from two-carbon precursors by way of testosterone and other C_{19}-steroid intermediates. Appreciable amounts of radiolabelled estradiol are present in homogenates from human, dog and cat testes after incubation with labelled precursors (Armstrong and Dorrington 1977). The transformation of exogenous androgens into estrogens takes place readily in placental and ovarian tissues; the pathways and enzymatic mechanisms therein have been extensively investigated (Engel 1973). Androstenedione and testosterone are respectively converted to estrone

Table 1. Estradiol-17β concentration in testicular and peripheral venous plasma (values are the mean ± standard deviation; figures in parentheses are the numbers of animals or individuals involved).

Species	Reference	Estradiol concentration (pg/ml)	
		peripheral	testicular
Rat	De Jong et al. (1973)	2.0±0.9 (12)	17.5±8.4 (43)
Dog	Kelch et al. (1972)	8.0±2.1 (9)	100±13.8 (4)
Monkey	Kelch et al. (1972)	17±10 (4)	50±20 (4)
Man	Kelch et al. (1972)	20±4 (8)	1049±161 (8)
	Baird et al. (1973)	32±15 (9)	2081±825 (9)
	Leonard et al. (1971)	32±21 (5)	948±200 (5)
	Longcope et al. (1972)	32±18 (8)	342±275 (8)
	Scholler et al. (1973)	50±28 (9)	1880±1240 (9)

and estradiol in a series of reactions collectively referred to as 'aromatization'. Hydroxylation and scission of the angular methyl group at carbon-10, and dehydrogenation of ring-A leads to the benzenoid structure characteristic of the estrogen molecule. Since 19-hydroxyandrostenedione and 19-hydroxytestosterone are effective precursors for estrogen formation, aromatization is thought to occur via the 19-oxo intermediates as shown in Figure 3. The several enzymes involved are collectively termed the 'aromatase complex' or 'aromatase'. The aromatase is associated with the microsomal fraction of tissue homogenates and involves a 'b-type' cytochrome-P-450 system (Wilson 1975).

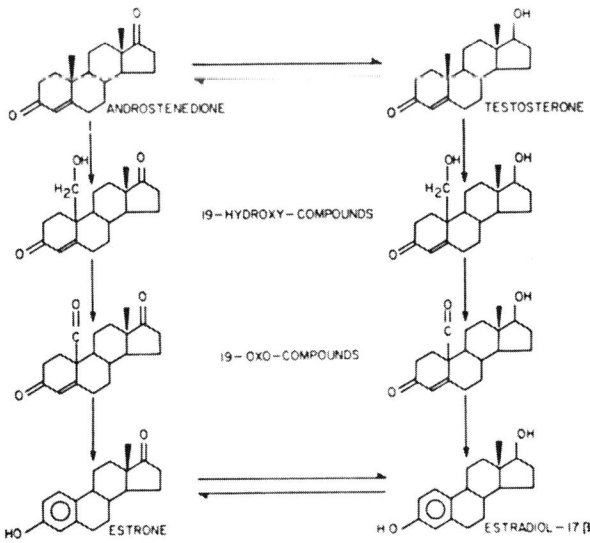

Figure 3. Biochemical intermediates in the conversion of androgens to estrogens by Sertoli cells. Nineteen-oxo-androstenedione and nineteen-oxo-testosterone are postulated intermediates, neither having been isolated from testicular preparation nor converted to estrone and estradiol in vitro.

The aromatase complex appears to be regulated by stimulatory and inhibitory influences which are not fully understood. Both testosterone and androstenedione, in addition to being secreted directly or aromatized to estrogens, may undergo metabolic inactivation involving saturation of the A ring by delta-4-steroid-5α-reductase in the testis. Since the latter is an irreversible process and ring-A saturated steroids cannot undergo aromatization, testicular metabolism by this means might constitute a regulatory mechanism in testicular estrogenesis by diverting androstenedione and testosterone away from the aromatase system. Furthermore, progesterone and its metabolites are effective inhibitors of $C_{17,20}$-lyase and consequently may suppress estrogen formation by limiting the rate of formation of aromatizable substrates. While aromatization by placental microsomes is competitively inhibited by 5α-reduced androgens such as dihydrotestosterone (DHT) and 5α-androstenedione, the aromatase substrate 19-nortestosterone also competitively inhibits both aromatization and the cytochrome-P-450 binding of androstenedione (Thompson and Siiteri 1973; Armstrong and Dorrington 1977). Whether or not such regulatory mechanisms for estrogen biosynthesis are present in the mammalian testis remains to be demonstrated. Follicle-stimulating hormone (FSH) is known to increase estrogen production by isolated Sertoli cells in the presence of an aromatizable substrate (Dorrington and Armstrong 1975). These findings suggest a regulatory role of steroids (including aromatase substrate) and gonadotropin in in-vitro estrogenesis. The precise mechanics of the aromatase complex and the physiological significance of these regulatory mechanisms in testicular estrogen production remain to be fully clarified.

2.2. Testicular cell types involved in estrogen biosynthesis

Both Sertoli and Leydig Cells have been implicated as sites of testicular estrogen biosynthesis. Prolonged administration of human chorionic gonadotropin to normal and hypogonadal men increases urinary estrogen secretion. Although Leydig cells appear to be stimulated, the seminiferous tubules regress after the hormonal treatment (Maddock and Nelson 1952). HCG treatment also results in parallel elevations in androgen and estrogen as well as an increase in interstitial cell numbers, further suggesting that interstitial cells may be involved in the synthesis of both classes of steroids (Leach et al. 1956). Leydig cell tumours are capable of synthesizing significant amounts of labelled estradiol-17β and estriol from radioactive steroid precursors (Pierrepoint et al 1966). However, the histogenesis of certain testicular interstitial androblastomas which were previously used extensively to demonstrate estrogen secretion by interstitial cells might have been of tubular origin. Thus, the conclusion that Leydig cells *per se* are the testicular source of estrogen needs to be considered with caution.

Feminization of male dogs and men with Sertoli cell tumours indicates that this cell type may be involved in estrogen biosynthesis (see Armstrong and Dorrington 1977). Furthermore, Sertoli cell tumours not only contain substantial amounts of biologically active estrogenic material but are also capable of synthesizing labelled estrogen from radioactive acetate or androstenedione in vitro. While HCG elicits a greater increase in testicular venous concentration of testosterone than estradiol-17β in intact adult rats, a marked reduction of the estradiol-17β testosterone ratio is observed after five days of gonadotropin treatment (De Jong et al. 1973). Estradiol-17β concentration is 9-15 times greater in interstitial tissue than in seminiferous tubules. During a three-hour incubation of testicular preparations, estradiol-17β concentration is significantly increased in the total testis and seminiferous tubules, but not in the interstitial tissue. In contrast, only the concentration of testosterone in the interstitial tissue and the total testis is increased during the incubation (De Jong et al. 1974). Thus it appears that (1) the two steroids are synthesized in different compartments of the testis; (2) interstitial cells produce testosterone; and (3) estrogen is synthesized in the seminiferous tubules.

Sertoli cells from testes of immature rats (18-20 days old) maintained in primary cultures for 48 h possess the capacity to synthesize low but detectable levels of estradiol-17β from testosterone; the amount of estradiol-17β synthesized is dramatically increased in the presence of both FSH and the androgen (Armstrong and Dorrington 1977). This response is specific to FSH since high concentrations of LH cause only a marginal stimulation. Under the influence of FSH, the Sertoli cells also synthesize significant amounts of estrone from testosterone but the quantity produced is only about 10% that of estradiol. The fact that cyclic AMP, its synthetic analogues as well as cholora toxin (an activator of adenylate cyclase), mimic the effect of FSH on estrogen synthesis by cultured Sertoli cells strongly suggests that cyclic AMP is involved in this steroidogenic process. Although cyclic AMP production by these cells in response to FSH stimulation is extremely rapid (within minutes), there appears to be a four-hour lag period in the estradiol response. Moreover, synthesis of new protein is necessary for the expression of its effect on estrogen synthesis by Sertoli cells (Dorrington et al. 1978).

The conclusion that the Sertoli cell is a target cell for FSH action is based on several lines of evidence (Means 1975; Steinberger 1975; Hansson et al. 1975; Fritz et al. 1975) including the demonstration that FSH binds specifically to Sertoli cells, induces morphological changes, increases cyclic AMP production, activates protein kinases and stimulates a variety of end responses. These responses include the production of plasminogen activator, androgen-binding protein and the incorporation of ^{3}H-thymidine into DNA in Sertoli cells.

Apart from testosterone, various intermediates involved in estrogen biosynthesis (Figure 4), such as androstenedione, 19-hydroxyandrostenedione and 19-hydroxytestosterone are good substrates for the testicular aromatase. Estradiol synthesis by cultured Sertoli cells is markedly stimulated by FSH or dibutyryl AMP in the presence of each of these C19 steroids. FSH thus regulates the conversion of androgens to estrogens by way of cyclic AMP, involving enzymatic conversion of 19-hydroxylated androgens to estrogens (Dorrington et al. 1978).

2.3. The two-cell hypothesis for testicular estrogen biosynthesis

Sertoli cells from immature rats do not synthesize significant amounts of estradiol in response to FSH when incubated in the absence of exogenous androgenic substrate, or in the presence of pregnenolone or progesterone (Dorrington et al. 1978). The inability of Sertoli cells to utilize pregnenolone or progesterone as substrate for aromatization suggests that the androgen used for estrogen synthesis in vivo may be produced elsewhere in the testis. Isolated seminiferous tubules are unable to synthesize testosterone from endogenous precursors or from exogenous 7α-^{3}H-cholesterol whereas interstitial tissue produces androgens under the same conditions (Cooke et al. 1972). While Sertoli cells have only a limited capacity to metabolize ^{14}C-pregnenolone to ^{14}C-testosterone, they do not synthesize significant quantities of androgen in vitro even in the presence of gonadotropins. Cell suspen-

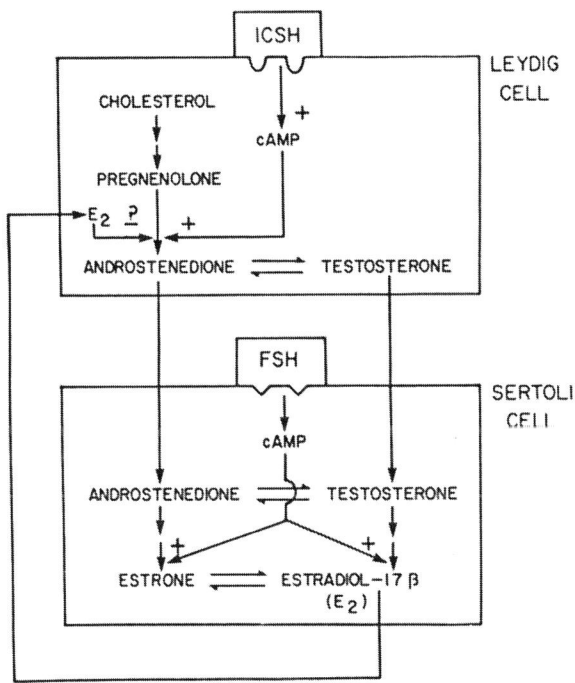

Figure 4. Hypothetic model for the cellular and biochemical sites of action of ICSH and FSH in the regulation of testicular estrogen biosynthesis (+: stimulation; −: inhibition).

sions rich in interstitial cells, however, synthesize testosterone and this is stimulated by LH (Moyle and Ramachandran 1973; Catt et al. 1974). Moreover, the endogenous production of pregnenolone and testosterone by mitochondria from interstitial tissue accounts for 92-97% of that synthesized by mitochondria from the whole testis (Van der Vusse et al. 1973). Since LH, but not FSH, increases the

cyclic AMP concentration of isolated interstitial cells of the testes, and only FSH stimulates the production of this nucleotide by either seminiferous tubules or Sertoli cells (Means 1975), cyclic AMP would seem to mediate the effects of LH and FSH on the production of testosterone and estradiol in the Leydig cells and Sertoli cells respectively.

The testosterone concentration in the testicular lymph which bathes the seminiferous tubules is almost as high as that in the testicular venous blood (Setchell 1970) and there does not appear to be a barrier against entry of testosterone and other steroids into the tubules (Parvinen et al. 1970). The high levels of testosterone present in isolated seminiferous tubules and the rete testis fluid seem then to be derived from the Leydig cells (Setchell 1970; Podesta and Rivarola 1974). These observations not only suggest that both Leydig cells and Sertoli cells participate in the biosynthesis of estrogens, but also that FSH is intimately involved in this process at a site that is quite distinct from that at which LH stimulated Leydig cell steroidogenesis. As shown in Figure 4, it is conceivable that testosterone and androstenedione formed by the Leydig cells under the influence of LH are transported through the lymph to the Sertoli cells, where they are converted to estradiol and estrone in the presence of FSH.

2.4. Age-related changes

Some limited human experimental data exists to suggest that estrogen secretion is age-dependent. Yet high estrogen levels are associated with decreased reproductive capacity. While the testes of very young boys and old men secrete more estradiol, estrone is secreted in larger amounts by the testes of pubescent boys as compared with other age groups. Estradiol levels are thus high in nonfertile men (i.e. young and old) and spermatogenesis is associated with high levels of estrone (Axelrod 1965). The possible physiological role of estrone in male reproduction remains to be determined.

Estrogen synthesis by the developing testis has been examined more extensively in laboratory animals. Sertoli cells isolated from five-days-old rats synthesize greatest amounts of estradiol-17β in vitro in the presence of exogenous testosterone and FSH, when compared with those from rats of other age groups. The aromatizing capacity of these cells decreases with age and by thirty days only very low levels of estradiol are produced. Likewise, production of estrone in response to FSH also decreases with increasing age (Dorrington et al. 1978). Testicular estradiol production in vivo, however, remains relatively constant during the first 21 days of postnatal life, after which time there is a decline with age.

A clear understanding of the control of testicular estrogen biosynthesis during sexual maturation is often complicated by the dynamic nature of the gonads, particularly with regard to the synthesis and availability of aromatizable precursors. In the rat, testicular testosterone concentration (Resko et al. 1968) and testosterone-synthesizing capacity (Payne et al. 1977) appear to be at their maximum in the early postnatal period and decline to low levels by 21 days of age. Thereafter, they increase again with the onset of puberty but progressively drop to low values in thirty and forty-day-old animals. During the twentieth to fortieth days of postnatal life, radioactive progesterone is converted by rat testes to radioactive androsterone, rather than to labelled testosterone (Ficher and Steinberger 1968). Moreover, testicular tissue (Ficher 1970) and isolated Sertoli cells (Dorrington and Fritz 1975) from twenty day-old rats convert testosterone and androstenedione to non-aromatizable androgens such as 5α-dihydrotestosterone, androstenediols and androsterone. FSH stimulates the activity of both 5α-reductase and 3α-hydroxysteroid dehydrogenase in Sertoli cells of immature (ten-day-old) rats (Welsh and Wiebe 1978). Steroid 5α-reduction, and thus the decline in availability of aromatizable substrates for estrogen biosynthesis, may be important for the rat testis during the period of transition from immature to mature function. In addition to the marked decline in the aromatizing capacity of Sertoli cells (Armstrong and Dorrington 1977), low testicular estrogen production in vivo by 35-day-old animals may, at least in part, be attributed to the low levels of aromatizable substrates.

Another complication arises fom the fact that both circulating FSH levels and the number of testicular FSH receptor sites also change dramatically with age. Circulating FSH concentrations in the rat remain low and relatively unchanged until 21 days of age. Thereafter the levels of gonadotropin increase dramatically to about threefold in the 35-day-old animals, and decline to normal adult values shortly after puberty (Payne et al. 1977). The total number of FSH receptor sites per Sertoli cell increases with age and is coincident with the increase in the circulating FSH titre (Steinberger et al. 1977; Payne et al. 1977). Sertoli cells also respond to FSH in cyclic AMP production in vitro in an age-related manner; greatest accumulation of cyclic AMP is evident in cells from eighteen-day-old animals. Despite increased FSH binding sites and availability of FSH to Sertoli cells, these FSH-induced cyclic AMP levels decrease rapidly between eighteen and thirty-six days of age (Steinberger et al. 1977). Sertoli cells from thirty-day-old rats are incapable of responding to FSH and dibutyryl cyclic AMP, in terms of estrogen synthesis in vitro (Armstrong and Dorrington 1977). The apparent decrease in the responsiveness of Sertoli cells to FSH in cyclic AMP production with increased age may only partially explain the decrease in the aromatizing capacity of the older Sertoli cells.

2.5. Physiological significance of Sertoli cell estrogens

It is generally agreed that the mammalian testis secretes 15-25% of the circulating estradiol, but several tissues including the brain, adrenals, adipose tissue, and liver are known to be peripheral sites of estrogen production (Baird et al. 1969; Bolt and Gobel 1972; Naftolin et al. 1971; Wu et al. 1970). It is thus conceivable that estrogen of testicular origin plays a quantitatively less important role in possible peripheral processes than the estrogens formed by extragonadal sources. What then is the physiological significance of testicular estrogen in the male?

Firstly, estradiol produced by the Sertoli cells may exert a local effect to modulate androgen production by the Leydig cells. Estradiol benzoate inhibits LH-stimulated testosterone production in vitro by isolated Leydig cells from immature rats (Van Beurden et al. 1977), and markedly reduces plasma and testicular concentrations of testosterone, but not LH levels, in adult rats (Chowdhury et al. 1974). Estrogen treatment also decreases the responsiveness of the adult testis to exogenous ICSH in vivo, presumably by interfering with the binding of ICSH to Leydig cell receptors (Moger 1976). The uptake of radiolabelled estradiol by interstitial cell nuclei (Stumpf 1969) and the presence of both cytoplasmic and nuclear receptors specific for estradiol in rat testicular interstitium (Brinkmann et al. 1972; Mulder et al. 1973) indicate that these are indeed estrogen target cells. Inhibition of Leydig androgen production and hence limitation of precursors for Sertoli cell aromatization may thus constitute an intra-testicular feedback mechanism of self-regulation (Figure 4).

Secondly, testicular androgens are necessary for normal spermatogenesis. Estrogens inhibit testicular androgenesis in vitro and in vivo (Bartke et al. 1977b; De Jong et al. 1975), and thus Sertoli cell estrogens may be indirectly involved in the local regulation of spermatogenesis. Sertoli cells from five-day-old rat testes possess a greater capacity to synthesize estrogen in vitro than cells from older animals; testicular production of estradiol in vivo is greatest in rats during early postnatal life. The level of specific estradiol receptors in the cytosol of interstitial tissue is also at a maximum during this postnatal period and declines thereafter as the rat approaches puberty (De Boer et al. 1976). The ontogenic decline in interstitial estradiol receptor protein thus parallels exactly the decrease in estradiol synthesis by developing Sertoli cells. It is also apparent that estradiol synthesis by Sertoli cells is maximal before the first wave of spermatogenesis is initiated and may presumably be important during prepubertal development.

3. CONCLUDING REMARKS

Whilst a comprehensive understanding of the endocrine functions of the testis is presently available, there are several gaps in our knowledge which merit continued attention. Regulation of testicular activity during intrauterine life and the ability of the fetal pituitary to produce gonadotropins during key phases of male organogenesis need further clarification. The precise importance of placental gonadotropins for testicular steroidogenesis in the human embryo is also far from being adequately appreciated.

Puberty may be much more than just a shift in androgen production in favour of testosterone and the roles of gonadotropin stimulation between pre-pubertal and postpubertal stages of development still need to be settled. Finally, the life-span of the human species is continuously increasing and there is an obvious need for more information on the changes in testicular activity and function with age in all mammalia. Information on the alterations with age in activities of essential testicular steroidogenic enzymes would be of great practical importance.

Nevertheless, tremendous advances have taken place in the last fifteen years. Perhaps most notable is the area of Sertoli cell functions and the ability of these rather unusual cells to biomanufacture steroid hormones. It may be some time, however, before the physiological roles of these estrogenic principles in spermatogenic events and the overall physiology of the hypothalamic-pituitary-testicular axis is fully appreciated.

ACKNOWLEDGEMENTS

Financial support was generously provided by the Dean's Fund, School of Medicine, University of Ottawa. The authors wish to acknowledge the assistance of Elizabeth McNally, Garry A. Kinson and David G. Gillan. NRCC No. 17259.

REFERENCES

Albeaux-Fernet M, Bohler CC, Karpas AE: Testicular function in the aging male. In: Geriatric endocrinology, Greenblatt RB (ed), New York, Raven, 1978, vol 5, 201.

Armstrong DT, Dorrington JH: Estrogen biosynthesis in the ovaries and testis. In: Regulatory mechanisms affecting gonadal hormone action, Thomas JA, Singhal RL (eds), Baltimore, University Park Press, 1977, 217.

Attal J: Levels of testosterone, androstenedione, estrone and estradiol-17β in the testes of fetal sheep. Endocrinol 85: 280, 1969.

Axelrod LR: Metabolic patterns of steroid biosynthesis in young and aged human testes. Biochim Biophys Acta 97: 551, 1965.

Baillie AH, Ferguson MM, Hart DM: Histological evidence of steroid metabolism in the human genital ridge. J. Clin Endocr Metab 26: 742, 1966.

Baird DT, Ano A, Melby JC: Adrenal secretion of androgens and oestrogens. J Endocr 45: 135, 1969.

Baird DT, Galbraith A, Fraser IS, Newsam JE: The concentration of oestrone and oestradiol 17β in spermatic venous blood in man. J. Endocr 57: 285, 1973.

Bartke, A: Effects of prolactin on spermatogenesis in hypophysectomized mice. J Endocr 49: 311, 1971.

Bartke, A, Hafiez AA, Bex FJ, Dalterio S: Hormonal interactions in regulation of androgen secretion. Biol Reprod 18: 44, 1978.

Bartke A, Musto N, Caldwell BV, Behrman HR: Effects of a cholesterol esterase inhibitor and of prostaglandin $F_{2\alpha}$ on testis cholesterol and on plasma testosterone in mice. Prostaglandins 3: 97, 1973.

Bartke A, Smith MS, Michael SD, Peron FG, Dalterio S: Effects of experimentally-induced chronic hyperlactinemia on testosterone and gonadotropin levels in male rats and mice. Endocrinol 100: 182, 1977a.

Bartke A, Williams II Kl, Dalterio S: Effects of estrogens on testicular testosterone production in vitro. Biol Reprod 17: 645, 1977b.

Beall D: The isolation of alpha-oestradiol and oestrone from horse testes. Biochem J 34: 1293, 1940.

Bolt HM, Gobel P: Formation of estrogens from androgens by human subcutaneous adipose tissue in vitro. Horm Metab Res 4: 321, 1972.

Brinkmann AO, Mulder E, Lamers-Stahlhofen GJM, Mechielson NJ, Van der Molen HJ: Binding of oestradiol by the nuclear fraction of rat testis interstitial tissue. FEBS Letters 26: 301, 1972.

Catt KJ, Tsuruhara T, Mendelson C, Ketelslegers JM, Dufau MI: Gonadotropin binding and activation of the interstitial cells of the testis. In: Hormone binding and target cell activation in the testis, Dufau ML, Means AR (eds), New York, Plenum, 1974, p 1.

Charreau EH, Attramadal A, Torjesen PA, Purvis K, Calandra R, Hansson V: Prolactin binding in rat testis: specific receptors in interstitial cells. Mol Cell Endocr 6: 303, 1977.

Chowdhury M, Tcholakian R, Steinberger E: An unexpected effect of oestradiol-17β on luteinizing hormone and testosterone. J Endocr 60: 375, 1974.

Christensen AK: Leydig cells. In: Handbook of physiology, sec 7; Endocrinology; vol 5: Male reproductive system, Greep RO, Astwood EB (eds), Baltimore, Williams and Wilkins, 1975, p. 59.

Christensen AK, Mason NR: Comparative ability of seminiferous tubules and interstitial tissue of rat testes to synthesize androgens from progestrone-4-^{14}C in vitro. Endocrinol 76: 646, 1965.

Cooke BA, De Jong FH, Van der Molen HJ, Rommerts FFG: Endogenous testosterone concentrations in rat testis interstitial tissue and seminiferous tubules during in vitro incubations. Nature 237: 255, 1972.

Davis JR, Langford GA, Kirby PJ: The testicular capsule. In: The testis, Johnson AD, Gomes WR, Vandemark NL (eds), New York, Academic Press, 1970, vol 1, p 282.

De Boer W, Mulder E, Van der Molen HJ: Effects of oestradiol-17β, hypophysectomy and age on cytoplasmic oestradiol-17β receptor sites in rat testis interstitial tissue. J Endocr 70: 397, 1976.

De Jong FH, Hey AH, Van der Molen HJ: Effect of gonadotropins on the secretion of oestradiol-17β and testosterone by the rat testis. J Endocr 57: 277, 1973.

De Jong FH, Hey AH, Van der Molen HJ: Oestradiol-17β and testosterone in rat testis tissue: effect of gonadotropins, localization and production in vitro. J Endocr 60: 409, 1974.

De Jong FH, Vilenbrock JHJ, Van der Molen HJ: Oestradiol-17β-treated intact adult male rat. J Endocr 65: 281, 1975.

Dorrington JH, Armstrong DT: Follicle-stimulating hormone stimulate estradiol-17β synthesis in cultured Sertoli cells. Proc Nat Acad Sci USA 72: 2677, 1975.

Dorrington JH, Fritz IB: Androgen synthesis and metabolism by preparations from the seminiferous tubule of the rat testis. In: Hormonal regulation of spermatogenesis, French FS, Hansson V, Ritzén EM, Nayfeh SN (eds), New York, Plenum, 1975, p 37.

Dorrington JH, Fritz IB, Armstrong DT: Control of testicular estrogen synthesis. Biol Reprod 18: 55, 1978.

Eik-Nes KB: Factors controlling the secretion of testicular steroids in the dog. J Reprod Fertil, suppl 2: 125, 1967.

Engel LL: The biosynthesis of estrogens, In: Handbook of physiology sec 7: Endocrinology; vol 2: Reproductive system: female, Greep RO, Astwood EB (eds), Baltimore, Williams and Wilkins, 1973, p 467.

Fawcett DW: Ultrastructure and function of the Sertoli cell. In: Handbook of physiology, sec 7: Endocrinology; vol 5: Male

reproductive system, Greep RO, Astwood EB (eds), Baltimore, Williams and Wilkins, 1975, p 21.

Feliner OO: Über die Wirkung des Placentar- und Hodenlipoids auf die männlichen und weiblichen Sexualorgane. Pflügers Arch 189: 199, 1921.

Ficher M: Metabolism of androstenedione and testosterone in testicular tissue of developing rats. Proc Ann Meeting Soc Study Reprod 4, 1970.

Ficher M, Steinberger E: Conversion of progesterone to androsterone by testicular tissue at different stages of maturation. Steroids 12: 491, 1968.

Frasier SD, Horton R: Androgens in the peripheral plasma of prepubertal children and adults. Steroids 8: 777, 1966.

Frasier SD, Gafford F, Horton R: Plasma androgens in childhood and adolescence. J Clin Endrocr Metab 29: 1404, 1969.

Fritz IB, Louis BG, Tung PS, Griswold M, Rommerts FG, Dorrington JH: Biochemical responses of cultured Sertoli cell-enriched preparations to follicle-stimulating hormone and dibutyryl cyclic AMP. In: Hormonal regulation of spermatogenesis, French FS, Hansson V, Ritzen EMM, Nayfeh SN (eds), New York, Plenum, 1975, p 367.

Goldzieher JW, Roberts IS: Identification of estrogen in the human testis. J Clin Endocr Metab 12: 143, 1952.

Haines WJ, Johnson RH, Goodwin MP, Kuizenga MH: Biochemical studies on hog testicular extract. J Biol Chem 174: 925, 1948.

Hansson V, Ritzén EM, French FS, Nayfeh SN: Androgen transport and receptor mechanisms in testis and epididymis. In: Handbook of physiology, sec 7: Endocrinology; vol 5: Male reproductive system, Greep RO, Astwood EB (eds), Baltimore, Williams and Wilkins, 1975, p 173.

Hooker CW, Pfeiffer CA: The morphology and development of testicular tumors in mice of the A strain receiving estrogens. Cancer Res 2: 759, 1942.

Johnson BH, Ewing LL: Follicle-stimulating hormone and the regulation of testosterone secretion in rabbit testes. Science 173: 635, 1971.

Kaplan SL, Grumbauch MM, Shepard TH: Gonadotropins in serum and pituitary of human fetuses and infants: abstract. Pediat Res 3: 512, 1969.

Kelch RP, Jenner MR, Weinstein R, Kaplan SL, Grumbach MM: Estradiol and testosterone secretion by human, simian and canine testes, in males with hypogonadism and in male pseudohermaphrodites with the feminizing testes syndrome. J Clin Invest 51: 824, 1972.

Laatikainen TE, Laitinen A, Vihko R: Secretion of neutral steroid sulfates by the human testis. J Clin Endocr Metab 29: 219, 1969.

Laatikainen T, Laitinen EA, Vihko R: Secretion of free and sulfate-conjugated neutral steroids by the human testis: effect of administration of human chorionic gonadotropin. J Clin Endocr Metab 32: 59, 1971.

Leonard JM, Flocks RH, Korenman SG: Estradiol (E$_2$) secretion by the human testis. Prog Endocr Soc 53 (113) 1971.

Lipsett MB: Steroid secretion by the gonads in man. In: Hormonal steroids, James VHT, Martini L (eds), Amsterdam, Excerpta Medica, 1971.

Longcope C, Widrich W, Sawin CT: The secretion of estrone and estradiol-17β by human testis. Steroids 20: 439, 1972.

Maddock WO, Nelson WO: The effects of chorionic gonadotropin in adult men. J Clin Endocr Metab 12: 985, 1952.

Maeir DM: Species variation in testicular ^{5}-3β-hydroxysteroid dehydrogenase activity: absence of activity in primate Leydig cells. Endocrinol 76: 463, 1965.

Marsh JM: The role of cyclic AMP in gonadal steroidogenesis. Biol Reprod 14: 30, 1976.

Means AR: Biochemical effects of follicle-stimulating hormone on the testis. In: Handbook of physiology, sec 7: Endocrinology; vol 5: Male reproductive system. Greep RO, Astwood EB (eds), Baltimore, Williams and Wilkins, 1975, p 203.

Moger WH: Serum testosterone response to acute LH treatment in estradiol treated rats. Biol Reprod 14: 115, 1976.

Moyle WR, Ramachandran J: Effects of LH on steroidogenesis and cyclic AMP accumulation in rat Leydig cell preparations and mouse tumor Leydig cells. Endocrinol 93: 127, 1973.

Mulder E, Peters MJ, Van Beurden WMO, Galdieri M, Rommerts FFG, Janszen FHA, Van der Molen HJ: Androgen receptors in isolated cell preparations obtained from rat testicular tissue. J Endocr 70: 331, 1976.

Naftolin FK, Ryan KJ, Petro Z: Aromatization of androstenedione by the diencephalon. J Clin Endocr Metab 33: 368, 1971.

Oshima H, Sarada T, Ochiai K, Tamaoki B: Effects of a synthetic estrogen upon steroid bioconversion in vitro in testes of patients with prostatic cancer. Invest Urol 12: 43, 1974.

Parvinen M, Hurme P, Niemi M: Penetration of exogenous testosterone, pregnenolone, progesterone and cholesterol into the seminiferous tubules of the rat. Endocrinol 87: 1082, 1970.

Payne AH, Kelch RP, Murono EP, Kerlan JT: Hypothalamic, pituitary and testicular function during sexual maturation of the male rat. J Endocr 72: 17, 1977.

Pierrepoint CG, Griffiths K, Grant JK, Stewart JSS: Neural steroid sulphation and vestrogen biosynthesis in vitro by a feminizing Leydig cell tumor of the testis. J Endocr 35: 409, 1966.

Podesta EJ, Rivarola MA: Concentration of androgens in whole testis, seminiferous tubules and interstitial tissue of rats at different stages of development. Endocrinol 95: 455, 1974.

Resko JA, Feder HH, Goy RW: Androgen concentrations in plasma and testis of developing rats. J Endocr 40: 485, 1968.

Rodriguez-Rigau L, Tcholakian RK, Smith KD, Steinberger E: Effect of in vitro estrogen administration on in vitro steroid bioconversion in human testes. In: The testis in normal and infertile men, Troen P, Nankin HB (eds), New York, Raven, 1977, p 457.

Saez JM, Bertrand J: Studies on testicular function in children: plasma concentrations of testosterone, dehydroepiandrosterone and its sulfate before and after stimulation with human chorionic gonadotropin. Steroids 12: 749, 1968.

Samuels LT, Short JG, Huseby RA: The effect of diethylstilbestrol on testicular 17α-hydroxylase and 17-desmolase activities in BALB/c mice. Acta Endocr 45: 487, 1964.

Scholler R, Grenier J, Castanier M, DiMaria G, Niaudet C, Millet D, Netter A: Concentrations de l'estradiol-17β, de l'estrone, et de la testosterone dans la veine spermatique de l'homme. CR Acad Sci Paris 276: 1329, 1973.

Serra GB, Perez-Palacios G, Jaffe RB: De novo testosterone biosynthesis in the human fetal testis. J. Clin Endocr Metab 30: 128, 1970.

Setchell B: Testicular blood supply, lymphatic drainage and secretion of fluid. In: The testis, Johnson AD, Gomes WR,

Vandemark NL (eds), New York, Academic Press, 1970, vol 1, p 101.

Steinberger A, Steinberger E: Replication pattern of Sertoli cells in maturing rat testis in vivo and in organ culture. Biol Reprod 4: 84, 1977.

Steinberger A, Heindel JJ, Walter J: Changes in Sertoli cell responses to FSH during sexual maturation. Proc NICHD Testis Workshop 4, 1977.

Steinberger E: Hormonal regulation of the seminiferous tubule function. In: Hormonal regulation of spermatogenesis, French, F.S., Hansson V, Ritzén EM, Nayfeh SN (eds), New York, Plenum, 1975, p 337.

Steinberger E, Steinberger A: Spermatogenic function of the testis. In: Handbook of physiology, sec 7: Endocrinology; vol 5: Male reproductive system, Greep RO, Astwood EB (eds), Baltimore, Williams and Wilkins, 1975, p 1.

Stumpf WE: Nuclear concentration of ^{3}H-estradiol in target tissues: dry mount autoradiography of vagina, oviduct, ovary, testis, mammary tumor, liver and adrenal. Endocrinol 85: 31, 1969.

Swerdloff RS, Odell WD: Modulating influences of FSH, GH, and prolactin on LH-stimulated testosterone secretion. In: The testis in normal and infertile men, Troen P, Nankin HR (eds), New York, Raven, 1977, p. 395.

Thompson EA, Siiteri PK: Studies on the aromatization of C-19 androgens. Ann NY Acad Sci 212: 378, 1973.

Thorner MO, Edwards CRW, Hanker JP, Abraham G, Besser GM: Prolactin and gonadotropin interaction in the male. In: The testis in normal and infertile men, Troen P, Nankin HR, (eds), New York, Raven, 1977, p 351.

Van Beurden WMO, Roodnat B, De Jong FH, Mulder E, Van der Molen HJ: Hormonal regulation of LH stimulation of testosterone production in isolated Leydig cells of immature rats. Proc NICHD Testis Workshop 4, 1977.

Van der Vusse GJ, Kalkman ML, Van der Molen HJ: Endogenous production of steroids by subcellular fractions from total rat testes and from isolated interstitial tissue and seminiferous tubules. Biochim Biophys Acta 297: 179, 1973.

Velle W: Urinary oestrogens in the male. J Reprod Fertil 12: 65, 1966.

Welsh MJ, Wiebe JP: Sertoli cell capacity to metabolize C_{19} steroids: variation with age and the effect of follicle-stimulating hormone. Endocrinol 103: 838, 1978.

Wilson JD: Metabolism of testicular androgens. In: Handbook of physiology, sect 7: Endocrinology; vol 5: Male reproductive system, Greep RO, Astwood EB (eds), Baltimore, Williams and Wilkins, 1975, p 491.

Wu CH, Flickinger CL, Archer DF, Touchstone JF: Estrogen formation in vitro by foetal liver, fetal adrenal gland and placenta of early human pregnancy. Am J Obstet Gynecol 107: 313, 1970.

Yanaihara T, Troen P: Studies of the human testis I: biosynthetic pathways for androgen formation in human testicular tissue in vitro. J Clin Endocr Metab 34: 783, 1972.

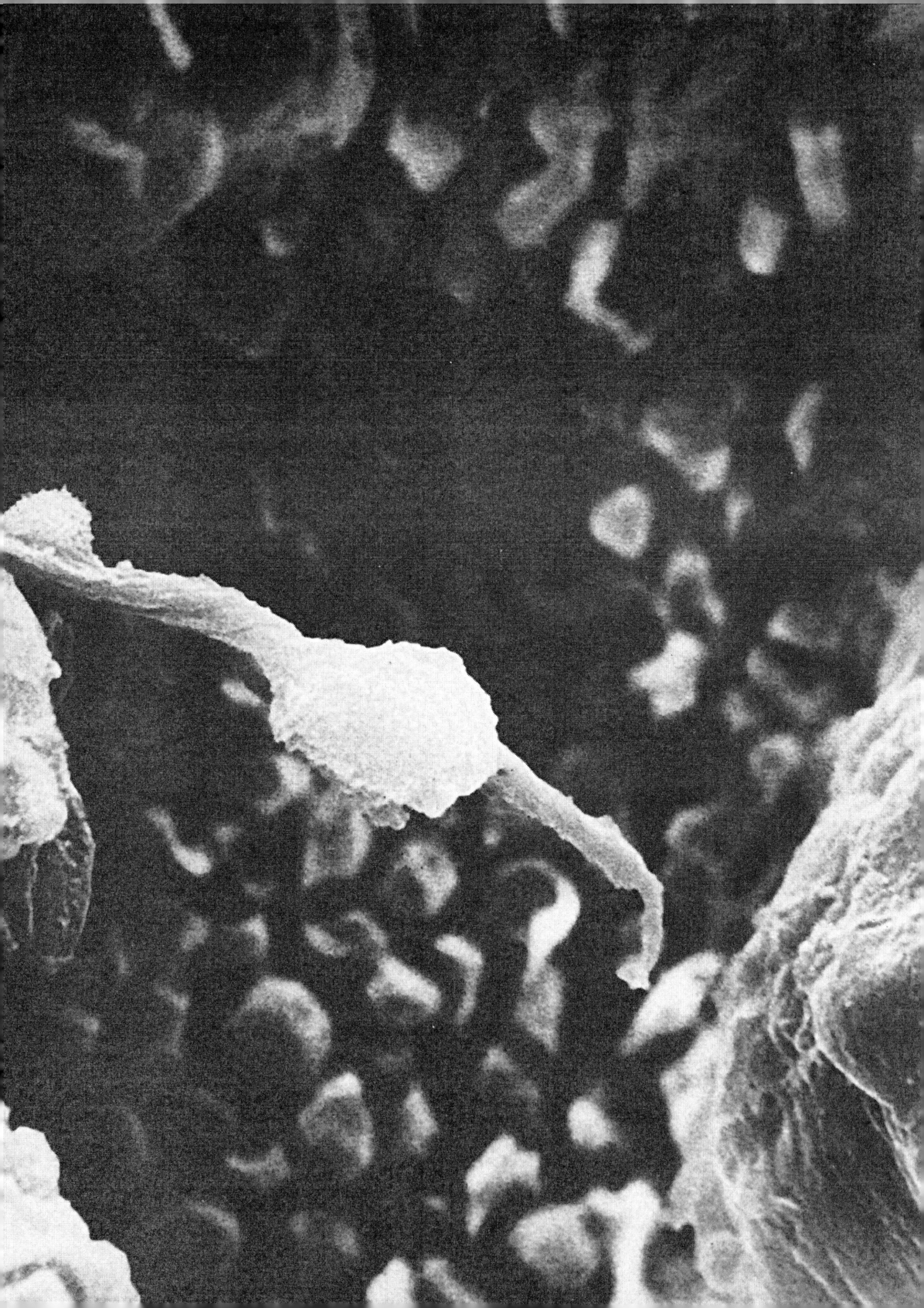

II. CRYPTORCHID TESTIS

10. NORMAL AND ABNORMAL TESTICULAR DESCENT IN SOME MAMMALS

C.J.G. WENSING, B. COLENBRANDER and H.W.M. VAN STRAATEN

The process of testicular descent has provided a classic problem of developmental anatomy since the time of John Hunter. It also possesses considerable clinical importance since anomalies of testicular position are frequently encountered in man and in several domestic species. In spite of the great attention the subject has received since Hunter's description of 1762 even recent accounts are still contradictory: the mechanisms involved are not completely understood. Several theories have been put forward to explain the changes in morphology involved in the movement of the testis from its site of origin in the genital ridge to its final resting place in the scrotum. Especially opinions on the role of the gubernaculum testis in the process differ. The results of recent research on the morphology of the process of testicular descent will be summarized. The information is confined to species with a strip-like cremaster muscle (e.g. pigs, dogs, cats, cattle, horses) since the process in species with a sac-shaped cremaster muscle (e.g. rodents), although in principle comparable, is morphologically different. A description of normal as well as of abnormal morphology of testicular descent will be followed by some notes on the regulation of this process.

1. NORMAL TESTICULAR DESCENT

The gubernaculum plays a crucial role in the migration of the testis (Wensing 1968; Wensing 1973a). It is a mesenchymal structure which, before the migration of the testis actually starts, runs from the caudal part of the testis towards the inguinal canal and ends in a knoblike expansion between the differentiating internal and external oblique abdominal muscles. Within the abdomen it is covered with peritoneum. The peritoneum invades the extra-abdominal part of the gubernaculum in a more or

less semicircular fashion at the level of the future internal inguinal ring. This evagination, which can be considered as the beginning of the vaginal process, divides the gubernaculum into three parts (Figure 1):

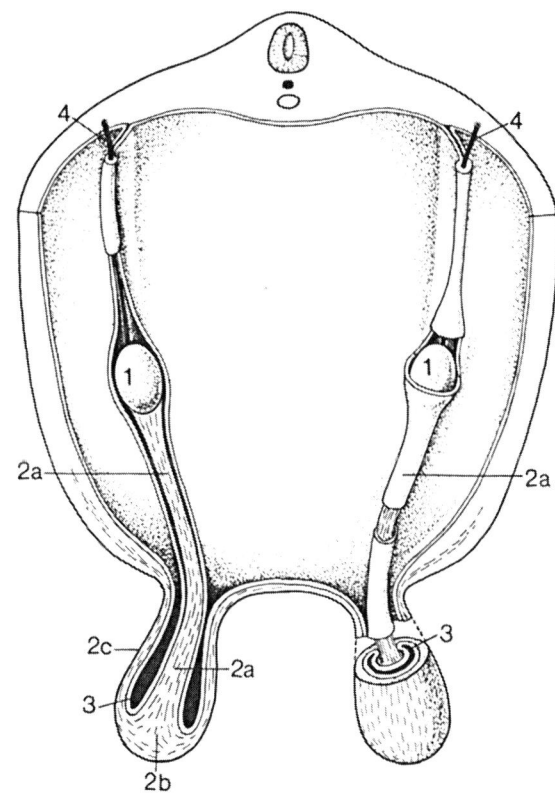

Figure 1. Schematic drawing of the testis and its gubernaculum. On the left side the gubernaculum is sectioned longitudinally: 1: testis; 2: gubernaculum; 2a: proper gubernaculum; 2b: infra-vaginal part of gubernaculum; 2c: vaginal part of the gubernaculum; 3: cavity of vaginal process; 4: testicular artery.

(a) proper gubernaculum: the intra-abdominal part and the extra-abdominal part suspended by the visceral peritoneal layer of the vaginal process;

(b) vaginal part of the gubernaculum: the extra-abdominal part surrounding the parietal layer of the vaginal process externally;

(c) infravaginal part of the gubernaculum: the caudal end of the gubernaculum which has not been invaded by the vaginal process.

In the early stages of testicular descent there is no organized connection between the caudal tip of the gubernaculum and the area of the future scrotum. The extra-abdominal part is easily recognizable as a separate entity within loose surrounding mesenchyme. The scrotal fascia, formed by the continuation of the external abdominal fascia and the aponeurosis of the external oblique abdominal muscle, extends and is connected with the bottom of the future scrotum (Figure 2a). The extra-abdominal part of the gubernaculum is contained within this scrotal fascia. A similar arrangement exists in female embryos of the same age but here the gubernaculum either develops only slightly (in the dog, for instance) or does not develop (in the pig) any further.

The changes in gubernacular morphology which are of utmost importance in the process of testicular descent can be divided into an outgrowth phase and a regression phase; we will deal with these phases consecutively.

1.1. Gubernacular outgrowth

The first and most marked change that takes place in gubernacular development is an outgrowth of its extra-abdominal part, which increases greatly in length as well as in volume. Due to this increase it is carried beyond the external inguinal ring into the region of the scrotum (Figure 3).

Concomitantly with the outgrowth reaction of the extra-abdominal part, the intra-abdominal part becomes shorter and during this process the testis approaches the internal ring. The alteration in the ratio of intra-abdominal and extra-abdominal parts of the gubernaculum is substantial during the outgrowth of this structure. The outgrowth of the extra-abdominal gubernaculum is mainly confined to that part covered by the visceral layer of the processus vaginalis, i.e. the extra-abdominal part of the proper gubernaculum and the infravaginal part (Figure 1). This outgrowth is caused partly by active cell division and partly by the increase of extracellular substance (Wensing 1973a). Major components of this extracellular substance are mucopolysaccha-

rides. The vaginal process closely follows the outgrowth of the extra-abdominal part of the gubernaculum and the fundus of the cavity is never more than a few millimetres distant from the caudal gubernacular tip. In consequence the vaginal process is an elongated cleft whose visceral and parietal walls are in close apposition at the time of passage of the testis through the inguinal canal (Figure 2b). As a result of the outgrowth of the extra-abdominal part of the gubernaculum four important events can be observed.

1. Migration of the testis from a position lateroventral to the metanephros to or at least in the direction of the internal inguinal ring takes place (Figure 3). It appears that the intra-abdominal part of the gubernaculum gradually becomes incorporated into the extra-abdominal part of the proper gubernaculum. Comparison can be made with a balloon that is placed with its neck within a restricted passage (inguinal canal) and then inflated. Inflation results in expansion of the free part of the balloon and as a consequence the originally constricted portion becomes gradually incorporated in the distended part. Occasionally the migration of the testis during the outgrowth phase has been explained by the degeneration of the mesonephros, the increase in size of the testis and other differences in relative growth (Wyndham 1943; Backhouse and Butler 1960). There is no reason to believe this to be true, since in several species (dog, cat) this migration occurs after the degeneration of the mesonephros while the increase in size of the testis is too insubstantial to explain a migration of 5-10 mm (Wensing 1968).

2. The shaping of the vaginal process takes place before the moment when the testis escapes from the abdomen, almost to the extent it has immediately after completion of the descent process.

3. The shaping of the cremaster muscle to an elongated strip-like shape inserting into the parietal wall of the vaginal process occurs. This is in fact an elongation of the caudal fibers of the internal oblique abdominal muscle (Figure 2a, b).

4. There is a dilation of the inguinal canal brought about by the outgrowth of the intra-inguinal part of the proper gubernaculum; this allows final passage of the testis (Figure 2b). The testis is able to move easily up and down the inguinal canal. When this stage is reached a simple increase in intra-abdominal

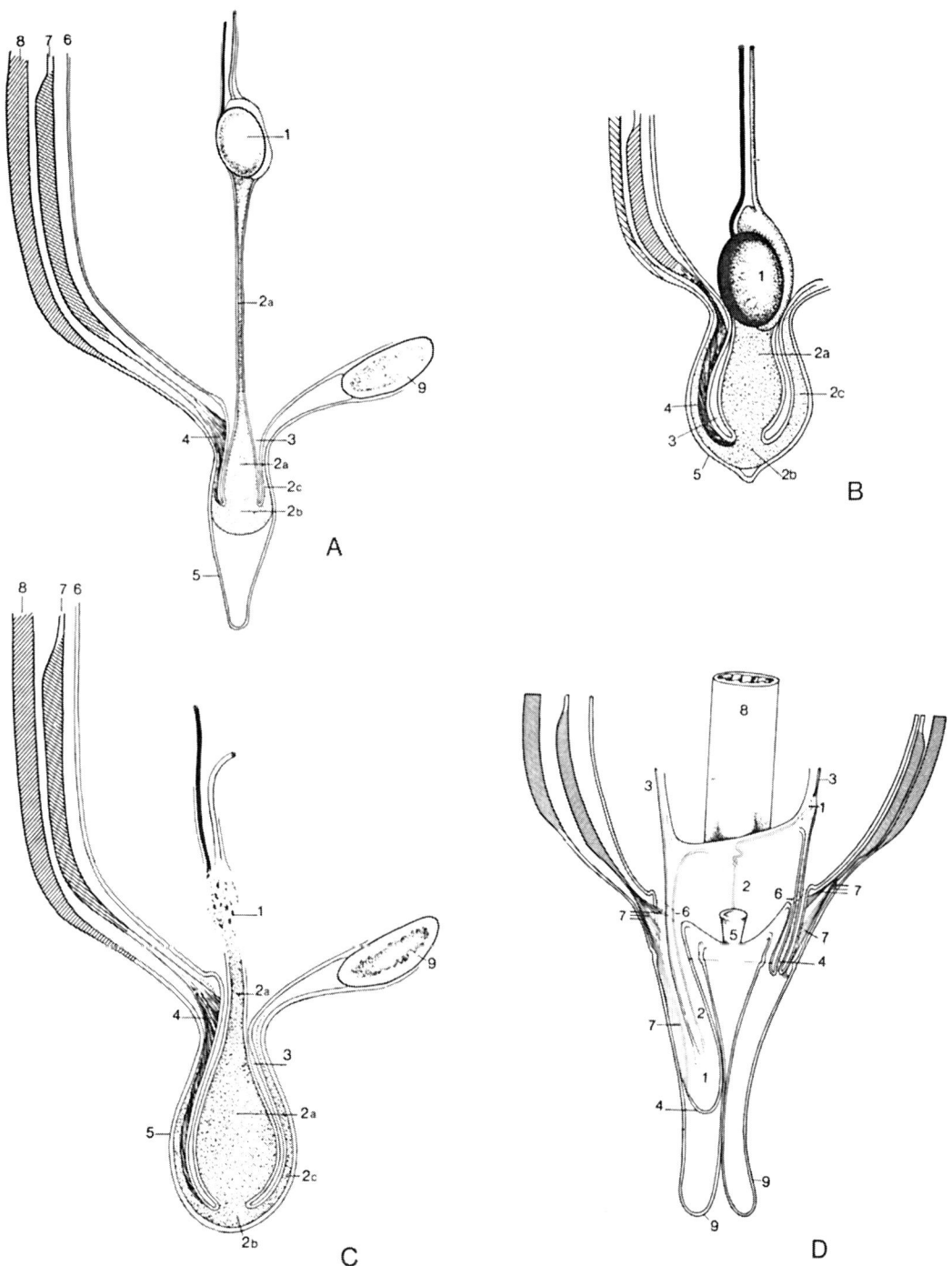

Figure 2. A: Testis, gubernaculum and scrotal fascia in the beginning of the outgrowth phase. 1: testis and epididymis; 2: gubernaculum; 2a: proper gubernaculum; 2b: infravaginal part; 2c: vaginal part; 3: cavity of vaginal process; 4: cremaster muscle; 5: scrotal fascia; 6: peritoneum; 7: internal oblique abdominal muscle; 8: external oblique abdominal muscle; 9: pelvic skeleton. B: Testis and gubernaculum at the end of the gubernacular outgrowth phase. 1: testis and epididymis; 2: gubernaculum; 2a: proper gubernaculum; 2b: infravaginal part; 2c: vaginal part; 3: cavity of vaginal process; 4: cremaster muscle; 5: scrotal fascia. C: Gubernacular outgrowth in a porcine freemartin. 1: ovarian remnants; 2: gubernaculum; 2a: proper gubernaculum; 2b: infra- vaginal part; 2c: vaginal part; 3: cavity of vaginal process; 4: cremaster muscle; 5: scrotal fascia; 6: peritoneum; 7: internal oblique abdominal muscle; 8: external oblique abdominal muscle; 9: pelvic skeleton. D: Anatomy of the inguinal area in an adult freemartin pig. The vaginal process on the left side contained abdominal viscera. The right vaginal process is underdeveloped. 1: connective tissue accumulation at the side of the gonad; 2: remnants of genital ducts; 3: gonad artery; 4: vaginal process; 5: bladder neck; 6: internal inguinal opening; 7: cremaster muscle; 8: rectum' 9: 'scrotal fascia'.

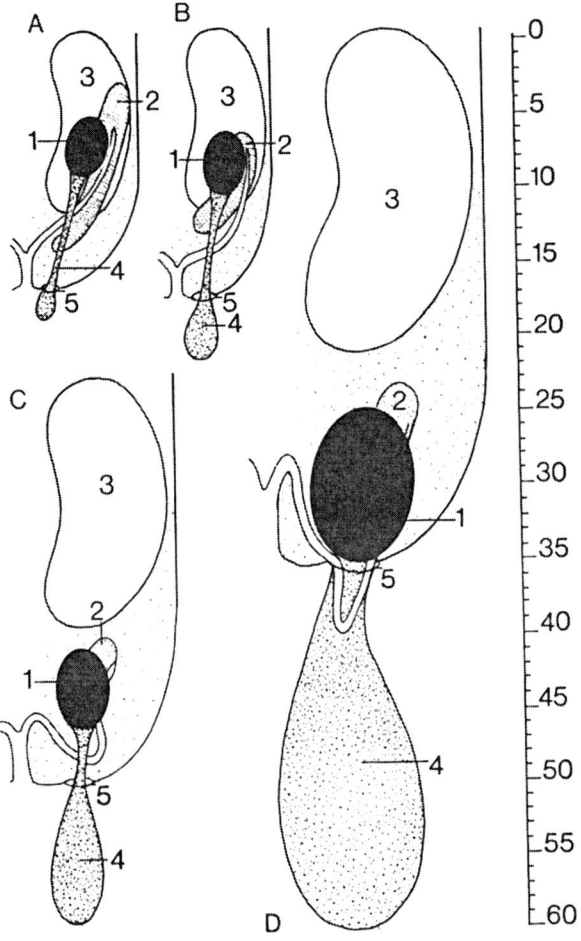

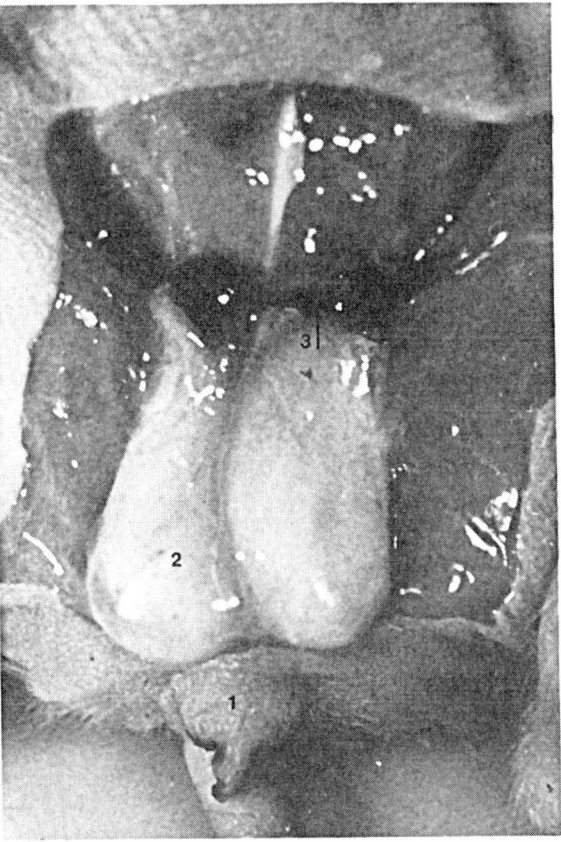

Figure 4. Dissection of the inguinal area in freemartin piglet two days postnatal. The extra-abdominal parts of the gubernaculum, hardly recognizable in normal females, show an excessive outgrowth reaction and extend to the vulva. 1: vulva; 2: gubernaculum; 3: external inguinal ring.

Figure 3. Four schematic drawings to scale of the changes in testis and gubernaculum morphology. The outgrowth phase of the gubernaculum and the change in relation between intra- and extra-abdominal parts is illustrated. 1: testis; 2: mesonephros; 3: metanephros; 4: gubernaculum; 5: internal inguinal opening (A: 45 days; B: 52 days; C: 63 days; D: 75 days).

pressure is enough to transport the testis through the canal.

All these events can take place even in the absence of the testis and epididymis in this morphological complex. Nature provides an elucidating example to illustrate this. In pigs occasionally the circulatory systems of a male and a female fetus are interconnected. In such females, called porcine freemartins, a complete regression of the ovary usually takes place. The gubernaculum, however, grows out in a male-like fashion and as a consequence the end ramification of the ovarian artery with gonadal remnants is moved to the internal inguinal opening (Figure 2c, Figure 4). A deep vaginal

process and a cremaster muscle are formed; the inguinal canal becomes dilated. The migration of the gonadal remnants and as a consequence the elongation of the ovarian artery appear to be due only to the extra-abdominal gubernacular outgrowth reaction since this and the disappearance of the ovary are the only two morphological structures that are at variance with normal development of all structures connected with gonadal descent (Colenbrander and Wensing 1975).

1.2. Gubernacular regression

The second important change that takes place in gubernacular morphology is the regression of mainly the proper gubernaculum and its infravaginal part (Figure 5). Regression starts, depending on the species, when the testis has reached the internal inguinal opening or shortly before it has

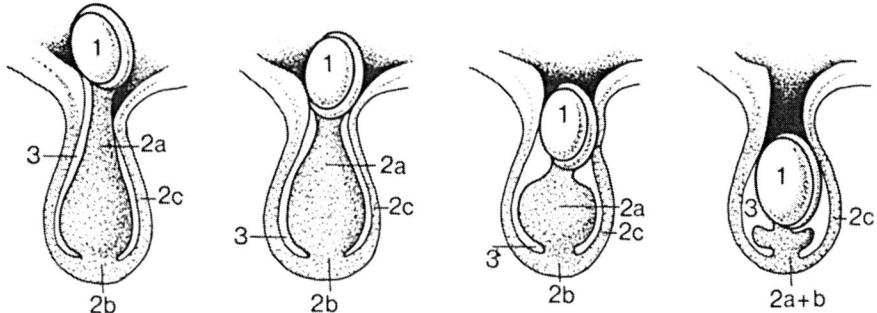

Figure 5. Four successive stages of gubernacular regression. The proper gubernaculum and the infravaginal part are converted into the proper testicular ligament and the caudal epididymal ligament. 1: testis and epididymis; 2: gubernaculum; 2a: proper gubernaculum; 2b: infravaginal part; 2c: vaginal part; 3: cavity of vaginal process.

attained this position (Backhouse and Butler 1960; Wensing 1968). The first signs of onset of this regression phase are the cessation of mitotic activity and the decline of the water-binding capacity of gubernacular tissue due to a decrease of the mucopolysaccharide concentration (Wensing 1973a). In the pig these signs can be noticed around 85 days post coitum. The regression process is at first gradual but later on the gubernaculum undergoes a rapid and radical transformation, between 100 days post coitum and two weeks after birth, with the loss of mucopolysaccharides and concurrent increase in collagen content. The proper gubernaculum and the infravaginal part are converted into the proper ligament of the testis and the caudal epididymal ligament (Figure 5).

At the start of the regression phase the testis is located on top of a large conus of mucoid connective tissue in a low intra-abdominal or in a high inguinal position. As the conus of mucoid tissue, in a manner of speaking, melts away, the testis descends gradually to the bottom of the vaginal process. In the porcine freemartin the regression phase of the gubernaculum takes place in a comparable fashion, usually causing further descent of the gonadal remnants and extra elongation of the ovarian artery (Figure 2d). A full development of the vaginal process, the cremaster muscle, and complete descent of the gonadal remnants take place when the inguinal canal is dilated to an extent allowing an indirect inguinal hernia to develop (Colenbrander and Wensing 1975). The mere filling of the vaginal process now seems to be all that is needed for full development of the vaginal process and the cremaster muscle. In cases where the inguinal canal

remains narrow the development of the vaginal process after gubernacular regression lags behind and becomes insubstantial (Figure 2d).

In summary gubernacular outgrowth and regression are responsible for the migration of the testis to the internal inguinal opening and later on to the scrotal area and for the final shaping of the vaginal process and the cremaster muscle.

2. ABNORMAL TESTICULAR DESCENT

According to the theory that gubernacular outgrowth and subsequent regression is essential for normal testicular descent there are three ways in which abnormality of the gubernaculum could affect testicular descent, through:

- absolute or relative failure of the outgrowth,
- excessive outgrowth,
- aberrant outgrowth causing the gubernaculum to extend into an unusual position.

Large numbers ($\pm$ 3000) of pig fetuses and neonates and a limited number of dog fetuses and neonates ($\pm$ 100) were screened in order to investigate abnormalities of testicular descent. A considerable number of pig fetuses with substantial abnormality of testicular descent were collected and examined. In the dog material only a few abnormalities were found, and since they fit well into the pattern found in the pig, the following description is mainly based on pig material (Wensing 1973c).

A complete absence of the gubernacular outgrowth reaction has not been reported but substantial bilateral underdevelopment was seen in a few cases. In these animals both testes were located intra-abdominally whilst in normal fetuses of comparable age the testes have already descended beyond the external inguinal opening. It is hard to conjecture what would have been the fate of these testes had the piglets been allowed to survive but it is quite possible that they would have descended in normal fashion but at a more leisurely rate. Unilateral underdevelopment was seen quite regularly. The testis connected with the underdeveloped gubernaculum always lags behind the contralateral one (Figure 6). Follow-up studies of a group of animals in which the extra-abdominal part of the gubernaculum was smaller at birth made it clear that either delayed descent or low abdominal cryptorchidism will be the final outcome (Wensing and Colenbrander 1973). An inguinal position of the testis is also possible but this abnormality has only been encountered in a few animals.

Abnormalities caused by excessive outgrowth of the extra-abdominal part of the gubernaculum were

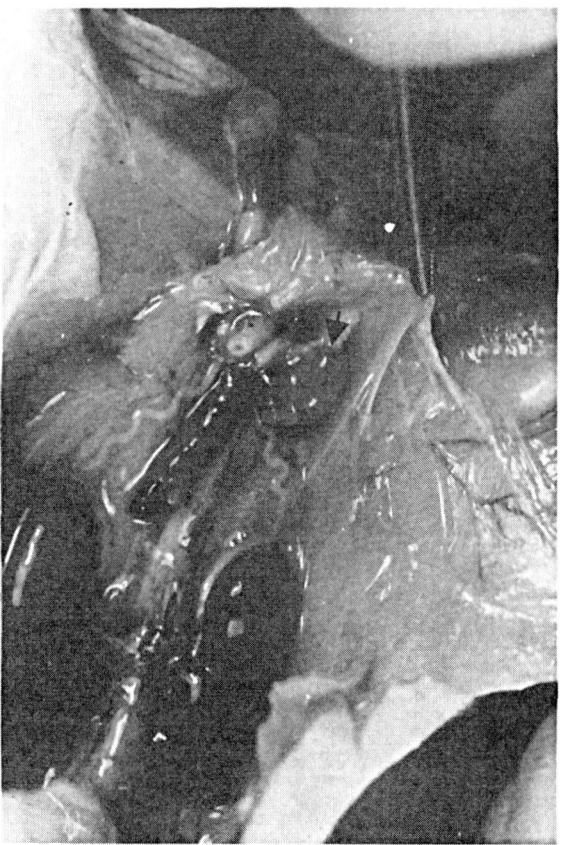

Figure 6. Pig fetus, 100 days: underdevelopment of the right gubernaculum. The abdominal cavity is opened. The right testis (arrow) is still located intra-abdominally.

regularly found, mostly unilaterally. By excessive growth the gubernaculum exceeds the normal size for that age by a substantial margin. The gubernaculum develops in the normal direction, that is, within the fascial pouch. Since the outgrowth reaction continues over a longer period and the regression of the gubernaculum did not appear to commence until several days after birth, although in normal piglets it precedes this event by several days, passage of the testis through the inguinal canal is delayed if it takes place at all. The initial large size of the gubernaculum results in a vaginal process with an unusually wide neck which predisposes to inguinal hernia. In a follow-up study it became evident that in several of these animals an inguinal hernia did in fact develop after the testis had descended through the inguinal canal.

Abnormal location of the gubernaculum takes three forms (Figure 7) which will be considered seriatim.

1. The extra-abdominal part of the gubernaculum does not expand beyond the inguinal canal. After swelling within the confined space it later thrusts back into the abdominal cavity. As a consequence the site of invagination of the vaginal process is lifted away from the internal inguinal ring and carried cranially (Figure 7a; Figure 8). The traction normally developed by the swelling reaction is now absent and thus the testis fails to leave its original position caudal to the kidney. The external cremaster muscle is insufficiently developed and remains within the canal, or may even extend intra-abdominally. This 'reversed swelling reaction' has been observed regularly in pigs and occasionally in dogs, mostly unilaterally. After the regression of the gubernaculum a permanent high-abdominal cryptorchidism will be the outcome. The topography of the cremaster muscle is indicative in these cases.

2. The outgrowth reaction takes place mainly but sometimes even entirely in the inguinal canal (Figure 7b). The outgrowth reaction in these animals is quite often excessive and continues for a longer period. If it is partly intra-abdominally but mainly intra-inguinally only slight displacement of the testis in the direction of the internal inguinal opening results. Further descent is impossible as long as the outgrowth reaction continues. In later stages of the fetal period the location of the testes in these animals is intermediate between the original position and the

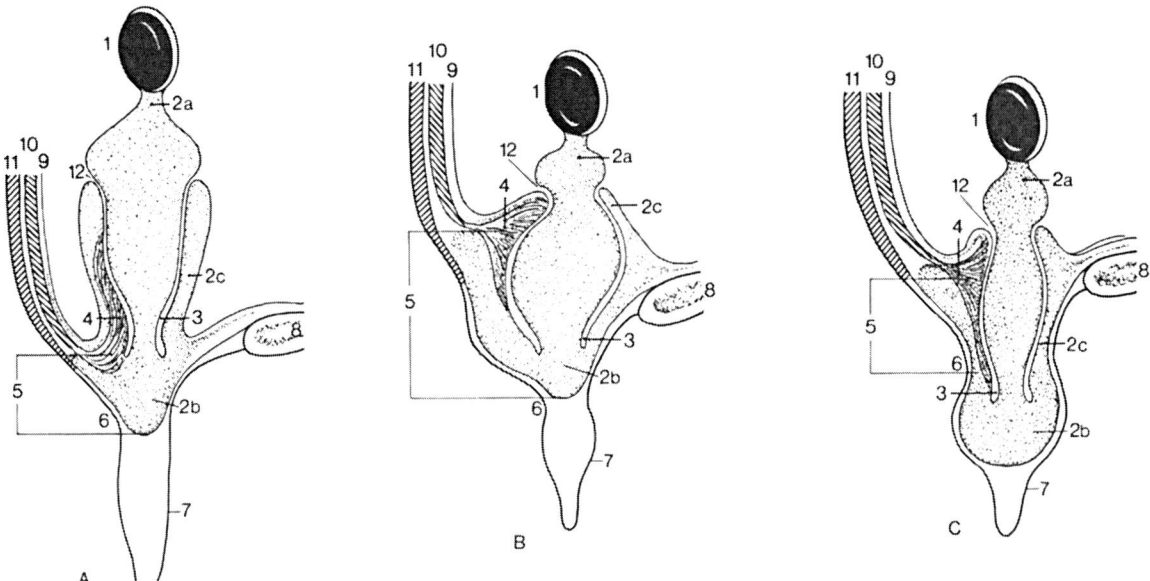

Figure 7. Some forms of abnormal gubernacular outgrowth. A: 'Reversed swelling reaction': the entrance (12) to the vaginal cavity is lifted away from the internal ring and the cremaster muscle (4) extends intra-abdominally. B: Outgrowth reaction mainly within the inguinal canal. The anatomical relations in this area (5) are gravely disturbed. C: Outgrowth reaction partly within the inguinal canal. The anatomical relations in the canal (5) are disturbed but there is also extension of the gubernaculum within the scrotal fascia. 1: testis and epididymis; 2: gubernaculum; 2a: proper gubernaculum; 2b: infravaginal part; 2c: vaginal part; 3: cavity of vaginal process; 4: cremaster muscle; 5: inguinal canal; 6: external inguinal ring; 7: scrotal fascia; 8: pelvic skeleton; 9: peritoneum; 10: internal oblique abdominal muscle; 11: external oblique abdominal muscle; 12: entrance to the vaginal cavity.

internal inguinal opening. In these cases the cremaster muscle is not or is insufficiently pulled out and remains within the inguinal canal (Figure 7b). If the reaction is more extra-abdominal, descent can progress further and the testis may even reach the internal inguinal opening. The entrance to the vaginal process stays at the internal inguinal opening. The cremaster muscle may develop slightly beyond the external inguinal opening (Figure 7c). The regression of the gubernaculum in these animals is usually delayed and commences shortly before or after birth; it allows some further descent of the testis. In a number of these animals the descent might become complete eventually, but it is also possible that the testis remains in a low abdominal or even an inguinal position. The initial large size of the gubernaculum in the inguinal area results after regression in a vaginal process with an unusually wide entrance which predisposes to inguinal hernia. In a large percentage an inguinal hernia in fact develops when or after the testis has descended through the canal. In these animals cryptorchidism, delayed descent and inguinal hernia appear to have their initial origin in gubernacular anomaly (Wensing 1973c; Wensing and Colenbrander 1973).

3. It is also possible that besides the main outgrowth within the inguinal canal the gubernaculum may extend between the aponeurosis of the external and the fleshy part of the internal oblique abdominal muscle and fail to pass through the external inguinal ring. The intra-abdominal part of testicular descent appears to have proceeded normally. Regression results in further descent of the testis to an ectopic position underneath the aponeurosis of the external oblique abdominal muscle. It goes without saying that the deviating gubernacular development can be due to disturbance in the regulation of gubernacular outgrowth or regression (Raynaud 1958; Jean 1973), but may also be due to an aberrant morphology of the structures surrounding the gubernaculum by which the gubernaculum is forced into an unusual position (Scorer 1964; Bierich 1967; Bergin et al. 1970; Shafik 1977).

3. REGULATION OF TESTICULAR DESCENT

The factors responsible for gubernacular outgrowth and regression are still obscure. Dependence of the process of testicular descent on androgens or

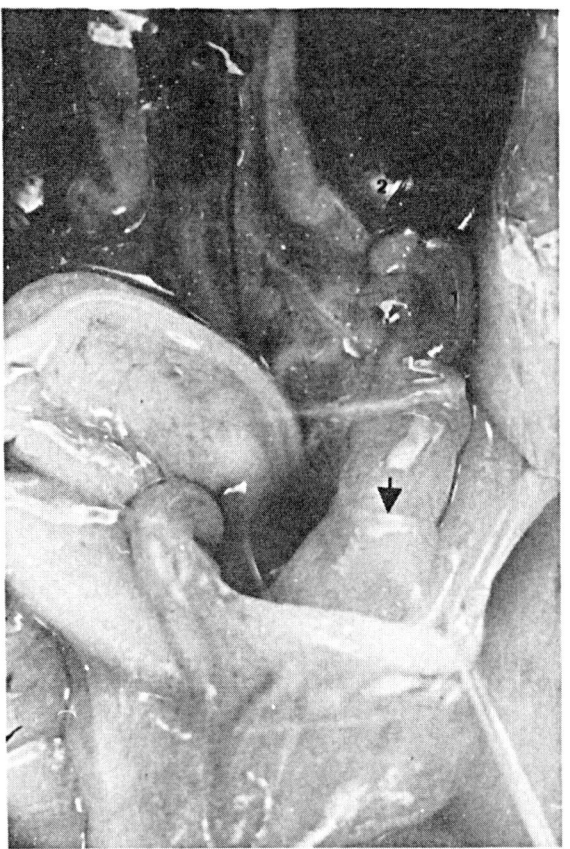 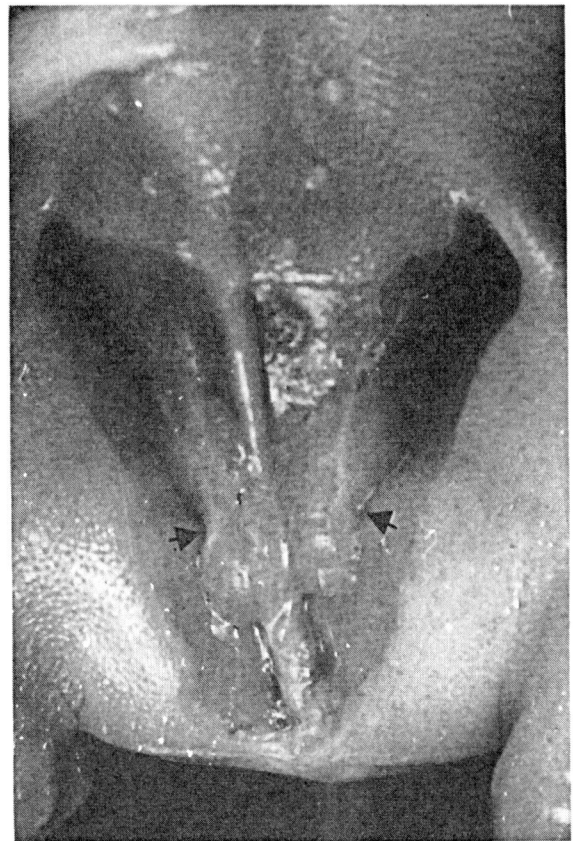

Figure 8. Unilateral 'reversed swelling reaction' within the abdomen. The left testis (1) is located just caudal to the kidney (2). The entrance to the vaginal cavity is marked by an arrow.

Figure 9. Abnormal outgrowth of the gubernacula within the inguinal region. Bilateral abnormal gubernacular location. Parts of the gubernacula extend into the scrotal fascia. The external inguinal openings are indicated by arrows.

gonadotropins is suggested (Engle 1932; Hamilton 1938; Backhouse 1964; Hadžiselimović and Herzog 1976; Reifer and Walsh 1977). Initial experiments either to initiate gubernacular outgrowth in females by androgen administration or to depress the reaction in males by administration of anti-androgens were unsuccessful (Frosberg et al. 1968; Wensing 1973b; Elger et al. 1977). A functional and morphological study of the development of the testis and a study of the role of the gonadotropins in this development in connection with testicular descent was carried out in the pig; the results are briefly summarized below.

3.1. Morphological and histomorphological development of the testis during descent

During and immediately after gonadal differentiation a first transient development of Leydig cells occurs; this takes place between four and seven

weeks post coitum (Moon and Hardy 1973). From the moment that sex cords are formed they increase in diameter until the seventh week post coitum. The rate of development for the testis and its components is low from seven to fourteen weeks post coitum – testicular growth lags behind body growth. A marked growth of the testis occurs between fourteen weeks post coitum and about three weeks post partum (Dierichs and Wrobel 1973; Moon and Hardy 1973; Van Straaten and Wensing 1977). This growth is mainly due to an increase in number and volume of the Leydig cells. The seminiferous tubules also show an acceleration in their development, but to a lesser extent.

During the crucial period of testicular descent in the pig fetus, the outgrowth of the gubernaculum takes place between seven and twelve weeks post coitum. Only immature Leydig cells are present – their cell volume and nuclear diameter are small and, histochemically, hydroxysteroid dehydrogenases are not detectable. From about fourteen weeks post coitum till about three weeks post partum the large volume of well-differentiated Leydig cells shows high activity of several hydroxysteroid dehydrogenases (Figure 10), indicating that steroid hormones can be actively produced (Van Straaten and Wensing 1978). This remarkable phase in testis development partly coincides with the regression of the gubernaculum.

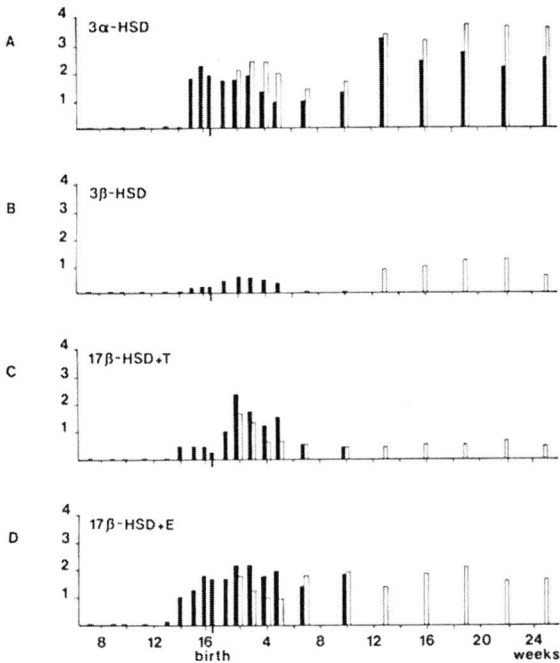

Figure 10. Enzyme histochemical data on Leydig cell development. Shortly after birth two types of Leydig cells can be distinguished: cells located between the individual seminiferous tubules and indicated as intertubular Leydig cells (shaded bars); and peritubular Leydig cells (unshaded). Substrates used: A: androsterone; B: dehydroepiandrosterone; C: testosterone; D: estradiol. Ordinate indicates intensity of the histochemical reaction.

3.2. *Changes in serum testosterone concentrations in the male pig during development*

Testosterone concentrations and testosterone secretion by testicular tissue in vitro is enhanced between 35 and 40 days post coitum (Steward and Raeside 1976). This secretion coincides with a high degree of differentiation of the fetal Leydig cells. Serum testosterone concentrations remain elevated until the end of the second month post coitum and decline thereafter, in parallel with the morphological and biochemical changes in the testis (Meusy-Dessolle

1974; Colenbrander et al. 1978). The principal function of the elevated concentrations of serum testosterone in this second month seems to be the differentiation of the male genital tract and the sexual differentiation of centres in the central nervous system. During gubernacular outgrowth and subsequent migration of the testis, serum testosterone levels are low (Colenbrander et al. 1978). This does not seem to support the postulation that testicular descent is dependent on increased concentrations of testosterone in the peripheral circulation (Backhouse 1964; Reifer and Walsh 1977). Serum testosterone concentrations rise in the perinatal period until the second and third week after birth (Booth 1975; Meusy-Dessolle 1975; Colenbrander et al. 1978) and decline thereafter (Figure 11). These changes are comparable with the changes in morphological differentiation and histochemical steroid activity of the testis.

3.3. *Changes in serum estradiol concentrations in the male pig during development*

Estradiol concentrations are very low or undetectable during the outgrowth phase of the gubernaculum. At about 85 days post coitum there is a remarkable increase in estradiol concentration which lasts till about 110 days post coitum after which there is a decline. At birth or immediately after birth the concentrations are again very low. A similar pattern of estradiol concentrations has been observed in female fetuses and neonates. It is not clear where this estradiol is synthesized. The increase in estradiol concentrations coincides with the onset of the regression phase of the gubernaculum.

3.4. *Changes in serum LH and FSH concentrations in the male pig during development*

In the period between 40 and 85 days post coitum serum LH was usually undetectable with the methods used, but at 85 days post coitum the concentrations increased and became substantially higher than concentrations in the maternal circulation. The high serum LH concentrations, which continued until the third week post partum (Colenbrander et al. 1977), were comparable to those of an adult female pig just prior to ovulation (Figure 12). This rise precedes the increase in number and in degree of differentiation of the Leydig cells. The

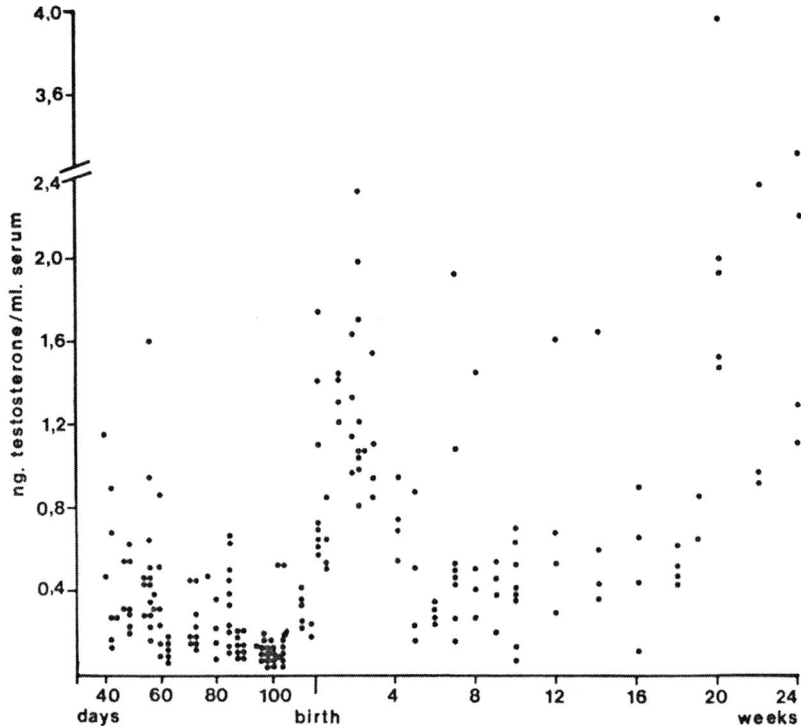

Figure 11. Serum testosterone concentrations in male pigs from 40 days post coitum to 24 weeks of age.

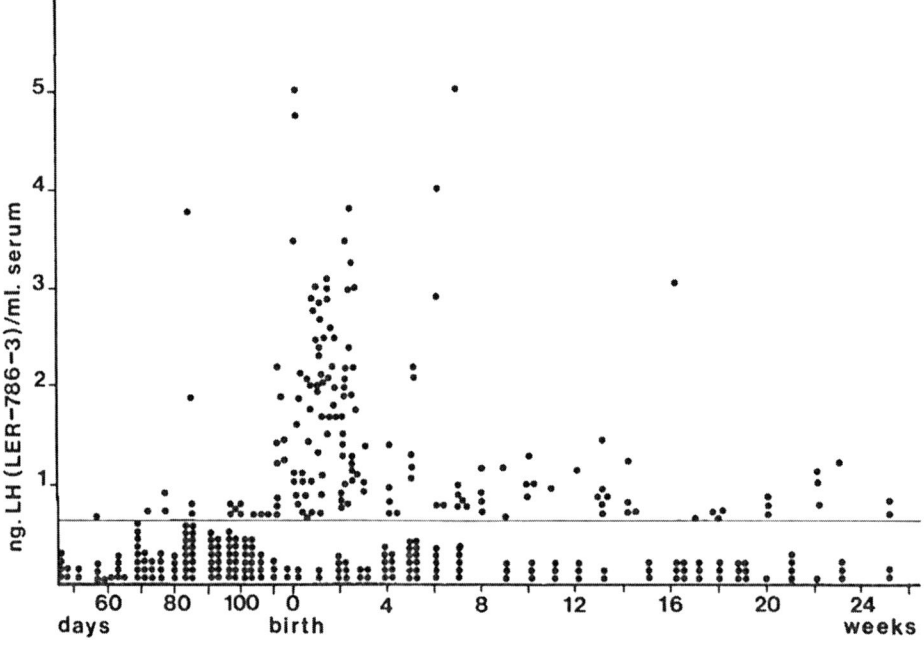

Figure 12. Serum LH concentrations in male pigs from 50 days post coitum to 25 weeks of age. The horizontal line shows the minimum detectable level (0.65 ng/ml).

progressive Leydig cell development in this period lags about one week behind the rise in serum LH. Therefore LH seems to be the initiating factor in this marked transitional Leydig cell development (Van Straaten and Wensing 1977, 1978). Hydroxysteroid dehydrogenase activity is very weak or absent between 40 and 85 days post coitum and serum testosterone concentrations are low during the period when fetal LH concentrations are minimal. They increase parallel with serum LH concentrations. The decrease in serum LH concentrations which starts in the third week after birth is accompanied by a regression of the Leydig cells, a decrease in hydroxysteroid dehydrogenase activity in the testis and a decrease in serum testosterone concentration (Figure 13).

In the period of the outgrowth of the gubernaculum (60-85 days post coitum) serum LH concentrations are undetectable; they increase afterwards. Moreover, since a similar increase in serum LH

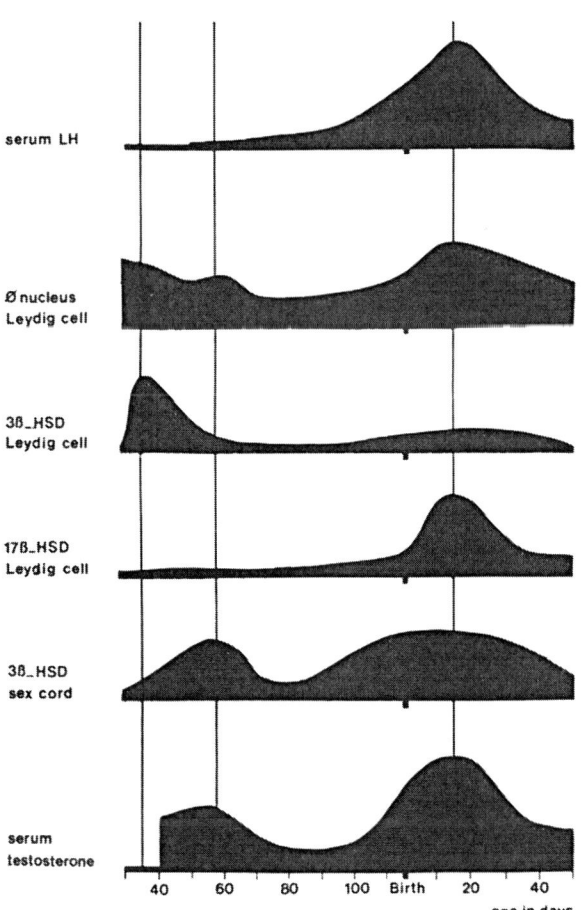

Figure 13. Comparison of a number of parameters related to testicular development in the pig.

concentrations appears in the female, in which gubernacular outgrowth does not take place, there appears to be little indication of a direct effect of LH on the outgrowth of the gubernaculum.

The serum FSH concentrations in the fetal and neonatal period more or less parallel LH concentrations (Colenbrander et al. 1980). They are low or undetectable during the outgrowth phase of the gubernaculum but increase substantially from 85 days post coitum onwards. Peak levels are reached during the first two weeks after birth.

3.5. *The effect of fetal decapitation on testis development and testicular descent*

Decapitation of the pig fetuses was performed at 42 days post coitum; fetuses were allowed to survive for periods between 10 and 70 days (to parturition). Both growth in length and increase in bodyweight were apparently unaffected in decapitated fetuses. The effect of fetal decapitation was prominent on the development of several endocrine organs (Colenbrander et al. 1979). The retarded increase in testicular weight is mainly caused by the lack of development of the Leydig cells. Only a few of these cells are present; they are small and enzyme-histochemically inactive. The smooth endoplasmatic reticulum, characteristic for steroid-producing cells, disappears, so it appears that the normally occurring marked proliferation and differentiation of Leydig cells after 80 days post coitum does not occur. This indicates that this development is dependent on pituitary hormone stimulation.

The influence of decapitation on other testicular components is less striking. Tubular length growth is disturbed but the tubular diameter is increased. This increase in diameter may be the result of the increase in number of germ cells per tubular transverse section. In the pig the development of germ cells is quantitatively undisturbed, indicating that germ cell development is quantitatively independent of gonadotropic hormone stimulation after 42 days post coitum.

The process of testicular descent appears to take place normally in the decapitated fetuses. The gubernaculum outgrowth is effected normally (Colenbrander et al. 1979). Although gubernacular outgrowth and testicular descent are independent of a functional hypophysis, it cannot be excluded that the regression of the gubernaculum is retarded to some extent. An intact hypothalamo-pituitary-gonadal axis is however not a prerequisite for a normal descent. Moreover, as Leydig cells are almost absent and, insofar as they are present, are histochemically inactive in decapitated fetuses, testicular androgens are not necessary for the descent of the male gonad.

4. CONCLUDING REMARKS

The experimental results made it clear that active Leydig cells and gonadotropins are not essential for normal testicular descent. The results obtained with the decapitated fetuses, in which normal descent takes place although testicular development is seriously hampered (Colenbrander et al. 1979), and the occurrence of a male-like gubernacular reaction in freemartins without a gonad (Colenbrander and Wensing 1975) create doubts about the significance of the testis itself in the process of testicular descent.

There are, however, indirect indications that the testis plays a role in gubernacular outgrowth. The Sertoli cells or the primitive germ cells may be the source of the factor(s) responsible for gubernacular outgrowth since in the decapitated fetuses these cells are not seriously affected.

Recent experiments (Bergh et al. 1978) and preliminary results in our own laboratory indicate that for the regression of the gubernaculum the presence of the testis is not essential although regression seems to be effected more slowly in animals in which the testes have been removed and also in patients with the testicular feminization syndrome (Wensing et al. 1975).

Whether the increase in estradiol concentration has any influence upon the onset of the regression phase of the gubernaculum remains a question that needs further investigation, but there are indications in that direction (Raynaud 1958; Jean 1973).

REFERENCES

Backhouse KM: The gubernaculum testis Hunteri, testicular descent and maldescent. Ann Roy Coll Surg Engl 35: 27, 1964.

Backhouse KM, Butler H: The gubernaculum testis of the pig. J Anat 94: 107, 1960.

Bergh A, Helander HF, Wahlqvist L: Studies on factors governing testicular descent in the rat, particularly the role of gubernaculum testis. Int J Androl 1: 342, 1978.

Bergin WC, Gier HT, Marion GB, Coffman JR: A developmental concept of equine cryptorchidism. Biol Reprod 3: 82, 1970.

Bierich JR: Moderne Gesichtspunkte zum Problem des Hodenhochstandes. Internist 8: 42, 1967.

Booth WD: Changes with age in the occurrence of C-19 steroid in the testis and submaxillary gland of the boar. J Reprod Fertil 42: 459, 1975.

Colenbrander B, Wensing CJG: Studies on phenotypically female pigs with hernia inguinalis and ovarian aplasia I: morphological aspects. Proc Kon Ned Akad Wetensch C 78: 33, 1975.

Colenbrander B, De Jong FH, Wensing CJG: Changes in serum testosterone concentrations in the male pig during development. J Reprod Fertil 53: 377, 1978.

Colenbrander B, Kruip TAM, Dieleman SJ, Wensing CJG: Changes in serum LH concentrations during normal and abnormal sexual development in the pig. Biol Reprod 17: 506, 1977.

Colenbrander B, Van Rossum-Kok CMJE, Van Straaten HWM, Wensing CJG: The effect of fetal decapitation on the testis and other endocrine organs in the pig. Biol Reprod, 1979.

Colenbrander B, Van de Wiel DFM, Wensing CJG: Changes in serum FSH concentration during fetal and prepubertal development in pigs. Proc VI Int Congr Endocr. Endocrinology 1980, Austr Acad Sci.

Dierichs R, Wrobel KH: Licht- und Elektronenmikroskopische Untersuchungen an den peritubulären Zellen des Schweinehodens während der postnatalen Entwicklung. Anat Embryol 143: 49, 1973.

Elger W, Richter J, Korte R: Failure to detect androgen dependence of the descensus testiculorum in foetal rabbits, mice and monkeys. In: Maldescensus testis, Bierich JR, Rager K, Ranke MB (eds), Munich, Urban and Schwarzenberg, 1977, p 187.

Engle ET: Experimentally-induced descent of the testis in the *Macacus* monkey by hormones from the anterior pituitary and pregnancy urine. Endocrinol 16: 513, 1932.

Frosberg JG, Jacobsohn D, Norgren A: Modifications of reproductive organs in male rats influenced prenatally or pre- and postnatally by an 'antiandrogenic' steroid (cyproterone). Anat Embryol 126: 175, 1968.

Gier HT, Marion GB: Development of mammalian testis and genital ducts. Biol Reprod 1: 1, 1969.

Hadžiselimović F, Herzog B: The meaning of the Leydig cell in relation to the etiology of cryptorchidism: an experimental electron-microscopic study. J Pediat Surg 11: 1, 1976.

Hamilton JB: The effect of male hormone upon the descent of the testis. Anat Rec 70: 533, 1938.

Hamilton JB, Hubert G: Effect of synthetic male hormone substance on the descent of testicles in human cryptorchidism. Proc Soc Exp Biol Med 39: 4, 1938.

Jean C: Croissance et structure des testicules cryptorchides chez les souris nées de mères traitées à l'oestradiol pendant la gestation. Ann Endocr 34: 669, 1973.

Meusy-Dessolle N: Evolution du taux de testosterone plasmatique au cours de la vie foetale chez le porc domestique. C R Acad Sci Paris 278: 1257, 1974.

Meusy-Dessolle N: Variations quantitatives de la testosterone plasmatique chez le porc mâle de la naissance à l'age adulte. C R Acad Sci Paris 281: 1875, 1975.

Moon YS, Hardy MH: The early differentiation of the testis and interstitial cells in the fetal pig, and its duplication in organ culture. Am J Anat 138: 253, 1973.

Raynaud A: Inhibition, sous l'effet d'une hormone oestrogène, du développement du gubernaculum du foetus mâle de souris. C R Acad Sci Paris 246, 176, 1958.

Reifer J, Walsh PC: Hormonal regulation of testicular descent: experimental and clinical observations. J Urol 118: 985, 1977.

Scorer CG: The anatomy of testicular descent: normal and incomplete. Brit J Urol 49: 357, 1962.

Scorer CG: The descent of the testis. Arch Dis Child 39: 605, 1964.

Scorer CG: The natural history of testicular descent. Proc Roy Soc Med 58: 933, 1965.

Shafik A: Anatomy and function of scrotal ligament. Urology 9: 651, 1977.

Steward DW, Raeside JI: Testosterone secretion by the early fetal pig testis in organ culture. Biol Reprod 15: 25, 1976.

Van Straaten HWM, Wensing CJG: Histomorphometric aspects of testicular morphogenesis in the pig. Biol Reprod 17: 467, 1977.

Van Straaten HWM, Wensing CJG: Leydig cell development in the testis of the pig. Biol Reprod 18: 86, 1978.

Wells LJ, State D: Misconception of the gubernaculum testis. Surgery 22: 502, 1947.

Wensing CJG: Testicular descent in some domestic mammals I: anatomical aspects of testicular descent. Proc Kon Ned Akad Wetensch C 71: 423, 1968.

Wensing CJG: Testicular descent in some domestic mammals II: the nature of the gubernacular change during the process of testicular descent in the pig. Proc Kon Ned Akad Wetensch C 76: 190, 1973a.

Wensing CJG: Testicular descent in some domestic mammals III: search for the factors that regulate the gubernacular reaction. Proc Kon Ned Akad Wetensch C 76: 196, 1973b.

Wensing CJG: Abnormalities of testicular descent. Proc Kon Ned Akad Wetensch C 76: 373, 1973c.

Wensing CJG, Colenbrander B: Cryptorchidism and inguinal hernia. Proc Kon Ned Akad Wetensch C 76: 489, 1973.

Wensing CJG, Colenbrander B, Bosma A: Testicular feminisation syndrome and gubernacular development in a pig. Proc Kon Ned Akad Wetensch C 78: 402, 1975.

Wyndham NR: A morphological study of testicular descent. J Anat 77: 180, 1943.

11. ETIOLOGY OF TESTICULAR DESCENT

F. Hadžiselimović and B. Herzog

Testicular descent is a process in which the gonads descend from the dorsal abdominal wall into the scrotum. Although it is the general opinion that this process develops similarly in most mammals, the etiology of this puzzling procedure is still controversial and to a great extent unknown.

No biological explanation of testicular descent has yet been found, but all those engaged in studying the etiology of human testicular descent come sooner or later to the *Gestaltungstheorie* [form theory] of Portman (1938). This theory maintains that mammals with completed descent are those where the head and anal pole have reached their highest development, in contrast to primitive and archaic mammals, who show no differentiation of the anal and frontal pole, and where testicular descent does not occur (Figure 1).

The gonads appear as an organ which forms externally on mammals and expresses the male sex in a new manner (Portmann 1965). There is no doubt that by calling attention to the sex pole, this latter acquires an ornamental character and signal effect (Portmann 1965; Starck 1975).

However, Portmann's theory cannot explain why, in the great majority of mammals, the scrotum is relatively inconspicuous and/or the visual sense is of minor importance in sex recognition (Ruibal 1957). As an example, the case of Chiroptera may be cited, where the scrotum may be enlarged and evident, yet visual clues probably play little if any part in sex recognition or mating (Ruibal 1957).

The majority of the evidence supports the theory that the evolutionary origin and primary function of the scrotum is the thermoregulation of the testes during spermatogenesis. The question is complicated by the fact that there are mammals whose testes remain completely within the abdomen, in the inguinal canal, or subintegumentally (Table 1), notwithstanding a basal body temperature of 37-38 °C in some cases.

Extensive investigations of the sensitivity of the descended testis to abdominal temperature and of its thermoregulation by the scrotum have so far failed to explain the adaptive significance of the scrotal

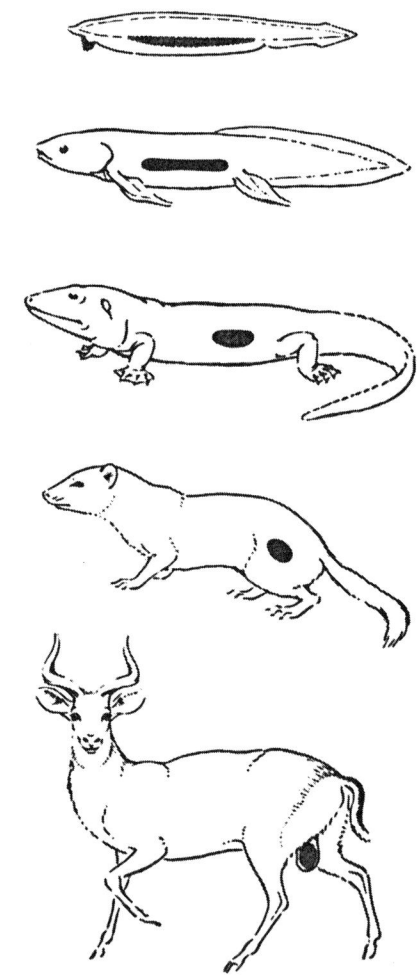

Figure 1. Gestaltungstheorie of testicular descent. Reproduced by kind permission of Prof. A. Portmann (Vergleichende Morphologie der Wirbeltiere, Beno-Schwabe & Co. Verl., Basel, Stuttgart, 1965).

Table 1. Classification of species according to scrotum development and differentiation.

Species	Naturally cryptorchid	Incomplete descent	Scrotal animals (complete descent)
Monotremata	all		
Marsupialia	Notoricidae	Vombatidae	Macropodidae
Insectivora	Macroscelidae Cententidae	Soricidae Tenrecidae Tupaiidae	
Paenungulata	Hyracoidae Probescidae Sirenia		
Pholidota		Manidae	
Edentata	Bradypodidae Myrmocephagidae	Dasipodidae	
Cetacea		Delphinidae Physeteridae Balenopteridae	
Chiroptera			Phylostomatidae
Lagomorpha			Muridae Leporinae
Rodentia		Chinchillidae	Seuridae
Carnivora		Phocidae	Canidae Ursidae Hyenidae
Ungulata		Rhinocerotoidae Tapiridae Hippopotamidae	Equidae Camelidae Cervidae Giraffidae Bovidae
Primata		Tupaiidae Lorisidae *Cheirogaleus*	Lemuridae Galgidae Cebidae Cercopithecidae Hylobatidae Pongidae Hominidae

state (Bedford 1978). It would appear from comparative anatomical and experimental studies that descent into the scrotum has been influenced primarily by the need for migration of the cauda epididymidis to the scrotal region. Testicular descent is seen as a purely mechanical event, which enables the cauda epididymidis to project from the body, but has no significance for the biological function of the testis as such (Bedford 1978). Summarizing all known theories about testicular descent – polarization (Müller 1938), ornamental (Portmann 1938), thermoregulatory (Moore and Quick 1924) and epididymis-linked polygynous state (Bedford 1978) – it may be said that it is not possible to establish a generally-accepted theory.

It should be stressed that the scrotum, and thus testicular descent, is a typical feature among mammals. It is found not only in Eutheria but is common also among marsupials, indicating that it is a parallel form of evolutionary development. It is characteristic that only mammals living on the ground may have a scrotum. However, in regard to evolution of mammals it is possible to distinguish that the scrotum and thus descent is common in evolutionarily younger species having also a differentiated stature.

Within all recent mammalian species we can observe mammals without testicular descent (testicond), those with incomplete testicular descent, and finally a group where the descent is complete (Table 1). Even within each mammalian species, all three forms of descensus are evident. As a rule, it can be said that mammals which are naturally cryptorchid are also evolutionarily older species. In Monotremata there is no testicular descent, while in marsupials all three types of descent occur (Weber 1928; Thenius and Hofer 1960; Kinzey 1971). Among Eutheria, insectivores are naturally cryptorchid or there is only partial descent (Table 1). Edentata, Pholidota and Cetacea are similar to Insectivora. In some families of Chiroptera, Dermoptera, Rodentia, Lagomorpha, Carnivora and in most Ungulata and Primata complete testicular descent is evident. From the embryological point of view, the testes in ruminants and man are descended completely at birth and have the best-developed scrotum compared with other mammals. The transient stage is, in most mammals, characterized by descent of the epididymis, while the testes remain in the inguinal region or intra-abdominally (Table 1).

Every animal form which usually has descended testicles shows to a certain extent cryptorchid and transitional stages of testicular descent. In the horse, cryptorchidism is common (Weber 1928); it is also observed in 6-9% of mice (depending on the strain) and 1-3% of men. In man we can observe a transitional stage, besides the true cryptorchid situation, where only the epididymis is descended (Figure 2).

1. ROLE OF THE MESONEPHROS

The mesonephros plays a key role in the ontogenetic process which leads to the descent of the testes. The differentiation of the Wolffian duct into the epididymis and ductus deferens on the one hand and the male type of mesonephros regression on the other is the motor of descent.

From the phylogenetic point of view, the epididymis is first regularly present in reptiles (Hildebrand 1974), where it is formed as a separate body. In birds, only a rudimentary epididymis is present, and finally, in mammals, the epididymis reaches the maximum degree of development. This degree of differentiation is directly proportional to the mode of cranio-caudal testis movement. For example, in Hyracoidae, where the testes remain in the abdomen, the epididymis has no cauda and the caput is only rudimentary. In comparison with the dog epididymis in which descensus has occurred, fewer coils are found in the sagittal section. Generally it can be said that this coiling of the epididymis is most highly developed in scrotal animals. In man, the whole epididymis (5 cm long when coiled), is about 6 metres long when stretched (Kinzey 1971).

But how can the evolution of species on the one hand and differentiation of the mesonephros, particularly the epididymis, ductus deferens and thus descent, on the other hand, be related? A hypothesis of a functioning hypothalamic-pituitary-gonadal axis, particularly in those mammals where testicular descent occurs, exactly at the time when this hormone-dependent development of the genital tract takes place, could be the explanation of this puzzling phenomenon.

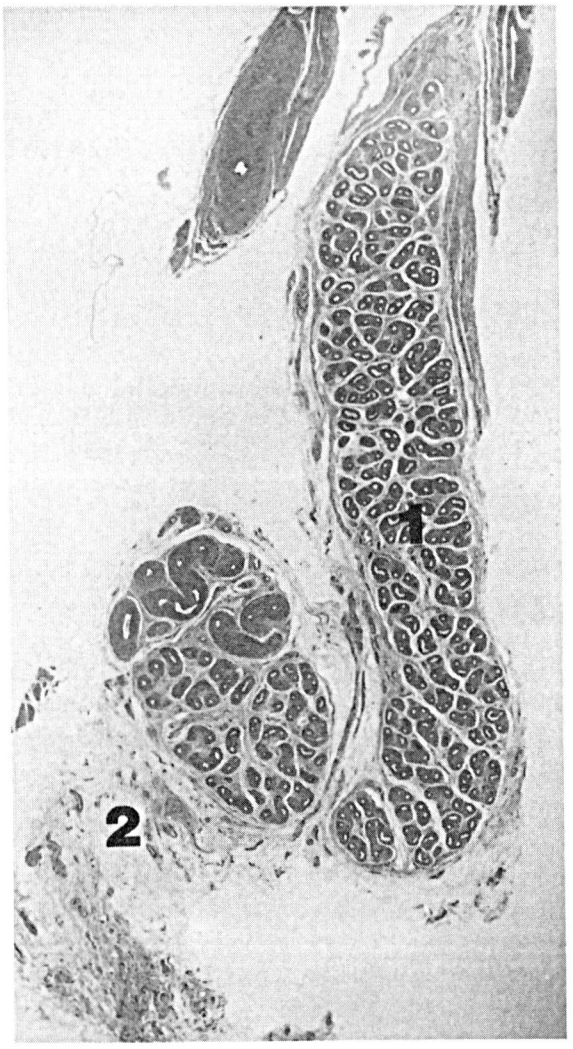

Figure 2. Incomplete descensus in human. Only epididymis (1) is descended; 2; gubernaculum.

2. TESTICULAR DESCENT IN MAN

In premature infants (26-29 weeks of pregnancy), the inguinal canals are almost vertical and there is communication between the processus vaginalis and the peritoneal cavity (Figure 3, Table 2). This communication is also present in babies born at term. In the sixth month of pregnancy, the gonads are still within the abdomen, lying dorsolaterally in the boomerang-shaped epididymis. The relation between the gonads and the epididymis remains the same during the whole process of descent. The peritoneum covers almost the entire testis, except for the dorsal side and caudal pole. The caput of the epididymis and, to a certain extent, the corpus epididymidis, are also almost entirely covered by the peritoneum. The cauda epididymidis lies completely retroperitoneally and is in direct connection with the caudal pole of the testis. The gubernaculum testis consists of a jellylike mass similar in consistency to the Wharton's jelly of the umbilical cord. The gubernaculum is in contact with the cauda epididymis; no direct connection between the gubernaculum and the testis can be observed during the late phase of descent.

The gubernaculum-gonad ratio is about 1:1.2 in the sixth month of pregnancy. Immediately after birth, when the gonads have descended, the ratio remains approximately the same. A few days post partum, the gubernaculum shrinks and increased vascularization can be observed. The innermost layer (the epiorchium) of the testicular sheath is a continuation of the peritoneum. It covers almost the entire testis, as well as the caput and a good portion of the corpus epididymidis. The peritoneum viscerale and parietale, with their connecting folds, can be clearly distinguished (Figure 4). The plexus pampiniformis lies almost entirely retroperitoneally.

The next layer, which is separated from the previous one by loose connective tissue, develops from the fascia transversalis. In contrast to the peritoneum, the fascia spermatica interna also surrounds the ductus deferens, the arteria spermatica, the plexus spermaticus, and the venae spermaticae with the plexus pampiniformis and the lymph vessels. This layer separates within the mesorchium area and partially penetrates the mesorchium and the mesoepididymis (Figure 4). The fascia cremasterica develops from the aponeurosis of musculus obliquus abdominis externus. Horizontally, it is ring-shaped and surrounds the testis and the epididymis as a closed unit. It contains the processus vaginalis, the testis, the epididymis and the gubernaculum. The remaining coverings of the testis are arranged as in adults.

There are many similarities between descent of the testes in man and in the mouse (Table 2). The epididymis of a newborn child, compared with that of a six-month premature baby, is like the epididymis in the mouse (fifteenth day of gestation and first day after birth), more clearly differentiated and compact. There are more coils and these lie closer together. The cauda epididymidis in the newborn

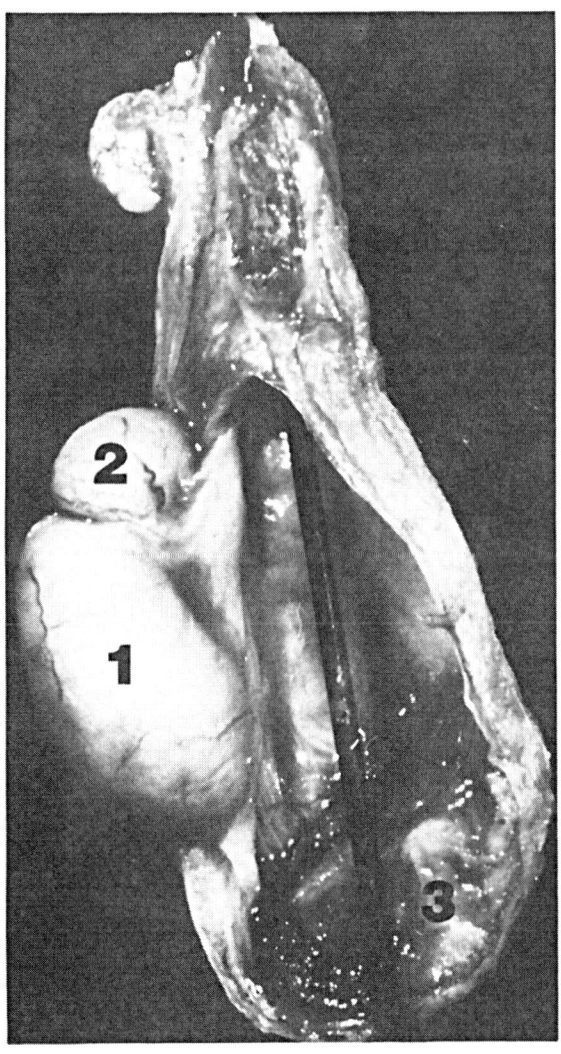

Figure 3. Descended testicle in newborn child. Testis (1) and caput epididymidis (2) are almost completely within the processus vaginalis. Gubernaculum (3) is in regression and there is no direct contact with testis. The processus vaginalis is still open (sonde).

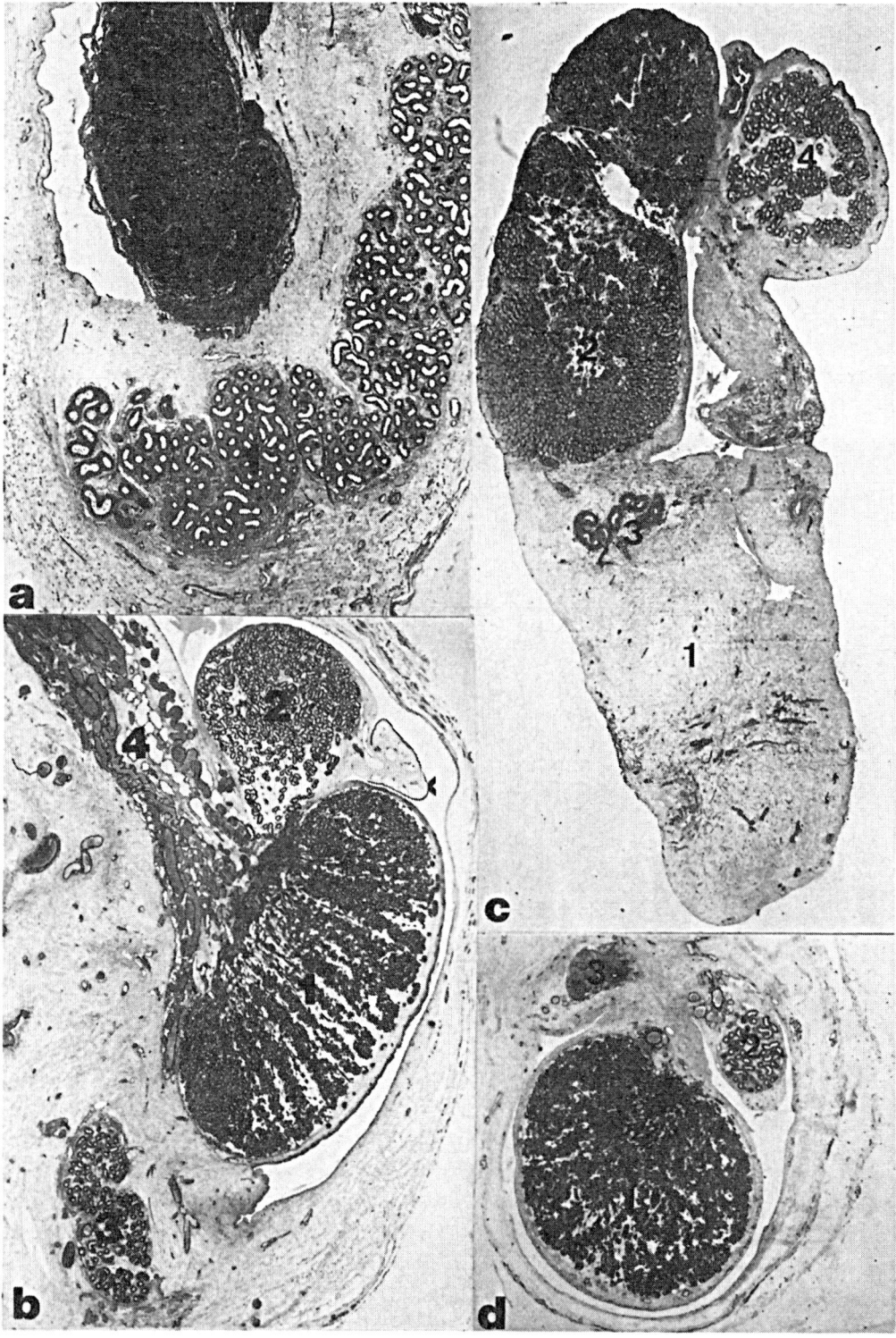

Figure 4. (a) Sagittal section of cauda epididymidis (1) in fully descended testis, showing a maximal development of coils. (b) Sagittal section of descended testis. Peritoneum (arrow) covers the testis (1) and caput epididymidis (2). Both cauda epididymidis (3) and plexus pampiniformis (4) are lying retroperitoneally. (c) Sagittal section of six-month-old fetus showing gubernaculum (1), testis (2), epididymis (3) The cauda epididymidis (3), compared with cauda in descended testis (a, b), appears undifferentiated. Craniocuadal differentiation is in progress. Caput epididymidis is developed (4). (d) Horizontal section of descended testis (1), corpus epididymidis (2). and ductus deferens (3).

Table 2. Correlations between testicular descent in mouse and man.

	Man	*Mouse*
1. Epididymis and ductus deferens descend before the testis	yes	yes
2. Epididymis (mesonephros) is in connection with testis over lig. testis inf.	yes	yes
3. Gubernaculum never inserts at testis but at epididymis (throughout whole descent)	yes	yes
4. Development of processus vaginalis	prenatal	postnatal
5. Caudo-cranial route of mesonephros differentiation	yes	yes
6. Descent within the processus vaginalis	yes	yes
7. Descent completed	birth	21 days postnatal
8. Processus vaginalis obliterated	yes	no

child is broader and reaches almost to the processus vaginalis (Figure 4). As the gonad grows, the cauda epididymidis moves to lie dorsally and laterally. While the majority of anatomists (Crelin 1973; Waldayer 1962; Kopsch 1955) stress that the descent is a retroperitoneal process, it actually occurs in the processus vaginalis, being attached to its dorsal wall.

3. SPECIAL POINTS WITH RELATION TO THE GUBERNACULUM

It seems very important to stress that the gubernaculum does not insert directly into the testis throughout the entire descent either in man or in the mouse. It always inserts into the epididymis, which is connected with the testis by testicular ligaments (superior and inferior). Its role in the control of descent is only in conjunction with the ligamentum diaphragmale. In the male, there is a marked regression of this ligament, while in the female the gubernaculum is more regressed.

Hunter (1762), Sonneland (1925) and Michel (1977) adhere to the concept that the gubernaculum or cremaster, or both, pull the testis into the scrotum. Backhouse (1964) and Starck (1975) describe a swelling of the gubernaculum within the inguinal canal, which promotes the development of the processus vaginalis and cremaster muscle. While some researchers (Wensing 1972) are of the opinion that a specifically infra-inguinal swelling of the gubernaculum is a main factor in testicular descent, later investigators deny the active traction force of the gubernaculum. The 'balloon-swelling' of the gubernaculum was not observed either in man or in the mouse (Forssner 1928; Eberth 1904; Wells 1943;

Hadžiselimović and Krušlin 1979; Hadžiselimović et al. 1978). On the contrary:

It becomes increasingly evident that the gubernaculum does not pull the testis into the scrotum. The view that retrogressive shrinkage of the gubernaculum pulls the testis downward is open to a serious criticism – the gubernaculum is not attached distally to an immovable structure. The gubernaculum functions chiefly, as its name implies, as a guiding agent for the testis. But there is experimental evidence that this structure is not absolutely necessary. In a small percentage of rodents, in which the gubernaculum was severed unilaterally during the prepubertal period, the testes subsequently descended into the scrotum (Wells 1943).

4. DISTURBANCE OF TESTICULAR DESCENT – CRYPTORCHIDISM

Cryptorchidism is a condition in which one or both testes lies outside the scrotum. It is the most common endocrine gland disturbance, 2.7% of all mature newborns being cryptorchid, while the percentage of cryptorchids among premature infants is as high as 31% (Scorer 1964). Operations on 351 patients, where HCG therapy was unsuccessful, revealed that 2% of testes were located intra-abdominally, 8.8% intracanalicularly, 10.9% at the anulus inguinalis superficialis, 74% epifascially (around the anulus inguinalis superficialis), 2.3% prescrotally, and 1.4% were anorchid (Bierich 1977).

Of those couples not using contraceptive methods, only eighty out of every hundred have children within the first two years of marriage. Forty percent of the failures are caused by the male partner; 6% of subfertile or infertile males have been found to be cryptorchid (Eisenhut and Hohenfellner 1964). In the case of bilateral cryptorchidism, the sterility rate is 91-100% (Nicole and Spindler 1964; Moorman 1972), while 60-85% of all unilateral cryptorchids are subfertile or infertile (Moorman 1972). In cryptorchids successfully treated with HCG, one third will, with a high degree of probability, be infertile; another third has to be considered subfertile, and only one third is likely to attain normal fertility (Knorr et al. 1977). In patients where HCG therapy has been successful, there is also a better fertility prognosis (Albescu et al. 1971), while successful treatment is three times more frequent in boys who respond normally to HCG (Forest 1977).

5. INTRAUTERINE GONADOTROPIN DEFICIENCY AS THE ETIOLOGICAL FACTOR IN CRYPTORCHIDISM

Premature descent of the testes in monkeys occurs upon treatment with pregnancy urine or a water-soluble extract of the anterior pituitary (Engle 1932). Testicular descent has been prevented in rodents by hypophysectomy (Rost 1933). Thus the introduction of hormonal therapy is the next logical step in the treatment of human cryptorchidism (Schapiro 1931).

The success of gonadotropin therapy is thought to be the result of increased androgen secretion (Backhouse 1964; Wells 1943). Androgen given alone is also successful in the treatment of cryptorchidism (Wells 1943; Hamilton 1938, 1941).

The finding of *atrophic Leydig cells* in cryptorchid newborns (Hadžiselimović and Herzog 1976) and the fact that Leydig cells in cryptorchid boys can be stimulated in vitro with LH to produce the same amount of cAMP as a normal gonad of the same age (Lloyd III et al. 1978) points to a gonadotropin deficiency as the cause of this disorder. Cryptorchid boys suffer from LH deficiency (Job et al. 1974), which lasts till puberty, after which the condition becomes rectified (Canlorbe 1978). Plasma testosterone levels are significantly lower in the early postnatal period (Gendrel et al. 1978). In infant Leydig cells, secretion of testosterone is *impaired* in cryptorchidism and normal in those with delayed testicular descent (Gendrel et al. 1978). On the other hand, experimentally cryptorchid mice with atrophy of the Leydig cells also have a reduced testicular testosterone content (Hadžiselimović 1977), indicating that a relationship exists between endocrine activity and the ultrastructural appearance of the Leydig cells.

The appearance of cryptorchid mouse Leydig cells is identical with the atrophied Leydig cells in cryptorchid newborn babies (Hadžiselimović 1977). The high temperature, which is thought to be the cause of atrophy of the Leydig cells, cannot explain the atrophic changes in newborn children with cryptorchidism and newborn cryptorchid mice. Neither can the functional and morphological pathology of the adult Leydig cells treated during pregnancy with estradiol be ascribed to the direct effect of estradiol. Further, the atrophic changes in the Leydig cells of newborn mice and changes in the mesonephros can be largely eliminated by simultaneous administration of HCG and estradiol. Such hormonal treatment can prevent cryptorchidism in mice (Hadžiselimović 1977; Rajfer and Walsh 1977). Intra-uterine injection of estradiol leads to impaired androgen secretion in the fetal testis, which in turn is responsible for delayed differentiation of the epididymis and ductus deferens and subsequently cryptorchidism (Figure 5). Because treatment with HCG, but not dihydrotestosterone, produces testicular descent without affecting the weight of the ventral prostate, it is assumed that high local concentrations of androgen are necessary to induce testicular descent in the rat (Rajfer and Walsh 1977).

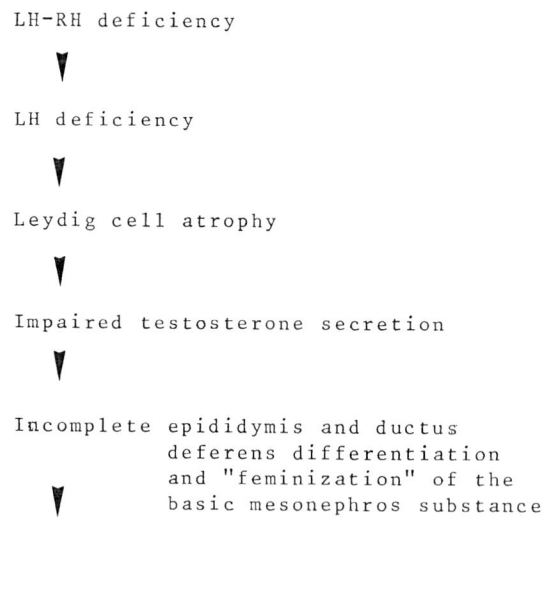

LH-RH deficiency

LH deficiency

Leydig cell atrophy

Impaired testosterone secretion

Incomplete epididymis and ductus
          deferens differentiation
          and "feminization" of the
          basic mesonephros substance

Cryptorchidism

Figure 5. LH-deficiency as a main factor in the etiology of cryptorchidism.

6. CLINICAL OBSERVATIONS CONNECTED WITH CRYPTORCHIDISM

Several clinical observations also point to a connection between gonadotropin insufficiency and cryptorchidism. In *Kallman's syndrome* (a condition in which there is a deficiency of LH-RH) cryptorchidism may often be observed (Bardin et al. 1969). In *congenital aplasia or hypoplasia of the pituitary gland*, the testes are intra-abdominal and there is an almost complete absence of interstitial cells (Steiner and Boogs 1965; Sedehi-Najad and Senior 1974). In *anencephaly*, the pituitary is usually hypoplastic, and such infants frequently have undescended testes (Ch'In 1938; Zondek and Zondek 1963); the Leydig cells, in the majority of cases, are hypoplastic and often there is anomaly of the epididymis (Zondek and Zondek 1963).

Since almost all cryptorchid boys have a normal puberty, it is clear that the underlying defect must be incomplete (Job et al. 1974). In this connection, it is important to mention that growth and bone age of cryptorchid patients do not differ from the normal population of the same age, which, in turn, supports the theory that the deficiency is an isolated one.

7. SOME REMARKS ON OTHER THEORIES ABOUT TESTICULAR DESCENT AND MALDESCENT

7.1. Mechanical theory

Surgeons, in particular, have always supported the theory that in most unilaterally cryptorchid boys, a malformation of the inguinal canal or a sheath between the scrotum and the inguinal region is the cause of this unfavorable testis position. In our experience, it is only possible in a very few cases that a proper mechanical barrier exists (two out of 66).

7.2. Abdominal pressure theory

This theory states that an increase in intra-abdominal pressure is the primary force causing the testis to leave the abdomen and enter the inguinal ring (Hunter 1962; Gier and Marion 1970; Josso 1977). It is obvious that intra-abdominal pressure, together with movements of the diaphragm, is one of the factors, but not a main factor, in descent.

7.3. Factor-X theory

Most proponents of this theory draw support from the work of Wensing and Colenbrander (1977). These investigators are of the opinion that a testicular factor other than androgen, the so-called factor X, is responsible for gubernacular swelling and descent. Wensing and Colenbrander performed their investigations on pigs, which, except in unilateral cryptorchidism, differ in many points from humans and mice in their cryptorchidism. They are fertile; there is no impairment of the hypothalamo-pituitary-gonadal axis; and administration of androgen cannot induce descent (Wensing and Colenbrander 1977). In contrast, 60% of human cryptorchids have a partial gonadotropin deficiency. And in man, the testes have been observed to descend in response to injection of androgens (Hamilton 1938, 1941; Thompson and Hackel 1939), just as they have in monkeys (Hamilton 1941), rats (Rajfer and Walsh 1978) and ground squirrels (Wells 1943; Wells and Overholser 1939). Even if the testis is removed from the tunica albuginea, together, presumably, with factor X, in the newborn monkey and then replaced by a paraffin ball, with the tunica albuginea afterwards reconstructed, testosterone administration causes descent of the paraffin testis into the scrotum (Martins 1938).

7.4. Heredity

Genetic influences appear to be of importance in the etiology of cryptorchidism in some instances. Recurrence is described in certain families (Johnston 1965). Defective gonadogenesis as an etiological factor in cryptorchidism is based on the observation of a total absence of germinal epithelium in some patients (Sohval 1954). Later investigators believe that testicular dysgenesis may play an important role in the etiology of certain cases of cryptorchidism. Satisfactory results following orchidopexy in bilateral cases support the view that the majority of undescended testes are not dysgenetic (Johnston 1965). Further, all biopsies from cryptorchid boys up to the age of one year showed germinal cells, in contrast to biopsies from cryptorchid boys aged from two to five years, 20% of which were completely without spermatogonia.

REFERENCES

Albescu JZ, Bergada C, Cullen M: Male fertility in patients treated for cryptorchidism before puberty. Fertil Steril 22: 829, 1971.

Backhouse KM: The gubernaculum testis Hunteri: testicular descent and maldescent. Ann Roy Coll Surg Engl 35: 15, 1964.

Bardin CW, Ross GT, Rifkind AB, Cargille CM, Lipsett MB: Studies of the pituitary-Leydig cell axis in young men, prepuberal boys and hypopituitary patients. J Clin Invest 48: 79, 1969.

Bedford M: Anatomical evidence for epididymis as a prime mover in the evolution of the scrotum. Am J Anat 152: 483, 1978.

Bierich JR: Treatment by human chorionic gonadotropin in maldescended testes. In: Maldescensus testis, Bierich JB, Rager K, Ranke MB (eds), Munich, Urban and Schwarzenberg, 1977 p 101.

Canlorbe P: Endocrine data in cryptorchid children: endocrinological aspects of cryptorchidism in pre-puberal children over one year and puberal adolescent. Int Symp Cryptorchidism, 1978.

Charny CW, Wolgin W: Cryptorchidism, London, Cassell, 1957.

Ch'In KY: The endocrine glands of anencephalic foetuses: a quantitative and morphological study of 15 cases. Chin Med J, suppl 2: 63, 1938.

Crelin ES: Functional anatomy of the newborn, New Haven, Yale University Press, 1973.

Eberth CJ: Die männlichen Geschlechtsorgane. In: Handbuch der Anatomie der Menschen, vol 7, sec 2, part 2, G. Fischer, Jena, 1904.

Eisenhut L, Hohenfellner R: Die Spätergebnisse der Kryptorchismusbehandlung und die resultierenden Folgerungen für die prophylaktische Medizin. Ann Paediat 203: 157, 1964.

Engle ET: Experimentally induced descent of the testis in the Macacus monkey by hormones from the anterior pituitary and pregnancy urine. Endocrinol 16: 513, 1932.

Forest MG: Plasma steroid hormones in prepubertal cryptorchid boys in basal state and after long-term gonadotropin stimulation. In: Maldescensus testis, Bierich JR, Rager K, Ranke MB (eds), Munich, Urban and Schwarzenberg, 1977, p 69.

Forssner H: Über den Descensus der Geschlechtsdrüsen beim Menschen. Acta Obstet Gynaec Scand 7: 379, 1928.

Gendrel D, Job JC, Roger M: Reduced postnatal rise of testosterone in plasma of cryptorchid infants. Acta Endocr 89: 372, 1978.

Gier HT, Marion GB: Development of the mammalian testis. In: The testis, Johnson AD, Gomes WR, Vandemark LN (eds), New York, Academic Press, 1970, p 2.

Hadžiselimović F: Cryptorchidism: ultrastructure of normal and cryptorchid testis development. Adv Anat Embriol Cell Biol 53: 3, 1977.

Hadžiselimović F, Herzog B: The meaning of the Leydig cells in relation to the etiology of cryptorchidism. J Pediat Surg 11: 1, 1976.

Hadžiselimović F, Krušlin E: The role of the epididymis in descensus testis and the topographical relationship between gonads, epididymis and testis from sixth month of pregnancy until immediately after birth. Anat Embryol 155: 191, 1979.

Hadžiselimović F, Herzog B, Krušlin E: The morphological background of estrogen-induced cryptorchidism in the mouse. Fol Anat Jugos 8: 63, 1978.

Hamilton JB: The effect of male hormone upon the descent of the testis. Anat Rec 70: 533, 1938.

Hamilton JB: Therapeutics of testicular dysfunction. JAMA 116: 1903, 1941.

Hildebrand M: Analysis of vertebrate structure, New York, John Wiley and Sons, 1974.

Hunter J: Observations on the state of the testis in the foetus and on the hernia congenita. In: Medical commentaries, Hunter W (ed), 1762, vol 1.

Job JC, Garnier PE, Chaussain JE, Tublanc JE, Canlorbe P: Effect of synthetic luteinizing hormone-releasing hormone on the release of gonadotropins in hypophysogonadal disorders of children and adolescents IV: undescended testes. J Pediatr 84: 371, 1974.

Johnston JH: The undescended testis. Arch Dis Child 40: 113, 1965.

Josso N: Development and descent of the fetal testis. In: Maldescensus testis, Bierich JR, Rager K, Ranke MB (eds), Munich, Urban and Schwarzenberg, 1977, p 3.

Kinzey WG: Male reproductive system and spermatogenesis. In: Comparative reproduction of nonhuman primates, Hafez ESE (ed), Springfield, Illinois, Charles C. Thomas, 1971, p 85.

Knorr D, Proschold U, Richter W: Fertility after treatment of maldescensus testis. In: Maldescensus testis, Bierich JR, Rager K, Ranke MB (eds), Munich, Urban and Schwarzenberg, 1977, p 95.

Kopsch FR: Rauber-Kopsch Lehrbuch und Atlas der Anatomie des Menschen II, Stuttgart, Georg Thieme, 1955.

Lloyd III JW, Stecker JF, Rakestraw MG: In vitro stimulation of adenosine 3', 5'-monophosphate in unilateral undescended testes of humans by follicle-stimulating hormone and luteinizing hormone. J Clin Endocr Metab 46: 158, 1978.

Martins T: La testostérone peut provoquer la descente de testicules artificiels de paraffine. C R Spc de Biol 131: 299, 1938.

Michel G: Kompendium der Embryologie der Haustiere, Jena, Gustav Fischer, 1977.

Moore CR, Quick WJ: The scrotum as a temperature regulator for the testes. Am J Physiol 68: 70, 1924.

Moorman JG: Histologische Untersuchungen bei der Lageanomalie des Hodens nach Behandlung mit humanem Chorion-Gonadotropin (HCG) im Tierexperiment und am klinischen Krankengut. Ann Univ Saraviensis 19(2), 1972.

Müller A: Individualität und Fortpflanzung als Polaritätserscheinung, Jena, Gustav Fischer, 1938.

Nicole R, Spindler B: Prognosis as to fertility following operations for cryptorchidism in children. Das Hormon 25: 6, 1964.

Portmann A: Article in: Individualität und Fortpflanzung als Polaritätserscheinung, Müller A, Jena, Gustav Fischer, 1938.

Portmann A: Einführung in die vergleichende Morphologie der Wirbeltiere, Basel, Schwabe, 1965.

Rajfer J, Walsch CP: Hormonal regulation of testicular descent: experimental and clinical observations. J Urol 118: 985, 1978.

Rost F: Versuche zum Descensus testiculorum. Langenbecks Arch Klin Chir 177: 680, 1933.

Ruibal R: The evolution of the scrotum. Evolution 11: 376, 1957.

Schapiro B: Ist der Kryptorchismus hormonell oder chirurgisch zu behandeln? Dtsch Med Wschr 38: 38, 1931.

Scorer CG: The descent of the testis. Arch Dis Child 39: 605, 1964.

Sedehi-Najad A, Senior B: A familial syndrome of isolated aplasia of the anterior pituitary. J Pediatr 84: 79, 1974.

Sohval RA: Histopathology of cryptorchidism. Am J Med 346, March 1954.

Sonneland SG: Undescended testicle. Surg Gynec Obstet 40: 535, 1925.

Starck D: Embryologie, Stuttgart, Georg Thieme, 1975.

Steiner MM, Boogs JD: Absence of pituitary gland, hypothyroidism, hypoadrenalism and hypogonadism in a 17-year-old dwarf. J Clin Endocr Metab 25: 159, 1965.

Thenius E, Hofer H: Stammgeschichte der Säugetiere, Berlin, Springer, 1960.

Thompson WO, Hackel NJ: Undescended testes: present status of glandular treatment. JAMA 112: 397, 1939.

Waldayer A: Anatomie des Menschen, vol 1, Berlin, Walter de Gruyter, 1962.

Weber M: Die Säugetiere, vols 1, 2, Jena, Gustav Fischer, 1928.

Wells LJ: Descent of the testis. Surgery 14: 436, 1943.

Wells LJ, Overholser MD: Sperm formation induced by androgens following anterior pituitary removal. Anat Rec 73 (suppl 2): 56, 1939.

Wensing CJG: Testicular descent in some domestic mammals III: Search for the factors that regulate the gubernacular reaction. Proc Kon Ned Akad Wetensch C 76: 196, 1972.

Wensing CJG, Colenbrander B: The process of normal and abnormal testicular descent. In: Maldescensus testis, Bierich JR, Rager K, Ranke MB (eds), Munich, Urban and Schwarzenberg, 1977, p 193.

Zondek HL, Zondek T: Observations on the testis in anencephaly with special reference to the Leydig cells. Biol Neonat 8: 329, 1963.

12. GERM CELL LINES IN THE NORMAL AND CRYPTORCHID TESTIS

Franco Cotelli, Marco Ferraguti, Marcello Gambacorta
and Carla Lora Lamia Donin

Various aspects of testicular pathology have been studied with electron microscopy in the last ten years. A finer morphological approach to the problem of cryptorchidism is now possible. Electron-microscopic studies enable a closer identification of the different cell types representing the maturation stages of the germ line in the normal prepuberal testis and an evaluation of possible differences occurring in the same cells in cryptorchid subjects. In addition to a quantitative numerical evaluation of the seminal line, carried out with the light microscope, the various cellular components and their possible morphological alterations, definitely ascertainable only at the ultrastructural level, can be accurately typified.

1. THE GERM CELL LINE IN NORMAL PRE-PUBERAL TESTIS

The germ cells of the germinal line both at the prepubertal and at adult age have been studied by Hadžiselimović (1977) and Rowley et al. (1971). There is a difference in the descriptions of germ cell morphology in the prepuberal (Hadžiselimović 1977) and adult (Rowley et al. 1971) normal testis. It is interesting to compare the observations of these authors (Table 1). Biopsies of scrotal testis from monolateral cryptorchids and the diagnoses of these authors point out essentially four types of spermatogonia in the age group of subjects we selected (from two to fourteen years); the presence of gonocytes has never been established. These four types are:

A. *Fetal spermatogonia* or *large spermatogonia*, which appear to be very large-sized cells, about 30-40 μm in diameter, with the major axis parallel to the basal membrane of the tubule, and a wide foundation on the membrane itself. The nucleus, either roundish or ovoid, is scarcely condensed, with some irregularities, and usually showing a single central nucleolus. Few organelles are present in the cytoplasm; mitochondria are well in evidence and may be gathered in small clusters connected by a rather electron-dense material and by thin RER chains. Cristae are either of the parallel or of the tubular type (Figure 1c).

B. A_p *spermatogonia* have a diameter of about 20-30 μm, are roughly round and are also in contact with the basal membrane. The nucleus is roundish in shape, and is in a slightly eccentric position, with fine granular chromatin and usually with a single, sometimes a double nucleolus peripherally located and possibly in contact with the perinuclear cisterna. In the cytoplasm, in addition to mitochondria either scattered or connected by the usual electron-dense material into groups, fairly sizeable vesicles of smooth reticulum, well-evidenced Golgi apparatus, glycogen granules, scattered microtubules and microfilaments can be found (Figure 1d).

C. A_d *spermatogonia* differ from A_p by a more condensed, but always granular chromatin and by the presence of a rarefaction zone of the nuclear matrix. One or two nucleoles are in eccentric position but without any contact with the perinuclear cisterna. Mitochondria can be grouped together and be in contact with the nuclear membrane. Lubarsch's crystals, arranged in two reciprocally orthogonal rows, are always present near the nucleus (Figure 2a, b).

D. *B spermatogonia* are derived from the *A* group. They are pyriform and with a contact area with the basal membrane. Occasionally cells showing a similar morphology can be observed in a more central position of the tubule. The cytoplasm is slightly more electron-dense, with scattered mitochondria, easily recognizable RER and SER vesicles, and Golgi area (Figure 2c).

Table 1. Morphological findings in germ cell lines of normal prepubertal testis (Hadžiselimović 1977) and adult scrotal testis (Rowley et al. 1971).

Hadžiselimović	Rowley et al.
Gonocytes	
Fetal spermatogonia	A_1 *spermatogonia*
flat, on the basal membrane	flat, on the basal membrane
mitochondria joined together	mitochondria joined together by bars near the nucleus
oval or round nucleus	flat nucleus irregular in shape
centrally-located nucleolus	peripherally-located nucleolus
Transitional spermatogonia	Lubarsch's crystals
oval nucleus	
peripherally-located nucleolus	A_d *spermatogonia*
A_p *spermatogonia*	flat
mitochondria joined together	mitochondria joined together by bars near the nucleus
round nucleus	lighter nuclear zone
peripherally-located nucleolus	peripherally located nucleolus
Lubarsch's crystals	Lubarsch's crystals
A_d *spermatogonia*	A_p *spermatogonia*
mitochondria joined together	round mitochondria far from the nucleus
lighter nuclear zone	peripherally-located nucleolus
peripherally-located nucleolus	
Lubarsch's crystals	
B spermatogonia	*B spermatogonia*
pear-shaped	pear-shaped
isolated mitochondria	isolated mitochondria
round nucleus	round nucleus
peripherally-located nucleoli	centrally-located nucleolus
Primary spermatocytes	*Primary spermatocytes*

Within the prepuberal germ cell line, spermatocytes are also present. These elements show a roundish shape, are about the same size as the type-B spermatogonia, and are located near the tubule lumen without any apparent contact with the basal membrane. The cytoplasm is scarcely electron-dense, with visible ribosomes, mitochondria, reticulum and Golgi apparatus. The nucleus is spherical with more or less regularly scattered chromatin. In the nuclei of cells at this stage, typical synaptinemal complexes of the meiotic phase are detected. Primary spermatocytes can be clearly identified from five years of age, even if in a reduced number. Only during the prepubertal age, starting from about the eleventh year, has a numerical increase of these elements been observed (Figure 2d). Similar observations have been reported by Scorer and Farrington (1971). Hadžiselimović (1977), however, has pointed out that these elements, present from four to seven years of age, disappear from eight to twelve, to reappear again at thirteen.

Mention of the so-called transitional gonia is precluded inasmuch as the time sequence and the modalities of differentiation for these forms appear to be difficult to determine at the moment.

2. GERM CELL LINES IN THE CRYPTORCHID TESTIS

Quantitative and qualitative classification of the germ cells is most significant for the evaluation of the future fertility or infertility of cryptorchid subjects. There is a standstill in development in the cryptorchid testis in comparison to the contralateral. This discrepancy accentuates progressively with age, starting from the earliest stages of development. Hedinger (1971, 1977), Hedinger et al. (1976), and Salle et al. (1968) confirm that the number of gonia in unilateral and bilateral cryptorchid subjects decreases with respect to the control testis after the second year of life. In about 50% of the studied cases, there is a reduction, or even an absence, of germ cell lines in the scrotal testis of monolateral cryptorchid subjects. Although Farrington (1969) and Mengel et al. (1977) evidence no significant differences between the scrotal testis in monolateral cryptorchid subjects and the testis of normal subjects, Hadžiselimović (1977) has confirmed that such differences exist.

Consequently the presence of lesions in the scrotal testis in monolateral cryptorchid subjects cannot either be denied or confirmed with any kind of

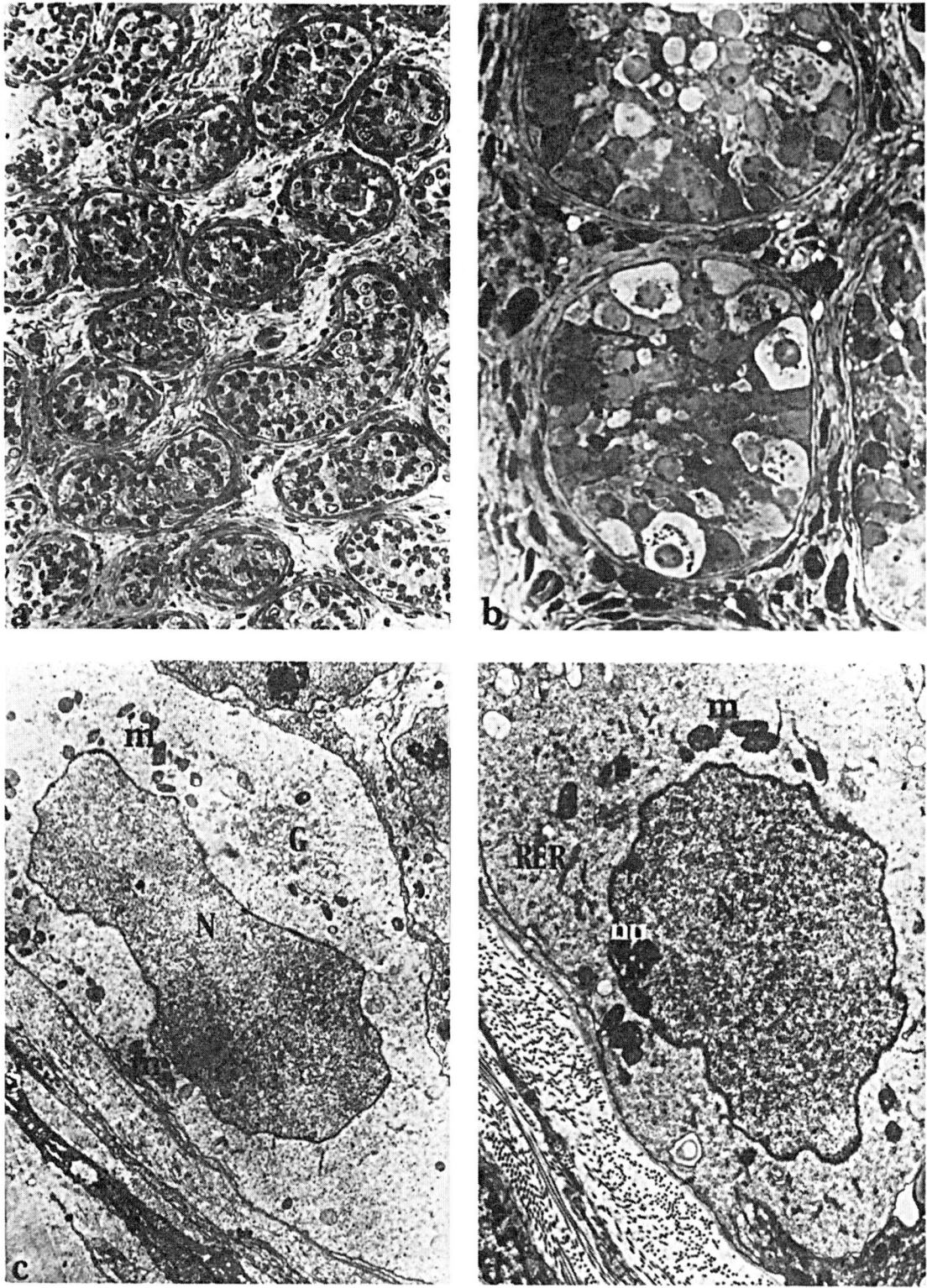

Figure 1. Normal testis. (a) Routine histology: normal morphology of prepubertal testis (× 125). (b) Semithin section: normal distribution of germ cells and Sertoli cells in seminiferous tubules (× 1200). (c) A₁ spermatogonia: the cell has a large contact with the basal membrane. N: nucleus; m: mitochondria joined together; G: Golgi area (× 4000). (d) A_p spermatogonia: N: roundish nucleus; nu: peripherally-located nucleolus; RER: rough endoplasmic reticulum; m: mitochondria. (× 8000).

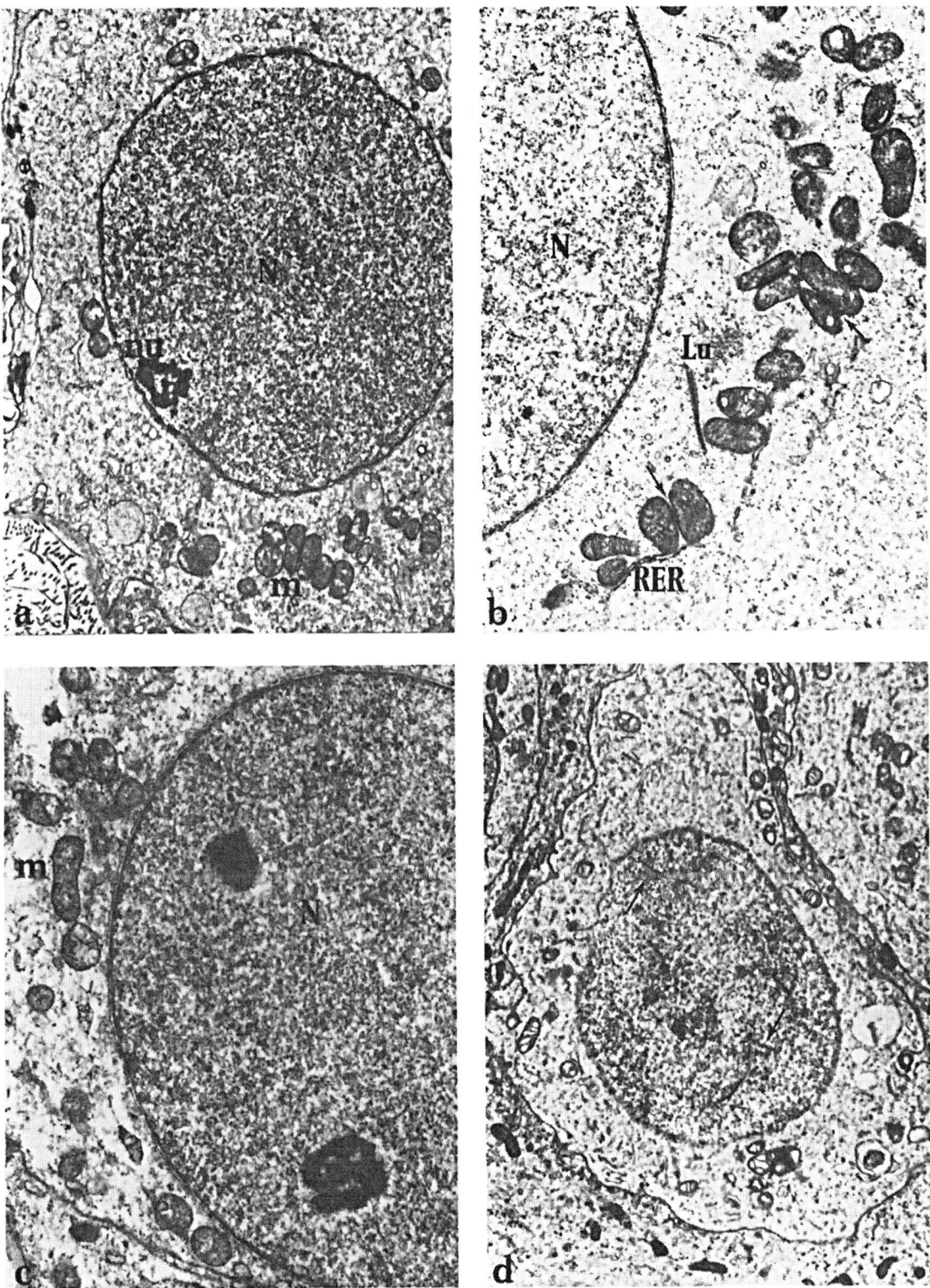

Figure 2. Normal testis. (a) a_d spermatogonia: N: roundish nucleus; nu: nucleolus eccentrically located, but not in contact with the perinuclear cisterna; m: mitochondria ($\times 8000$). (b) Enlargement of a portion of A_d spermatogonia with mitochondria joined together by bars of electron-dense material (arrow) and strains of RER; Lu: Lubarsch's crystals; N: nucleus ($\times 11500$). (c) B spermatogonia: N: roundish nucleus; m: single mitochondria scattered in cytoplasm near to the perinuclear cisterna ($\times 15000$). (d) Primary spermatocyte. In the nucleus it is possible to recognize the synaptinemal complex (arrows) typical of this stage ($\times 7000$).

certainty. If lesions are present, this could explain the fertility reduction of monolateral cryptorchid subjects at adult age (Bergada 1974). Two explanations for the subfertility of the monolateral cryptorchid are possible:

(1) a possible embryological injury whether or not accompanied by testicular retention;

(2) a possible secondary injury on the contralateral caused by the undescended testis.

When artificial cryptorchidism is produced in test animals by surgical means, lesions on the normally-positioned testis can be observed (Shirai et al. 1966).

The most apparent lesion in the testis of patients affected by either monolateral or bilateral cryptorchidism is the decrease or the total absence of the germ cells quota in the seminiferous tubules. The age of the appearance of such lesions is debatable, but the majority of authors now agree that at three years of age at the latest, these lesions have already appeared. This statement is particularly important to a precise indication of the most favorable moment for therapeutic intervention. Mengel and Moritz (1974), on the basis of a large number of cases, hold that the lesions appear at the end of the second year and progressively increase during the years immediately following. On the other hand, Knecht (1976), comparing biopsies of cryptorchid testis with normal ones, states that during the first year of life the number of germ cells and their tubular distribution are already inferior and becoming increasingly so during the second year. Tubules with a smaller diameter are present and spermatogonia are completely absent. The same germinal line elements are observed in cryptorchid testis and in normal ones, although their distribution appears quite variable (Cotelli et al. 1976; Gambacorta 1978). *Fetal* or *large spermatogonia* are elements more readily found in subjects up to six or seven years of age; they show the same morphology as that observed in the normal testis. These elements can show some slight vacuolization, and occasionally, binucleated elements may be observed. Relations with the basal membrane seem to remain roughly unaltered, but some inner blebs can be identified in certain instances (Figure 3d).

The numerical decrease of germ line elements in the cryptorchid testis with respect to the scrotal seems to involve mainly *spermatogonia of the A group*. In some of these elements the morphology appears normal, but in a fair percentage of cases

degenerative nucleo-cytoplasmic alterations begin to appear in correspondence to this development stage (Figure 3c; Figure 4a, b).

B gonia and primary spermatocytes have not been observed in the cryptorchid at the ultrastructural level (Hadžiselimović 1977). With the light microscope cells which could possibly be identified as spermatocytes are rarely seen.

Degenerating and abnormal cells in the seminiferous tubules of the retained testis appear in greater numbers than in the normally placed testis. In particular, besides the degeneration of Sertoli cells, all kinds of elements of the germinal line show symptoms of variously graded affections. Vacuolizations and progressive darkening of cytoplasm with marked asymmetry of the Golgian function are quite common. Sometimes a real degeneration of the cells with a possible phagocytosis of their remains by the Sertoli cells is present. This phenomenon, described by Hadžiselimović (1977), is apparent mainly in tubules lacking lumen. The degenerate elements show nuclear pycnosis often associated with karyorrhexis. Cytoplasmic remnants appear strongly vacuolized and contain remainders of cellular organelles (Figure 4d).

In all the groups considered (2-14 years) binucleated or trinucleated elements of the germinal line can be found. These cells can be ascribed to the different kinds of gonia (L - A types). Occasionally such binucleated or trinucleated elements are also observed in the normally-placed testis but there their frequency is certainly inferior to that observed in the cryptorchid testis (Figure 4c). Normally elements of the germinal line cannot be found in tubules showing the internal onionlike structures created by calcium salts, the 'psammoma bodies' (Gambacorta 1978).

3. STATISTICAL EVALUATION

The considerable difficulty met in interpreting testicular biopsies before puberty has necessitated the consideration of this material statistically, using semithin sections and routine histology under the light microscope (Figure 1a, b; Figure 3a, b).

Gothié et al. (1966) identified a diminishing of the tubular diameters in cryptorchid subjects. Salle et al. (1968) also reached the same conclusion, stating that the lesions appear to be more serious in bilateral cryptorchids than in monolateral. Farrington (1969)

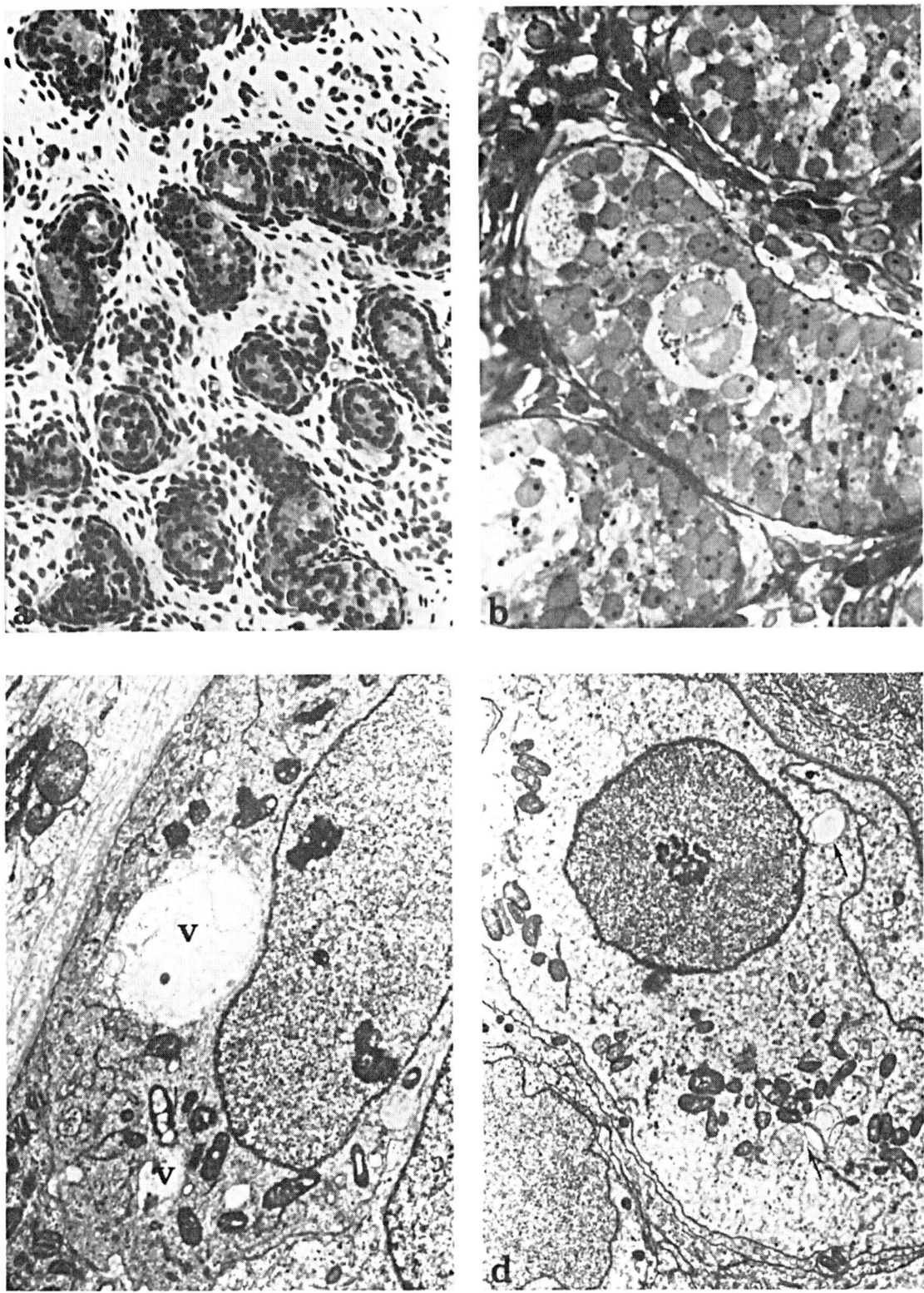

Figure 3. Cryptorchid testis. (a) Routine histology: typical morphology of cryptorchid testis with marked increase of connective tissue (× 125). (b) Semithin section: decrease of number of germ cells and presence of abnormal binucleated spermatogonia in seminiferous tubules. (× 1200). (c) A-type spermatogonia with abnormal morphology and large cytoplasmic vacuolizations (v) (× 6500). (d) A$_1$ spermatogonia. The morphology is quite normal, but it is possible to observe a lighter vacuolization (arrow) of the cytoplasm (× 6000).

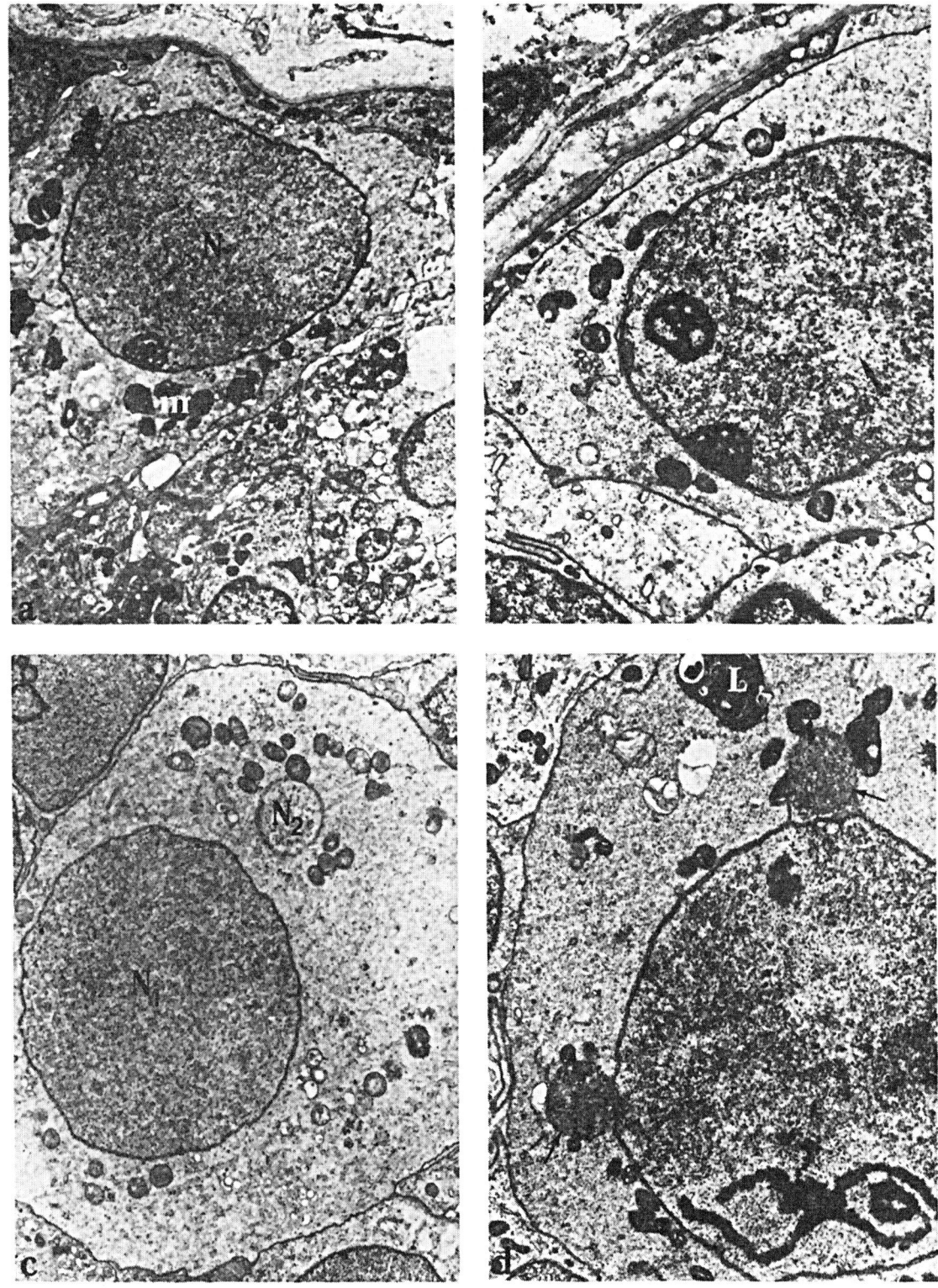

Figure 4. Cryptorchid testis. (a) A_p spermatogonia. N: nucleus; nu: nucleolus; m: mitochondria ($\times$ 5000). (b) A_d spermatogonia with clearer zones, arrowed in the nucleus ($\times$ 9000). (c) Binucleated spermatogonia of the A type. N_1, N_2: nuclei ($\times$ 5000). (d) Abnormal A-type spermatogonia with membranous bodies (arrow) joined to the nucleus. L: lipofuscin-like bodies ($\times$ 8000).

confirms the diminishing of the tubular diameters and of the number of spermatogonia in cryptorchid monolateral subjects, but finds a fundamental identity between the scrotal and the normal control testicle. Mengel and Moritz (1974) point out a significant difference in tubular diameter and the number of gonia, starting from two years of age onwards. Knecht (1976) reports a decrease in gonia plus an irregularity in their distribution in seminal tubules of retained testis within an age range from birth to two years in serial sections. The scrotal and cryptorchid testes show hypotrophy of the germinal line with respect to the norm; the fault becomes worse with time. Hadžiselimović (1977), in a range from one to thirteen years, confirmed what had already been reported.

The study of 123 biopsies of monolateral and bilateral cryptorchid subjects and of 93 scrotal testicles of monocryptorchid subjects confirms the presence of a marked hypotrophy in the undescended testis, considered both at the level of tubular diameters and in regard to number of germinal cells per section of the seminiferous tubule (Gambacorta 1978). The data are collected in tables in order to make a quick comparison easier. In the cases where tubular testicular structures were present, the cells of the germinal line existed in all the cases as far as the scrotal testis was concerned but in the cryptorchid contralateral their presence was established only in 78% of the cases. Furthermore, considering the quantity of germinal cells existing inside the single tubules it is noticeable that more than half of the cryptorchid testicles show a markedly reduced germinal line. In the cases examined, the picture in bilateral cryptorchids seems to be quite different from that in monolateral cryptorchid, an increase in the proportion of cases with complete atrophy of the germinal line having been observed (45%). Plurinucleated gonia have been noted in the scrotal testis but are more frequent in the cryptorchid. The endotubular psammoma bodies have also been observed more frequently in the cryptorchid than in the scrotal testis, particularly in individuals affected by bilateral cryptorchidism. In such subjects the tubules containing the psammoma bodies never hold any germinal cells. Plotting the data collected on the average tubular diameters of the scrotal and those of the cryptorchid testis, a constant inferiority of tubular diameters of the cryptorchid becomes evi-

dent (Figure 5). Furthermore, the difference in diameter remains constant from two- to twelve years of age, when diameters of tubules in the scrotal testicles show a rapid and sudden increase, a phenomenon not observed in the cryptorchid testis: this fact leads to the conclusion that the lesions already exist in the second year of life and do not undergo any further modification until the onset of puberty. A similar illustration has been drawn from data obtained by the consideration of elements of the germinal line. In this particular instance a distinct difference between the scrotal and the cryptorchid testis has again been identified, a difference perhaps greater than that which other authors have observed. Cell frequency in the scrotal/cryptorchid germinal line is estimated at a rate of approximately 5 to 1. This investigation also shows the persistence of the lesions during the whole age range considered (Figure 6).

4. CONCLUDING REMARKS

The pathogenesis of cryptorchidism has not yet been clarified – opinions reported disagree to a great extent. It is still uncertain whether the lesions in the cryptorchid testicles should be attributed to a genetic cause, to endocrinological disturbances induced during the embryonic life, or to its anomalous position. Among the various harmful characteristics manifested by the cryptorchid testicle, diminution or complete lack of germinal line cells is that which appears to be most significant in regard to the successful functioning of the organ. The literature is rather controversial in this respect, however. The lesions involve the cells of the germinal line either from the first weeks of life onward (Hadžiselimović 1977; Hedinger et al. 1976) or during later ages (Cotelli et al. 1976; Farrington 1969). According to Gambacorta (1978), the numerical decrease in germinal cells in the cryptorchid testicle occurs at the end of the first year of life. Morphological alterations of the cells in the germinal line are possible, and apparently normal elements together with others showing symptoms of an incipient degenerative phenomenon have been observed. This factor is quantitatively more significant in the undescended testis than in the normally-placed ones. There is also a disagreement whether the scrotal testis of monolateral cryptorchid subjects

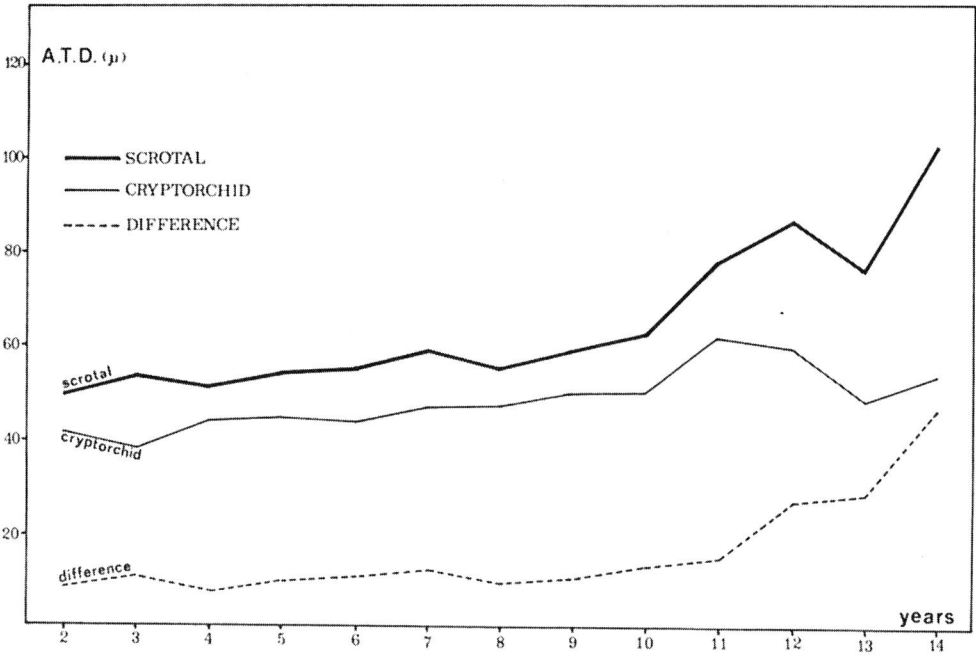

Figure 5. Average tubular diameter in scrotal and cryptorchid testis plotted against years of age, and their mathematical difference. A constant inferiority of the tubular diameter of the cryptorchid with respect to the scrotal testis is evident. The difference remains constant over much of the age range.

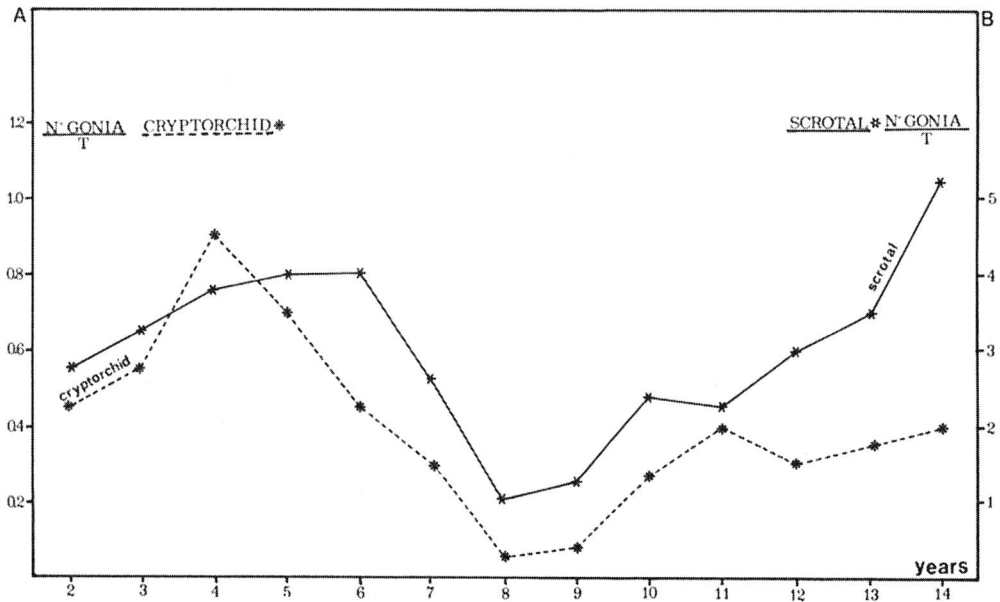

Figure 6. Average number of spermatogonia for tubule section in cryptorchid (A scale, left) and scrotal (B scale, right) testis, related to age. It is possible to identify a distinct difference in the number of germ cells between scrotal and cryptorchid testicles. This rate is approximately 5:1.

conforms to the norm or departs from it in a fair percentage of the cases. This may be due to the great biological variability of this organ, even before puberty, and to the extreme difficulty (material, social, moral) in securing normal human testicular biopsies for ultrastructural studies.

Studies on testicular morphology during the prenatal period are necessary in order to clarify the etiopathogenesis of cryptorchidism and to establish the presence of possible lesions when the testicles are physiologically placed in the abdominal cavity or thereabouts.

ACKNOWLEDGEMENT

This study was partly supported by grant 77.01659.04.115.3607 from Consiglio Nazionale delle Ricerche, Rome.

REFERENCES

Bergada C: Cryptorchidism and fertility. In: Male fertility and sterility. Mancini RE, Martini C (eds). New York, Academic Press, 1974, p 311-325.

Cotelli F, Faleri M, Ferraguti M, Gambacorta M: Aspetti ultrastrutturali del criptorchidismo. Ras It Chir Ped 19: 3-8, 1976.

Farrington GH: Histologic observations in cryptorchidism: the congenital germinal cells deficiency of undescended testis. J Pediat Surg 4: 606-613, 1969.

Gambacorta M: Valutazioni statistiche del criptorchidismo. In: International symposium on cryptorchidism. Bierich JR, Giarola A (eds). New York, Academic Press, 1978.

Gothié S, Canlorbe P, Lange JC: Etude histologique expérimentale et clinique du testicule cryptorchide. Ann Pédiatr 42: 262-269, 1966.

Hadžiselimović F: Cryptorchidism: ultrastructure of normal and cryptorchid testis development. Adv Anat Embryol Cell Biol 53: 3-72, 1977.

Hedinger C: Über den Zeitpunkt frühest erkennbarer Hodenveränderungen beim Cryptorchidismus des Kleinkindes. Verh Dtsch Ges Path 55: 172-175, 1971.

Hedinger C: The histopathology of the cryptorchid testis. In: Maldescensus testis. Bierich JR, Ranke M, Rager F (eds). Munich, Urban and Schwarzenberg, 1977, p 29-37.

Hedinger C, Fukuda T, Grosskurth P: Ultrastructure of developing germ cells in the fetal human testis. Cell Tiss Res 161: 55-70, 1976.

Knecht H: Tubulusstruktur und Keimzellverteilung in frühkindlichen Kryptorchen und normalen Hoden. Beitr Path 159: 249-270, 1976.

Mancini RE, Rosemberg E, Cullen M, Lavieri JC, Vilar O, Bergada C, Andrada JA: Cryptorchid and scrotal human testis I: cytological, cytochemical and quantitative studies. J Clin Endocr Metab 25: 927-942, 1965.

Mengel W, Moritz P: Licht und elektronenmikroskopische Studien am retinierten Hoden. Z Kinderchir 15: 102-105, 1974.

Mengel W, Hecker C, Moritz P: The treatment of the maldescended testis under special consideration of the moment of surgical treatment. In: Maldescensus testis. Bierich JR, Ranke M, Rager F (eds). Munich, Urban and Schwarzenberg, 1977, p 111-115.

Rowley MJ, Berlin JD, Heller CG: The ultrastructure of four types of human spermatogonia. Cell Tiss Res 112: 139-157, 1971.

Scorer CG, Farrington GH: Congenital deformities of the testis and epididymis. London, Butterworth, 1971.

Salle B, Hedinger C, Nicole R: Significance of testicular biopsies in cryptorchidism in children. Acta Endocr 58: 67-76, 1968.

Shirai M, Matsuskita S, Kagayama M, Ichijo S, Takuchi M: Histological changes of the scrotal testis in unilateral cryptorchidism. Tohoku J Exp Med 90: 363-371, 1966.

13. FUNCTIONAL MORPHOLOGY OF CRYPTORCHID LEYDIG AND SERTOLI CELLS

F. Hadžiselimović and B. Herzog

1. LEYDIG CELLS IN CRYPTORCHID BOYS

1.1. Development of normal Leydig cells

The development of the Leydig cells can be divided into three phases: (1) infantile, (2) prepubertal, and (3) pubertal phases (Figure 1). In each of these stages, Leydig cells have a typical appearance and their morphology is closely connected with the development of the hypothalamo-pituitary-gonadal axis.

1.1.1. Fetal Leydig cells. Immediately after birth, there is a rise in plasma testosterone values, with a peak about the second month (Forest et al. 1973; Winter and Faiman 1972). Testosterone remains high until the sixth month of life, when it falls to the prepubertal values (Forest et al. 1973). It is not possible from the plasma values alone to make any conclusions about the origin of this testosterone. A peripheral conversion of testosterone from its precursor or a direct origin from the Leydig cells is possible (Winter and Faiman 1972). The first hypothesis has had priority to date, because developed Leydig cells were observed only until the second month after birth (Mancini et al. 1965). The ultrastructural appearance of the Leydig cells within the first year of life, however, would support the second hypothesis, namely that testosterone originates directly from the Leydig cells rather than from peripheral conversion.

Immediately after birth, there are typical *fetal* or *infantile Leydig cells* in the interstitium (Figure 1). These are polygonal in shape, with a large, round nucleolus located eccentrically in the cytoplasm. The smooth endoplasmic reticulum and lipoid droplets are characteristic features of the Leydig cells at this stage, the amount of smooth endoplasmic reticulum being lower than in adult and greater than in juvenile

Leydig cells. The peripherally-situated rough endoplasmic reticulum is also one of the characteristic structures of infantile Leydig cells. The numerous lipid droplets are surrounded with concentric lamellae of smooth endoplasmic reticulum. An abundance of crista-type mitochondria of various sizes is dispersed throughout the cytoplasm, which reaches its peak of development around the age of two to three months.

From the sixth month to the end of the first year, involutional changes take place in the Leydig cells. These can in some cases also be observed in the second year. The nucleus becomes irregular and deep invaginations of the nuclear envelope begin to appear. In the first involutional phase, the number of lipid droplets seems to be increased (Figure 2); the nuclear chromatin is located more peripherally; and some of the Leydig cells show signs of phagocytosis. The smooth endoplasmic reticulum is greatly reduced, as is also the Golgi apparatus and mitochondria content. Generally it can be said that with completion of the first year of life, the transformation of the Leydig cells from infantile to juvenile Leydig cells has taken place. This points to a close parallel between the appearance of the Leydig cells and testosterone plasma values.

1.1.2. The prepubertal stage. Juvenile Leydig cells can be seen in the interstitium from the second until the twelfth year. They are mainly found in groups of two to six cells. On the whole, they are smaller than the neonatal Leydig cells, with a polygonal shape and microvilli covering the cell surface (Figure 1). The chromatin is homogeneously distributed, while the heterochromatin is found on the nuclear periphery. The nucleolus is very well-developed, with an easily distinguishable pars amorpha and reticularis. Smooth endoplasmic reticulum is also present; the lipid droplet content is reduced; and a few small

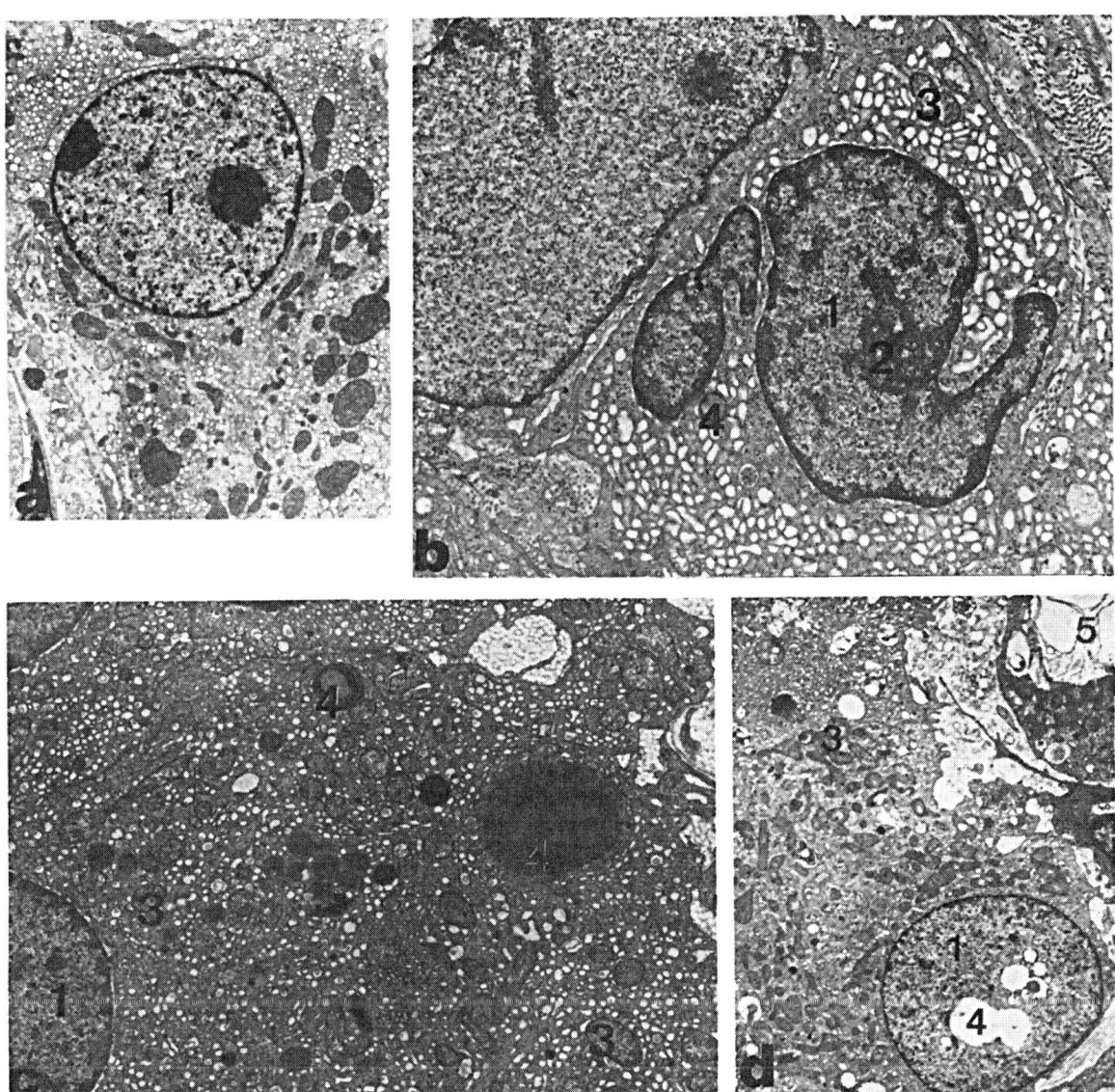

Figure 1. Three phases of Leydig cell development. (a) Fetal (infantile) Leydig cells, ×4400. (b) Prepubertal (juvenile) Leydig cells, ×3000. (c) Pubertal Leydig cells (×3200): nucleus (1), nucleolus (2), mitochondria (3). (d) Atrophic Leydig cell of a two-week-old cryptorchid testicle. The nucleus (1) has fenestrations (4). Nearby is a degenerating Leydig cell (5) with vacuoles in the cytoplasm (×4400).

mitochondria can be observed in the cytoplasm. Very rarely, microbodies can be seen, generally at the cell periphery. No Reinecke's crystalloid is discernible

The second type of Leydig cell, which is also observed in the interstitium throughout the whole period of childhood, is the so-called 'precursor' Leydig cell – Figure 3 (Fawcett and Burgos 1960). These precursors are fusiform in shape, having a longish nucleus with several invaginations and pe-ripherally-situated chromatin. A loose reticular nucleolus can be observed on the nuclear periphery.

The cytoplasm has a small Golgi apparatus and few mitochondria of the crista type. Poorly-developed rough endoplasmic reticulum is found, particularly in the cell processes. In the vicinity of the nucleus, a small number of lipid droplets may be noted. The cell membrane exhibits micropinocytotic vesicles. The ground cytoplasm has fine filaments less than 50 Å in diameter lying parallel to each other.

1.2. Development of cryptorchid Leydig cells

In research into cryptorchidism, particular atten-

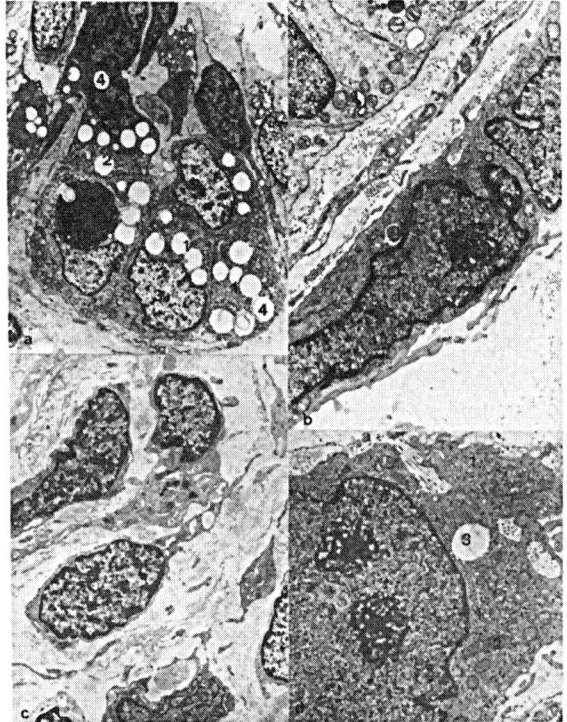

Figure 2. (a) Involutional changes in the infant Leydig cells: fetal Leydig cell (1); juvenile Leydig cell (2). The nucleus (3) becomes irregular with deep invaginations. The numbers of lipid droplets (4) seem to be increased (× 2890). (b) Precursor Leydig cell (fibroblast type-II) with elliptical nucleus (1) and developed nucleolus (2), × 2890. (c) Atrophic prepubertal cryptorchid Leydig cells (× 2720). (d) Transitional stage between precursor and juvenile Leydig cells. Note a paucity of smooth endoplasmic reticulum, many polyribosomes, and a great amount of rough endoplasmic reticulum (1). 2: mitochondria; 3: lipid droplets (× 2890).

tion has always been paid to the germ cells as the most important parameter in assessing the quality of the testicular tissue. The other testis components, especially the Leydig and Sertoli cells, have only been sporadically investigated, because it was believed that these two cell types were normal until shortly before puberty (Mancini et al. 1965; Sohval 1954; Gothié et al. 1966).

An absence of Leydig cells has, however, been noted in cryptorchid newborns (Hayashi and Harrison 1971), while Leydig cells found in cryptorchid boys of up to one year are vere different in appearance from those of boys of the same age with normally descended testicles (Hadžiselimović and Herzog 1976). The cryptorchid cells are generally atrophic and in the interstitium there are more degenerating Leydig cells (Figure 1, Figure 2).

This atrophy of the cryptorchid Leydig cells is present throughout childhood, it being caused by impaired stimulation (Hadžiselimović and Herzog 1976; Lloyd III et al. 1978) rather than by a hereditary disturbance (Kleinteich and Schickedanz 1976) or only secondary damage (Van Straaten et al. 1978). The reduction in both nucleus and cytoplasm size is sometimes so advanced that the cytoplasm appears as a thin rim surrounding the nucleus (Figure 2). There are also more nuclear invaginations and the amount of smooth endoplasmic reticulum is greatly reduced.

The lower the LH response to LH-RH stimulation in cryptorchid boys, the more such atrophic changes are visible in the Leydig cells. In cryptorchid boys without any LH response to LH-RH, the interstitium is wide and only a few Leydig cells can be observed. The only criterion in this stage of atrophy distinguishing the Leydig cells from fibroblasts is the nucleus. Generally, the Leydig cell nucleus is larger and more polygonal, with typical chromatin dispersion over the entire nucleus; there is more heterochromatin lying peripherally. The nucleolus is also more prominent (Figure 2).

1.3. Leydig cells after LH-RH and/or HCG stimulation

It is well known that HCG therapy leads to a significant increase in plasma testosterone and development of the Leydig cells (Bergada and Mancini 1973). If hormone therapy is discontinued, the tubulus returns to the immature state after a few months (Sniffen 1952).

1.3.1. Recruitment of Leydig cells. Treatment with LH-RH or HCG produces similar changes in the Leydig cell ultrastructure. After hormonal treatment, the Leydig cells are better developed and a great number of maturation stages are observed. There are more type-II fibroblasts (Hadžiselimović and Seguchi 1974), described as precursor Leydig cells – see Figure 2 (Fawcett and Burgos 1960). Transitional stages between fibroblast-II and the juvenile Leydig cells are frequently seen (Figure 2). These cells have a better-developed cytoplasm and more polyribosomes and glycogen granules are present. The rough endoplasmic reticulum is dispersed over the entire cytoplasm; the mitochondria are larger and have intermitochondrial granules. The cell surface shows many micropinocytotic vesicles and microvilli. The nucleus has an oval

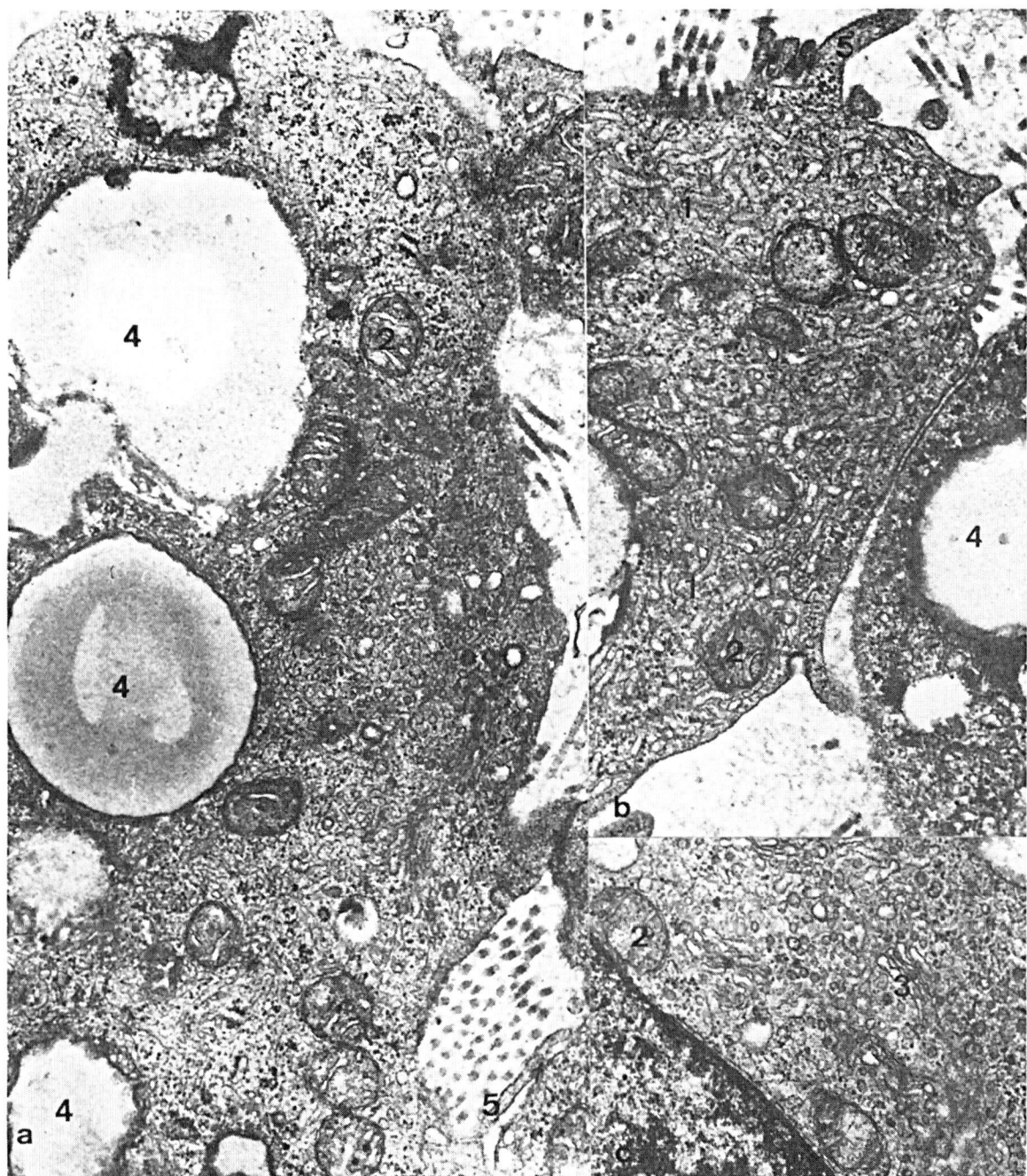

Figure 3. Leydig cells of LH-RH treated boy (a, b, c). The changes are identical to those observed after HCG treatment. Note the great amount of smooth endoplasmic reticulum (1). 2: mitochondria: 3: developed Golgi apparatus: 4: lipid droplets, membrane-bounded in various stages of development: 5: microvilli (× 7200).

contour and the invaginations of the nuclear envelope are less pronounced. Two well-developed nucleoli lie eccentrically within the nucleus (Figure 2). Finally, in precursor Leydig cells after stimulation with LH-RH or HCG, large membrane-bounded vacuoles can be observed.

1.3.2. Stimulated juvenile Leydig cells. Within the interstitium, especially around the blood vessels, there are juvenile Leydig cells (Figure 3). These stimulated juvenile Leydig cells are polygonal and, unlike the fetal and adult types, their nuclei retain their irregular shape. Characteristic changes take place in the cytoplasm. The most striking feature, as in most steroid-secreting cells, is the abundant smooth endoplasmic reticulum, located concentrically around the lipid droplets. These membrane-bounded lipid droplets, in various stages, are also a typical feature of LH-RH or HCG-stimulated Leydig cells.

The mitochondria are generally larger and of mixed type, with more numerous tubuli. The Golgi apparatus is prominent. At the cell border, micropinocytotic vesicles are found. Crystalloids are absent (Figure 3). An increase in the amount of smooth endoplasmic reticulum, microfilaments; enlargement of the Golgi apparatus; and, finally, an increase in the tubular content of mitochondria, are typical signs of increased gonadotropin stimulation of the Leydig cells.

The recruitment and the process of differentiation is centrifugal, i.e., precursor cells are in the vicinity of the tubuli, whereas better-developed Leydig cells are situated more deeply in the interstitium. The interstitial development and tubular enlargement after LH-RH or HCG treatment is a real maturational process.

2. ENDOCRINE PROFILE IN CRYPTORCHID BOYS

The period from the second to the sixth year of life is of particular interest in the evaluation of endocrine parameters, since 20-30% of cryptorchid boys from the age of two onwards have no spermatogonia, and the secondary changes in the Sertoli and Leydig cells take place only after age six. The mean number of spermatogonia per tubular cross-section is 0.39 ± 0.66 as compared to 1.4 ± 0.3 in normal boys aged two to six years.

Cryptorchid boys can be divided into two groups: (1) those without any detectable spermatogonia; and (2) those with a reduced number of spermatogonia $(0.44 \pm 0.71, SD)$. In Table 1 the values of basal and peak LH and FSH in patients with and without spermatogonia are compared. Basal LH and the maximum response to LH-RH are significantly lower in the group without spermatogonia.

LH response is diminished in cryptorchid newborns and in prepubertal boys (Job et al. 1977). A relationship between LH function and the number of spermatogonia is strongly suggested by the absence

of spermatogonia in the case of low LH response and the low LH response in boys with absence of spermatogonia. This obviously points to a connection between testicular descent, the development of spermatogonia, the endocrine testis function, and gonadotropin, particularly LH.

In the first year, cryptorchid boys (uni- or bilateral) always have germ cells (Figure 4). Since it is generally the case that cryptorchid adults with a bad spermiogram also had a low spermatogonia count (Figure 5), HCG or LH-RH treatment must be carried out at the end of the first year. If this is not successful, orchidopexy should be performed within the next three months.

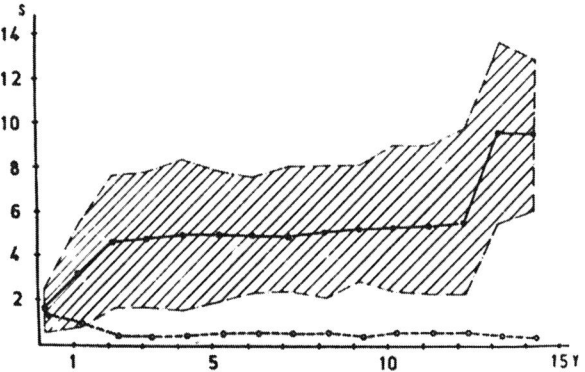

Figure 4. Mean and simple standard deviation (shaded area) of spermatogonia content per seminiferous tubule of 252 orthotopic testicles (continuous line) and 1197 congenitally dystopic testicles (broken line). The difference in spermatogonia count is significant for all age groups except the first year (from Kleinteich et al. 1979).

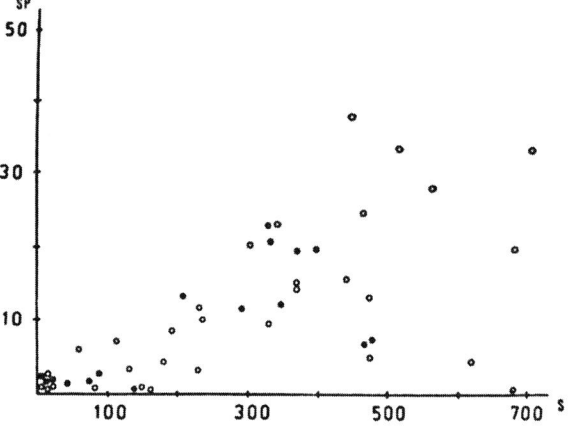

Figure 5. Correlation between sperm density (millions/ml) and total spermatogonia content (millions/testis) of both testicles of 32 adults operated for unilateral (circles) and 16 adults operated for bilateral (spots) congenital dystopy (from Kleinteich et al. 1979).

Table 1. Spermatogonia in cryptorchid boys correlated to LH and FSH plasma values.

	No. of patients	basal	LH (mIU/l) peak	basal	FSH (mIU/l) peak
No spermatogonia	7	1.7 ± 0.6	2.7 ± 1.9	1.1 ± 0.9	2.1 ± 1.0
With spermatogonia	25	4.1 ± 2.1	7.7 ± 4.1	1.4 ± 1.2	5.3 ± 3.5
Significance		p < 0.005	p < 0.005	Not significant	p < 0.05

3. SERTOLI CELLS IN CRYPTORCHID BOYS

3.1. Development and different types of normal Sertoli cells

The Sertoli cell is the most common cell in the infant seminiferous tubule. It is smaller than the spermatogonia and changes its form several times before puberty (Hadžiselimović 1977). Four different types of Sertoli cells can be distinguished in children: fetal *Sf, Sa, Sb* and *Sc*-type cells (Figure 6, Figure 7). *Sa*-type Sertoli cells develop from the fetal Sertoli cells in the first year of life. With increasing age, *Sb*-type cells, which develop from the *Sa* type, are more frequently encountered. The transition to the *Sc*-type cells takes place suddenly: with the appearance of the lumen, only *Sc*-type cells are found in the tubulus. Throughout the entire period of childhood, no division of the Sertoli cells was ever observed. The number of Sertoli cells per cross-section of tubulus decreased continuously in normal testicles from the first year until puberty (Hadžiselimović 1977).

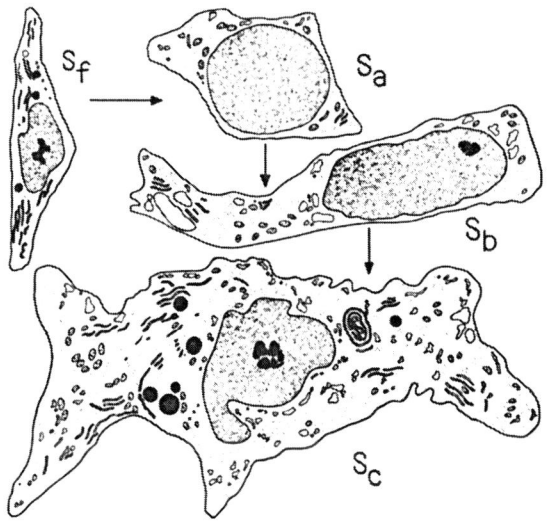

Figure 6. Diagram of a Sertoli cell development. Sf: fetal Sertoli cell; Sa:*Sa* type; Sb:*Sb* type; Sc:*Sc* type; arrow; route of transformation.

3.2. Development of cryptorchid Sertoli cells

In cryptorchid testicles, too, the Sertoli cells are the most frequently encountered in the seminiferous tubule. On the basis of their morphology, two types can be distinguished before puberty, namely types *Sa* and *Sb*. The fetal Sertoli cells, which in normal testicles persist until the third month post natum, are already absent as early as two weeks after birth.

The *Sa* type, with its large, round nucleus and only slightly differentiated cytoplasm, shows hardly any qualitative differences from the *Sa*-type cells of normal testicles, until puberty (Figure 7). The *Sb* type, on the other hand, is much rarer and these cells have less smooth endoplasmic reticulum and fewer lipid droplets than those in normal testicles of the same age.

Morphometric assessment of the Sertoli cells up to the age of six reveals no significant difference in number or individual cell volume. The number of Sertoli cells per cubic centimetre of testicular tissue in normal testicles is 1.44×10^6, while in cryptorchid testicles the figure is 1.617×10^6. The single-cell volume in normal testicles is 491 μ^3 and in undescended 429 μ^3. The differences in both the number and single-cell volume of the Sertoli cells are not significant.

In puberty, the transformation of the Sertoli cells to the *Sc* type is only partially completed. In most boys, either in puberty or immediately afterwards, the Sertoli cells remain stationary at the *Sa* stage (Figure 7). In particular, their nucleus retains its round form and few uncharacteristic cell organelles can be found in the entire cytoplasm. No crystalloid of Charcot-Böttcher is present and the number of lipid droplets is reduced (Hadžiselimović 1977).

Enzyme activity is reduced in the case of unilateral cryptorchidism and hypogonadotropic hypogonadism, suggesting that Sertoli cell maturation may never occur (Hodgen 1977).

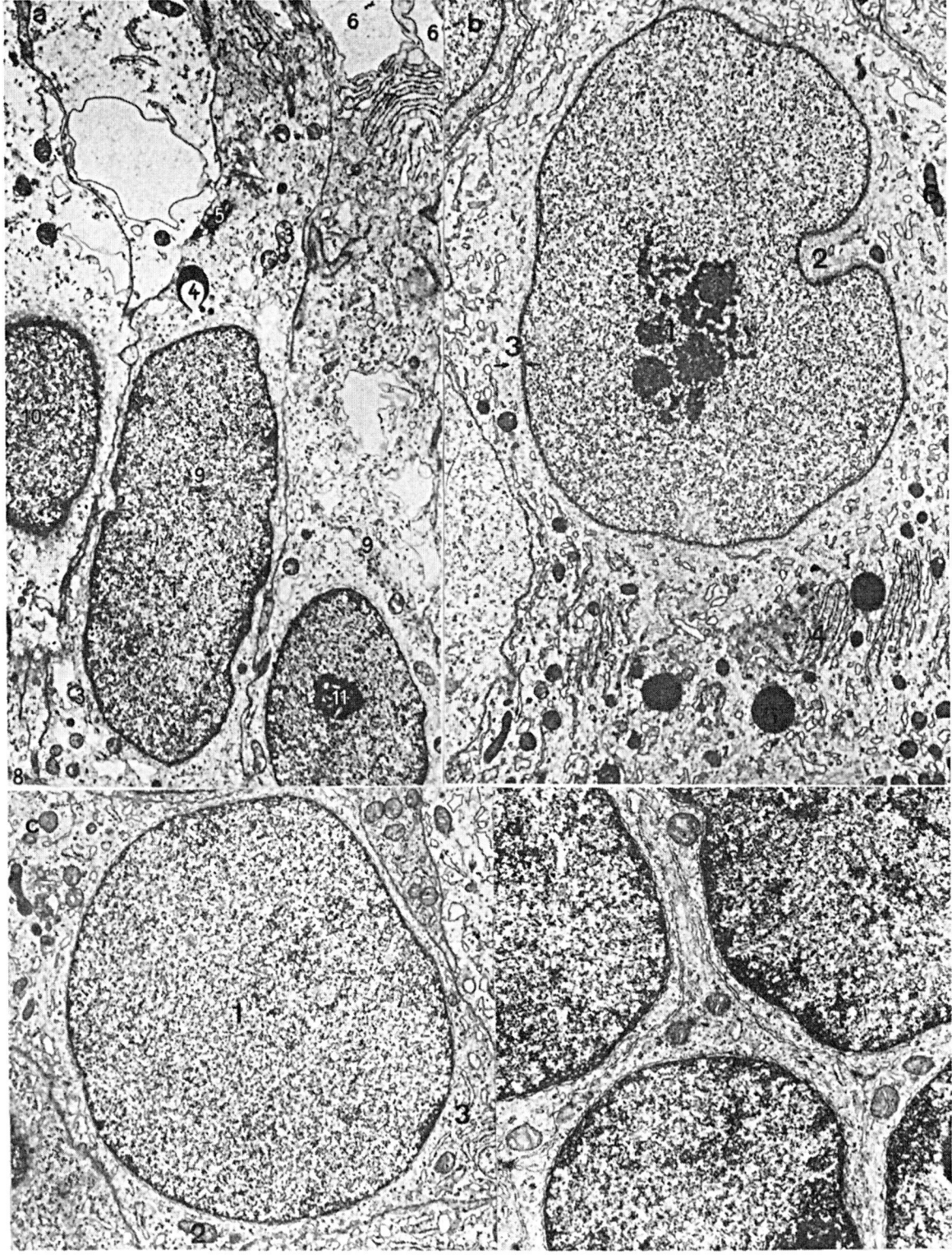

Figure 7. (a) *SB* type of Sertoli cells (9); transitional stage between *Sa* and *SB* (10); nucleus (1); nuclear invagination (2); mitochondria (3); lipid droplet (4); centrosome (5); vacuoles (6); and rough endoplasmic reticulum (7) are localized typically as vacuoles in the apical part of the cell. 11: nucleolus (×2805). (b) *Sc* Sertoli cell: 1: nucleus; 2: nuclear invagination; 3: cytoplasm 'halo'; 4: rough endoplasmic reticulum; 5: lipid droplet; 6: mitochondria (×4250). (c): *Sa* Sertoli cell: 1: nucleus; 2: mitochondria; 3: rough endoplasmic reticulum (×4250). (d): *Sa* cryptorchid Sertoli cells (×2890).

REFERENCES

Bergada C, Mancini RE: Effect of gonadotropins on the induration of spermatogenesis in human prepuberal testis. J Clin Endocr Metab 37: 935, 1973.

Fawcett DW, Burgos MH: Studies on the fine structure of the mammalian testis II: the human interstitial tissue. Am J Anat 107: 245, 1960.

Forest MG, Cathiard AM, Bertrand JA: Total and unbound testosterone levels in the newborn and in normal and hypogonadal children: use of sensitive radio-immuno-assay for testosterone. J Clin Endocr Metab 36: 1132, 1973.

Gothié S, Canlorbe P, Lange JC: Étude histologique, expérimentale et clinique du testicle cryptorchide. Ann Pédiat 42: 262, 1966.

Hadžiselimović F: Cryptorchidism: ultrastructure of normal and cryptorchid testis development. Adv Anat Enbryol Cell Biol 53: 3, 1977.

Hadžiselimović F, Herzog B: The meaning of the Leydig cell in relation to the etiology of cryptorchidism. J Pediat Surg 11: 1, 1976.

Hadžiselimović F, Seguchi H: Razvoj testisa u djece. Fol Anat Jugos 1: 67, 1974.

Hayashi H, Harrison RG: The development of the interstitial tissue of the human testis. Fertil Steril 22: 351, 1971.

Hodgen GD: Enzyme markers of testicular function. In: The testis, Johnson AD, Gomes WR (eds). New York, Academic Press, 1977, vol 4, p 401.

Job C, Gendrel D, Safar A, Roger M, Chaussain JL: Pituitary LH and FSH and testosterone secretion in infants with undescended testes. Acta Endocr 85: 644, 1977.

Kleinteich B, Schickedanz H: Der Spermatogoniengehalt kongenital-dystoper und operativ verlagerter Hoden bei Kindern und Jugendlichen. Z Urol 69: 819, 1976.

Kleinteich B, Hadžiselimović F, Hesse V, Schreiber G: Kongenitale Hodendystopien. In: Moderne Pädiatrie. Leipzig, Georg Thieme, 1979.

Lloyd III JV, Stecker JF, Rakestraw MG: In vitro stimulation of adenosine 3', 5'-monophosphate in unilateral undescended testes of humans by follicle and luteinizing hormone. J Clin Endocr Metab 46: 158, 1978.

Mancini RE, Rosemberg E, Cullen M, Lavieri JC, Vilar O, Bergada C, Andrada JA: Cryptorchid and scrotal human testis I: cytological, cytochemical and quantitative studies. J Clin Endocr Metab 25: 927, 1965.

Sniffen CR: Histology of the normal and abnormal testis at puberty. Ann N Y Acad Sci 55: 609, 1952.

Sohval RA: Histopathology of cryptorchidism. Am J Med 16: 346, 1954.

Van Straaten HWM, Ribbers-de Ridder R, Wensing CJG: Early deviations of testicular Leydig cells in the naturally unilateral cryptorchid pig. Biol Reprod 19: 171, 1978.

Winter JSD, Faiman C: Pituitary-gonadal relations in male children and adolescents. Pediatr Res 6: 126, 1972.

14. ESTROGEN-INDUCED CRYPTORCHIDISM IN ANIMALS

F. Hadžiselimovic, B. Herzog and E. Krušlin

1. NORMAL DESCENT IN THE MOUSE

Ontogenesis of the genital apparatus of the mouse shows a repetition of some phylogenetic stages (Figure 1). At the *eleventh* day of gestation, the gonads are situated in the urogenital anlage. By the *thirteenth* day this is clearly distinguished from the mesonephros. The gubernaculum extends from the caudal pole of the mesonephros to the inguinal region, where it terminates in a small prominence. The testis is held dorsolaterally by the mesonephros for its entire length and the gonad appears to be embedded in the mesonephros. By the *fifteenth* day the gubernaculum has become larger. The cranial pole derives from the mesonephros and its caudal pole is attached by a funnel-shaped formation to the inguinal region. The cranio-caudal differentiation of the mesonephros develops further in a caudal direction. The ligamentum diaphragmale is still present, but more elongated and lying against the dorsal abdominal wall. The transabdominal movement of the testis occurs as early as the *seventeenth* day of gestation, when the gubernaculum changes its shape and is pushed against the lower abdominal wall. The caudal pole of the mesonephros becomes somewhat smaller, because the ductus deferens has separated from the mesonephros. The epididymis has more coils.

At the *nineteenth* day the gubernaculum is thread-like, inserting in the region of the future scrotum, an incudiform formation inverted in the abdominal cavity. Immediately after birth, the gubernaculum is recognizable as a small thread. The epididymis is already formed and the processus vaginalis is visible. The testis has terminated its transabdominal movement and now lies lateral to the bladder neck, in the vicinity of the ventral abdominal wall. On the *third* postnatal day, the testis sinks into the processus vaginalis and the ductus deferens and epididymis move in front of the gonad. The actual scrotum is already developed.

At the *seventh* day, the processus vaginalis becomes deeper and wider. The cauda epididymidis lies deep in the processus vaginalis and has more coils. Only remnants of the gubernaculum are visible. This is the period where the testes become larger. The caput epididymidis is at the level of the anulus inguinalis profundus. At the *fourteenth* day the caudal scrotal tip is inverted and infolded. Between the scrotal tip and the caudal epididymis, there is still a short connection, a remnant of the gubernaculum.

At the *twenty-first* day, the gubernaculum has attained its final structure – a threadlike connection between scrotum and epididymis. The epididymis is fully developed and the testis lies in the scrotum.

It is possible to divide descent in the mouse into two phases, prenatal and postnatal. The *prenatal phase* is characterized by intra-abdominal testicular movement, with differentiation of the mesonephros into epididymis and ductus deferens. The *postnatal phase* is characterized by testicular growth and evagination of the processus vaginalis peritonei. The epididymis and ductus deferens continue to differentiate.*

2. ESTROGEN-INDUCED CRYPTORCHIDISM

Cryptorchidism can be produced in rats and mice by treating gravid females with estrogen at the thirteenth day of gestation (Greene et al. 1938). Raynaud (1942) repeated these experiments and postulated that cryptorchidism is the result of gubernacular atrophy, which in turn is the result of direct estrogen action on gubernacular growth. The

* This part is a summary of Krušlin's dissertation performed at the laboratory of the University Children's Hospital, Basel.

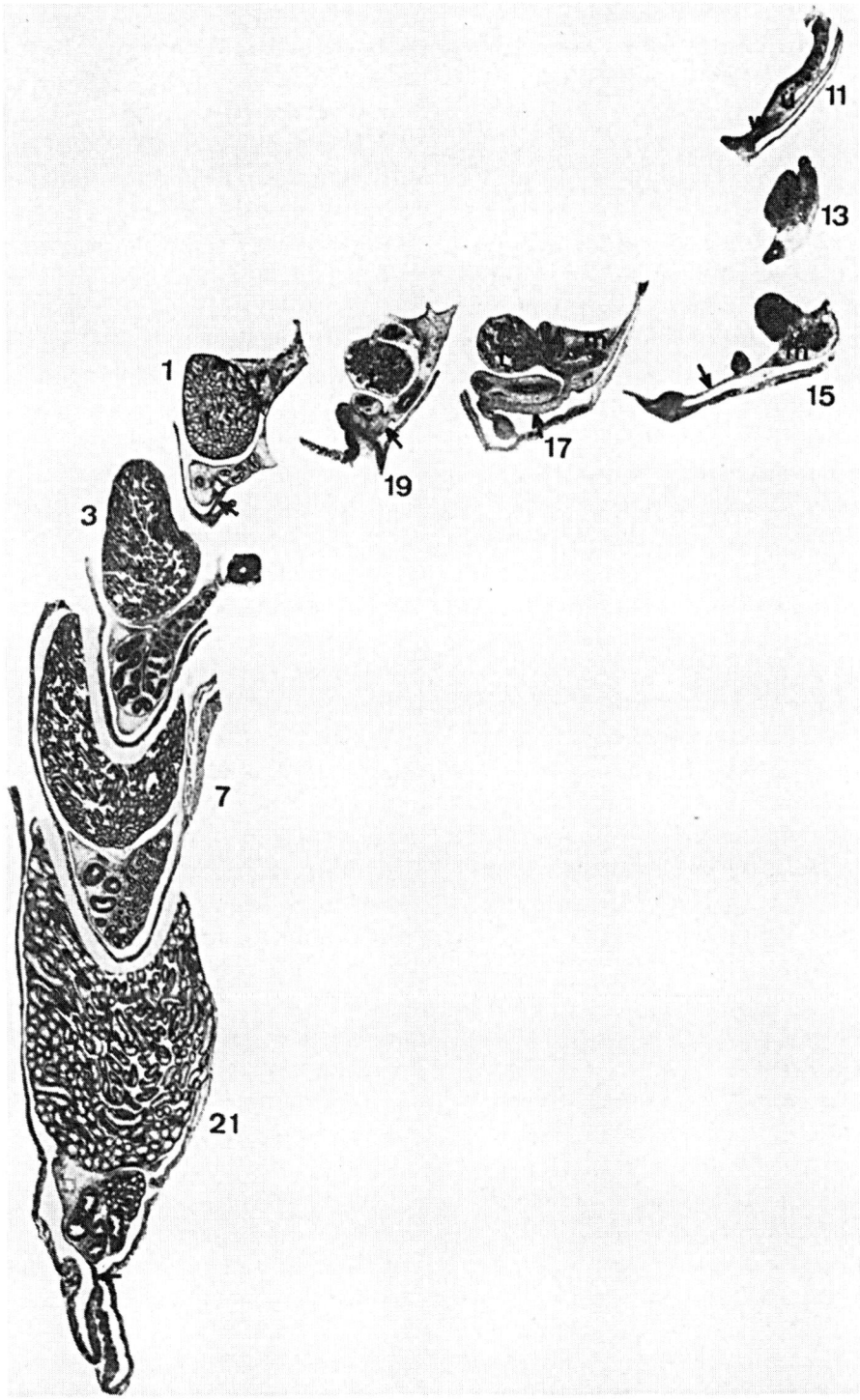

Figure 1. Photomontage of testicular descent in the mouse. The course of descent is S-shaped from dorsal-superior to ventral-inferior. Eleventh day of gestation, thirteenth, fifteenth, seventeenth, nineteenth as well as first third, seventh and twenty-first days after birth are presented. (u) urogenital anlage, (w) Wolffian duct, (t) testis, (m) mesonephros and gubernaculum (arrow) in their ontogenetic development can be followed. The magnification of all states is the same (13,5 ×) so that the relative development of gonadal growth and cranio-caudal epididymis and ductus deferens differentiation is comparable. Note: the gubernaculum never inserts directly in the testis, and there is no extra-abdominal swelling of gubernaculum. The excessive testicular enlargement starts postnatally.

importance of these experiments was in the opportunity to induce cryptorchidism without being forced to produce it by replacing already descended gonads in the abdomen.

2.1. Appearance of Leydig cells in newborn mice

The Leydig cells from the control mice are easily recognizable, generally lying in groups of three to nine cells in the interstitium. Their cytoplasm is polygonal in appearance, with an eccentrically-situated round nucleus, having two to three nucleoli. A typical feature of the nucleus of the Leydig cell is the peripherally located chromatin. In the cytoplasm of one-day-old control mice, numerous lipid vacuoles are seen, clustered together in groups. The Leydig cells in the mouse are notably smaller than those in man (Figure 2).

One day after birth the estrogen-treated mice show small, isolated Leydig cells in the interstitium, lying no longer in groups, but singly. They have a narrow cytoplasm, in which lipid droplets are seldom present. Besides these atrophic Leydig cells, the interstitium also contains degenerated Leydig cells having vacuoles. The entire cytoplasm is, to a large extent, filled with large, empty vacuoles. These highly-degenerate Leydig cells are observed only in estrogen-treated cryptorchid mice. The mice treated with HCG and estrogen simultaneously have Leydig cells which tend to remain together in groups. Compared with normal control testicles, the Leydig cells of HCG and estrogen-treated mice have noticeably fewer lipid droplets.

The ultrastructure of the Leydig cells in the control mice at birth corresponded to the descriptions in the literature (Burrows 1936; Raynaud 1942; Aoki 1968; Russo 1971). They have an oval nucleus, with heterogeneous chromatin, situated mainly on the periphery, and loose reticular nucleoli. The most noticeable feature of the polygonal cytoplasm is the abundance of glycogen and ribosomes. The smooth endoplasmic reticulum is moderately well developed: rough endoplasmic reticulum is seldom encountered on the cell periphery. The spherical lipid droplets lie mostly in groups, rarely singly, and are not in contact with the mitochondria. These latter are numerous, mostly round and of the tubulus type. Intramitochondrial granules are rarely found. The poorly-developed Golgi apparatus is found in the vicinity of the nucleus and also on the cell periphery.

The Leydig cells of cryptorchid mice whose dams were treated with estrogen differ markedly from those of the control mice and those of the mice whose dams received HCG and estrogen simultaneously. The cytoplasm is, on the whole, smaller, with a nucleus which is elliptical or fusiform, rather than oval, and exhibiting invaginations. The chromatin is distributed in groups, still lying mainly around the periphery. One to two loose reticular nucleoli lie on the periphery and form connections with the nuclear membrane. The typical feature of the Leydig cell – its smooth endoplasmic reticulum – is seldom seen here. Glycogen particles are not so abundant as in normal animals on the first day after birth. The mitochondria are smaller, mostly round, although some are longish in shape. The Golgi apparatus is small and seldom visible in the cytoplasm. The lipid droplets are reduced in number and have no contact with the mitochondria. In advanced atrophy of the Leydig cells, the endoplasmic reticulum is replaced by vacuoles. The mitochondria shrink and cytolysosomes appear in the dark cytoplasm.

The mice treated with HCG and estrogen have Leydig cells which show signs of stimulation in the cytoplasm. The mitochondria are more numerous, larger than those of the control animals, and have a tendency to form groups. Intramitochondrial granules are frequently visible. Lipid droplets in contact with the mitochondria are less common. The smooth endoplasmic reticulum is more highly developed, lying in vesicular and tubular form in the cytoplasm. The rough endoplasmic reticulum, too, is more frequently encountered and the glycogen forms larger agglomerations. The Golgi apparatus is also larger and more differentiate.

Leydig cells of adult control mice are polygonal in shape, with an eccentrically-located nucleus, which varies in form, but is often ovoid. The interstitial cell surface contains irregular microvilli, intercellular canaliculi and special septate-type functions (Blackburn et al. 1973). The smooth endoplasmic reticulum is the most striking feature of the Leydig cells, occupying the greater part of the cytoplasm and being mostly tubular in form. There are usually areas in the cytoplasm where the smooth endoplasmic reticulum is organized into closely-packed, fenestrated cisternae. Occasionally, the lamellae of the smooth endoplasmic reticulum form lamellae in the paracrystalline areas (Figure 3). In the vicinity of the concentric rows of smooth

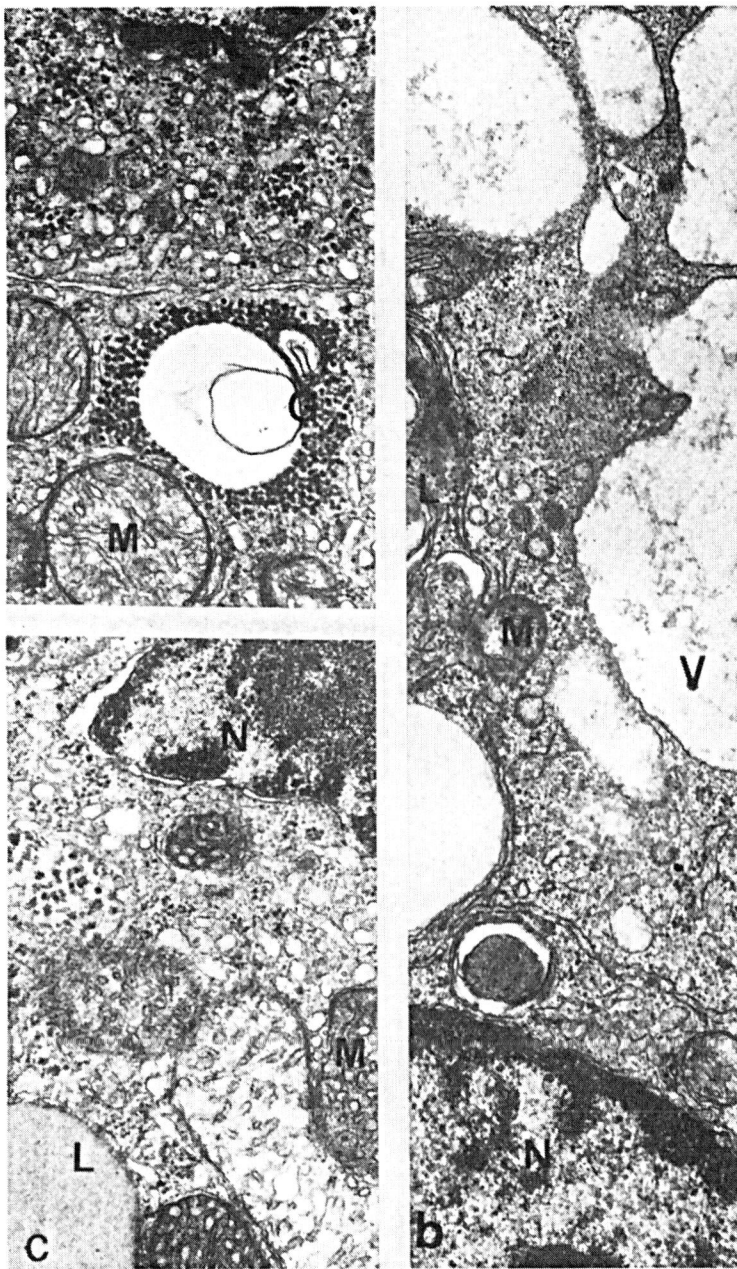

Figure 2. (a) Electron-microscopic view of the Leydig cells treated with estrogen and
HCG during pregnancy. There is an abundance of smooth endoplasmic reticulum. M:
mitochondria: N: nucleus: G: glycogen (×31,000). (b) Ultrastructure of estrogen-
treated Leydig cells: V: vacuoles: M: small mitochondria: N: nucleus. L: lipid droplets
(×31,000). (c) Cytoplasm of control Leydig cells: L: lipid droplets, smooth endoplasmic reticulum: M: mitochondria. N: nucleus (×31,000).

endoplasmic reticulum, there are many granules,
2500 Å in diameter, round or oval in shape and
bounded by a membrane, with homogeneously
dispersed electron-dense contents.

An accumulation of these granules is also seen
around the intercellular canaliculi. The mitochondria are about 1 μm in diameter, generally rod-
shaped. They are mostly of the crista type, but some
tubuli are also present, some of them with intramitochondrial granules. The numerous membrane-
bounded lipid droplets are arranged in concentric
circles around them. Pigment granules, presumably

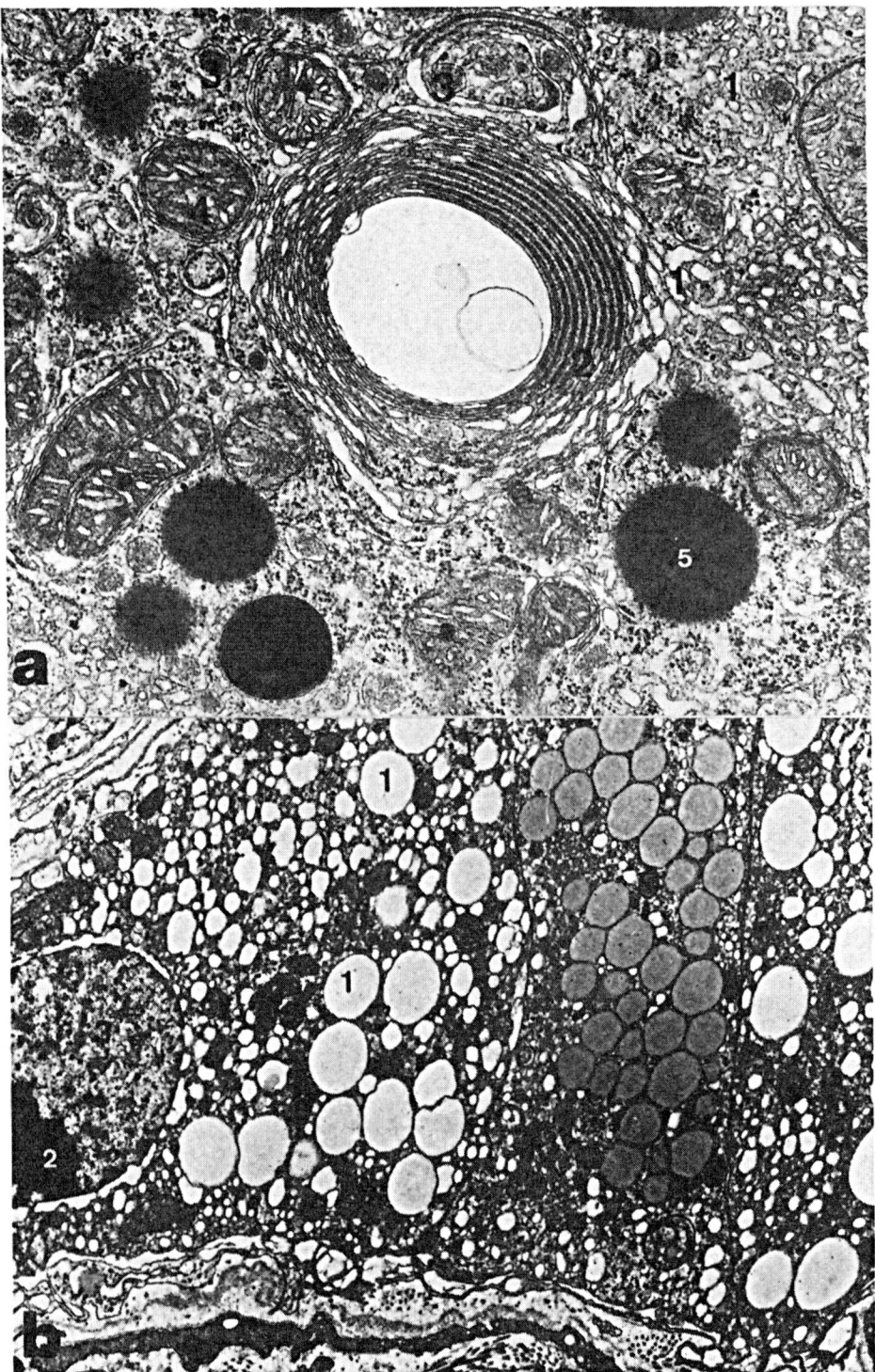

Figure 3. (a) Normal Leydig cell cytoplasm. Smooth endoplasmic reticulum (1) lies in tubular and vacuolar form in cytoplasm. Occasionally the lamellae of smooth endoplasmic reticulum form concentric rows (2). In the vicinity of the concentric rows of smooth endoplasmic reticulum there are many granules (3), usually 2,500 Å in diameter, which contain homogeneously dispersed electron-dense material. 4: mitochondria; 5: lipid droplets. The arrow indicates intramitochondrial granules ($\times$ 18,200). (b) Leydig cells of E_2B-treated adult mice ($\times$ 9300). The smooth endoplastic reticulum is enlarged and builds vacuoles (arrows). The lipid droplet (1) content seems to be increased. The prominent nucleolus (2) is situated peripherally in an eccentrically-located nucleus (3).

lipofuscin, are also occasionally seen in the cytoplasm. Adjacent to the nucleus is a prominent centrosomal region. The perinuclear region is relatively free of smooth endoplasmic reticulum and contains ribosomes and glycogen granules. No crystalloids are observed in mouse Leydig cells.

The Leydig cells of E_2B mice are generally different in appearance from those of control animals. The epitheloid cells are usually smaller, with a characteristic cytoplasm, in which the smooth endoplasmic reticulum is replaced by many vacuoles of various sizes, scattered throughout. These cells have an increased lipid content (Figure 3). The nucleus is eccentric, often with a prominent nucleolus and more differentiated than that in control Leydig cells. The granules, 2500 Å in diameter, frequently observed in control Leydig cells, are here almost completely absent. The glycogen and ribosome content is greatly reduced. The mitochondria are of the crista type and generally smaller. Many pigment inclusions, presumably lipofuscin, are accumulated in the cytoplasm. The cell surface is not differentiated and there are only rudimentary microvilli. These cells often degenerate, and many nuclei without cytoplasm and large numbers of plasma bodies are visible in the interstitium.

2.2. Testosterone content of the testis

The testosterone content of newborn cryptorchid mouse testes was 49 pg/testis, whereas the newborn controls had a testosterone content of 106 pg/testis. The weight difference of the newborn E_2B mice and the control mice was not significant.

The total testicular testosterone content in adult controls was 72.5 ng/testis and in E_2B intrauterine estrogen-treated adult mice 19 ng=testis. There is no significant difference between the mean weight of control mice (1.29 g) and that of E_2B mice (1.26 g).

2.3. Pituitary LH content of newborn mice

The pituitary LH content in E_2B and E_2B and HCG-treated mice was significantly lower than in control mice. E_2B mice had 93.7 mIU/ml; E_2B+HCG mice had 91.5 mIU/ml; control mice had 119.1 mIU/ml.

2.4. Changes in the mesonephros

E_2B administered at the thirteenth or fourteenth day

of gestation leads to unilateral or bilateral cryptorchidism in 75-100% of all male newborn mice (Greene et al. 1938; Burrows 1936; Raynaud 1942; Hadžiselimović and Herzog 1976; Hadžiselimović 1977). In control mice, the testes are located, immediately after birth, between the ventral abdominal wall and the bladder neck (Figure 4). The intra-abdominal movement is terminated. In contrast, in E^2B cryptorchid mice, the testes remain in a dorsal position, lying usually at the level of the fifteenth embryonal day in control animals. E^2B and HCG-treated animals have, in a majority of cases (80%), testes descended lik the control mice. The position of the testicles in E_2B and E_2B and HCG-treated animals was proportional to the degree of mesonephros development. The more differentiated the epididymis and ductus deferens, the further the gonad descended.

In one-day-old control mice, the mesonephros is transformed into epididymis and ductus deferens and there are only remnants of the Müllerian duct. The stromal cells of the mesonephros are fusiform and lie singly in the interstitium, forming the interstitium of the epididymis and the outer layer of the ductus deferens. These cells have an elongated nucleus, with peripherally situated chromatin. Their mitochondria, of the crista type, are distributed throughout the thin cytoplasm. In newborn cryptorchid mice treated with E_2B at the thirteenth or fourteenth day of gestation, the epididymis has a completely different appearance. The stroma, which consists of mesenchymal cells, is abundant and the cells are larger and polygonal in shape. Generally, they are less reduced in size and degree of differentiation than the mesenchymal cells of control mice. The individual tubules of the epididymis are very few in number and have a multilayered epithelium. The microvilli are better developed and secretion of material into the lumen is more common than in the epididymal tubules of the control mice. The stroma of the epididymis of E_2B and HCG-treated mice appear similar to that of control animals. The individual tubules of the epididymis and ductus deferens are almost the same as in the control mice.

3. CONCLUDING REMARKS

The genetic findings in mutant mice with hypogonadism due to LH-RH deficiency suggest that the

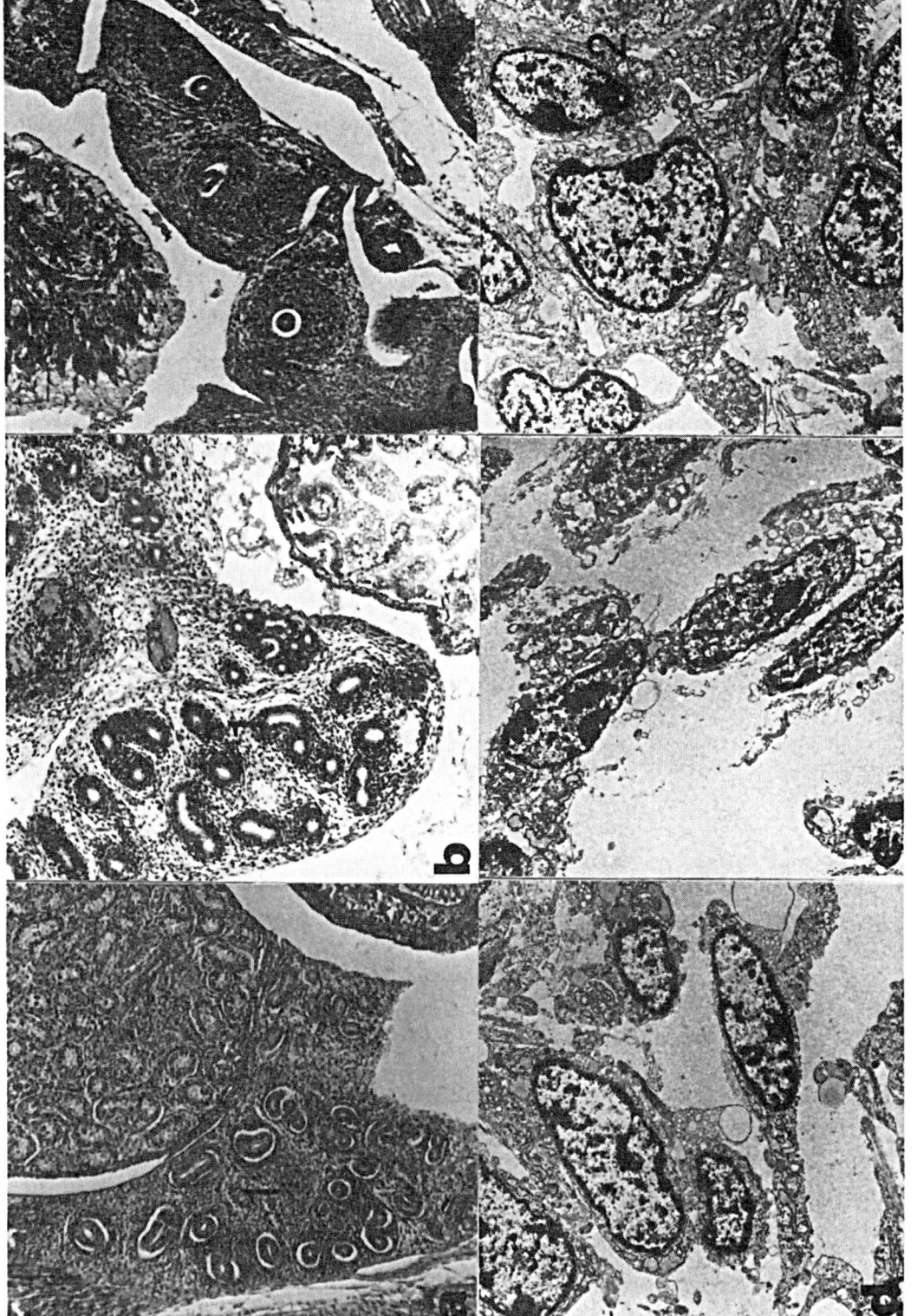

Figure 4. (a) Descended gonad in E_2B+HCG-treated mouse. The epididymis is differentiated (1) showing more coils than in the E_2B-treated mouse (sagittal section). (b) Epididymis (1) of one-day-old control mouse (frontal view). (c) Sagittal section of epididymis in one-day-old E_2B mice (1), testis lying posteriorly to the bladder. Depletion of androgens causes differentiation of the mesonephros stroma and inhibits development of the Wolffian duct. (d) Mesenchymal cells in E_2B+HCG-treated animals. ($\times 1.530$). (e) The mesenchymal cell (1) in one-day-old control mice ($\times 1.530$). (f) Mesenchymal cells in E_2B-treated animals are larger and polygonal in shape. 2: tubulus ($\times 1.530$).

mutant is akin to Ewer's series of men who had familial monotrophic pituitary insufficiency, transmitted as an autosomal recessive LH-RH deficiency. These mice are cryptorchid and sterile (Cattanach 1977). In testicular feminization in the mouse, there is a lack of androgen-dependent differentiation of the male genitalia, due to end-organ insensitivity to androgens. Affected mice have male genotypes, female phenotypes and cryptorchid testes (Blackburn et al. 1973). The administration of E_2B hinders the transformation of the Wolffian duct and produces 'feminization' of the mesonephros, with subsequent cryptorchidism. This should not be regarded as a direct effect of estrogen on the mesonephros, but rather as a consequence of the androgen deficiency brought about by insufficient stimulation of the Leydig cells by gonadotropins. Simultaneous administration of HCG and E_2B prevents atrophy of the Leydig cells in the critical phase of genital development; the Wolffian duct differentiated into the ductus deferens and epididymis, and descensus took place. The stroma of the mesonephros plays a key role in the critical phase of genital development.

The androgens seem to have an inhibiting action on stroma development, while depletion of androgens promotes differentiation of the stroma and inhibits differentiation of the Wolffian duct.

In cryptorchid boys, the anomalies in the epididymis-testis area are well known to surgeons. When the processus vaginalis is patent, the testis and its vessels are suspended within it by a peritoneal mesentery and the Wolffian derivatives are usually abnormally disposed (Scorer 1974; Johnston 1965). The epididymis may be separated considerably from the testis and its globus minor may be elongated towards the scrotum (Johnston 1965). On occasion, the abnormalities are more gross: in some cases the epididymis may be malformed and the vasa efferentia absent (Badenoch 1946). The vas deferens may be atretic proximal to the epididymis. In cases where orchidectomy is performed, because other therapy has been unsuccessful, histological tests show that the cryptorchid epididymides also have fewer coils and are generally underdeveloped. These changes contribute significantly to the incidence of infertility (Figure 5).

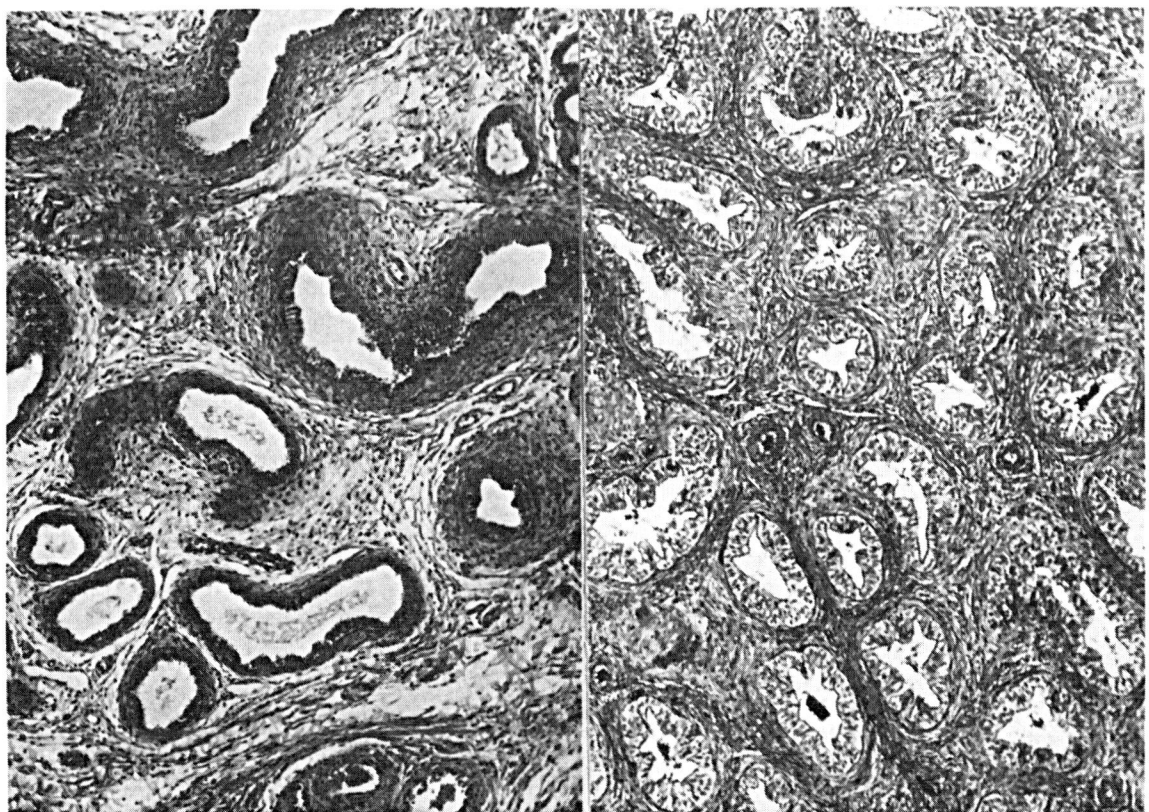

Figure 5. Left: Corpus epididymis of cryptorchid man shows fewer tubuli (1) and is generally underdeveloped in contrast (*right*) corpus epididymis of man with normal descended epididymis (× 16).

REFERENCES

Aoki A: Hormone-induced differentiation of granular endo-plasmic reticulum in the interstitial cells of the mouse testis. Protoplasma 66: 263, 1968.

Badenoch AW: Failure of the urogenital union. Surg Gynec Obstet 82: 471, 1946.

Blackburn WR, Kying WC, Bullock L, Bardin CW: Testicular feminization in the mouse: studies of the Leydig cell structure and function. Biol Reprod 9: 9, 1973.

Burrows H: The influence of oestrogenic compounds in causing hernia and descent of the testis in mice. Brit J Surg 23: 658, 1936.

Cattanach BM: Gonadotrophin-releasing hormone deficiency in a mutant mouse with hypogonadism. Nature 269: 338, 1977.

Greene RR, Burill MW, Ivy AC: Experimental intersexuality: the production of feminized male rats by antenatal treatment with estrogens. Science 88: 130, 1938.

Hadžiselimović F: Cryptorchidism: ultrastructure of normal and cryptorchid testis development. Adv Anat Embryol Cell Biol 53: 3, 1977.

Hadžiselimović F, Herzog B: The meaning of the Leydig cell in relation to the etiology of cryptorchidism. J Pediat Surg 11: 1, 1976.

Johnston JH: The undescended testis. Arch Dis Child 40: 113, 1965.

Raynaud A: Modification expérimentale de la différentiation sexuelle des embryons des souris par action des hormones androgènes et oestrogènes, Paris, Herman, 1942.

Reifer J, Walsh CP: Hormonal regulation of testicular descent: experimental and clinical observations. J Urol 118: 985, 1978.

Russo J: The fine structure of the Leydig cell during postnatal differentiation of the mouse testis. Anat Rec 170: 343, 1971.

Russo J, Rosas JC: Differentiation of the Leydig cell of the mouse testis during the fetal period: an ultrastructural study. Am J Anat 130: 461, 1971.

Scorer GC: The descent of the testis. In: Scientific foundation of pediatrics, Davis AJ, Dobbing J (eds), London, Heinemann, 1974.

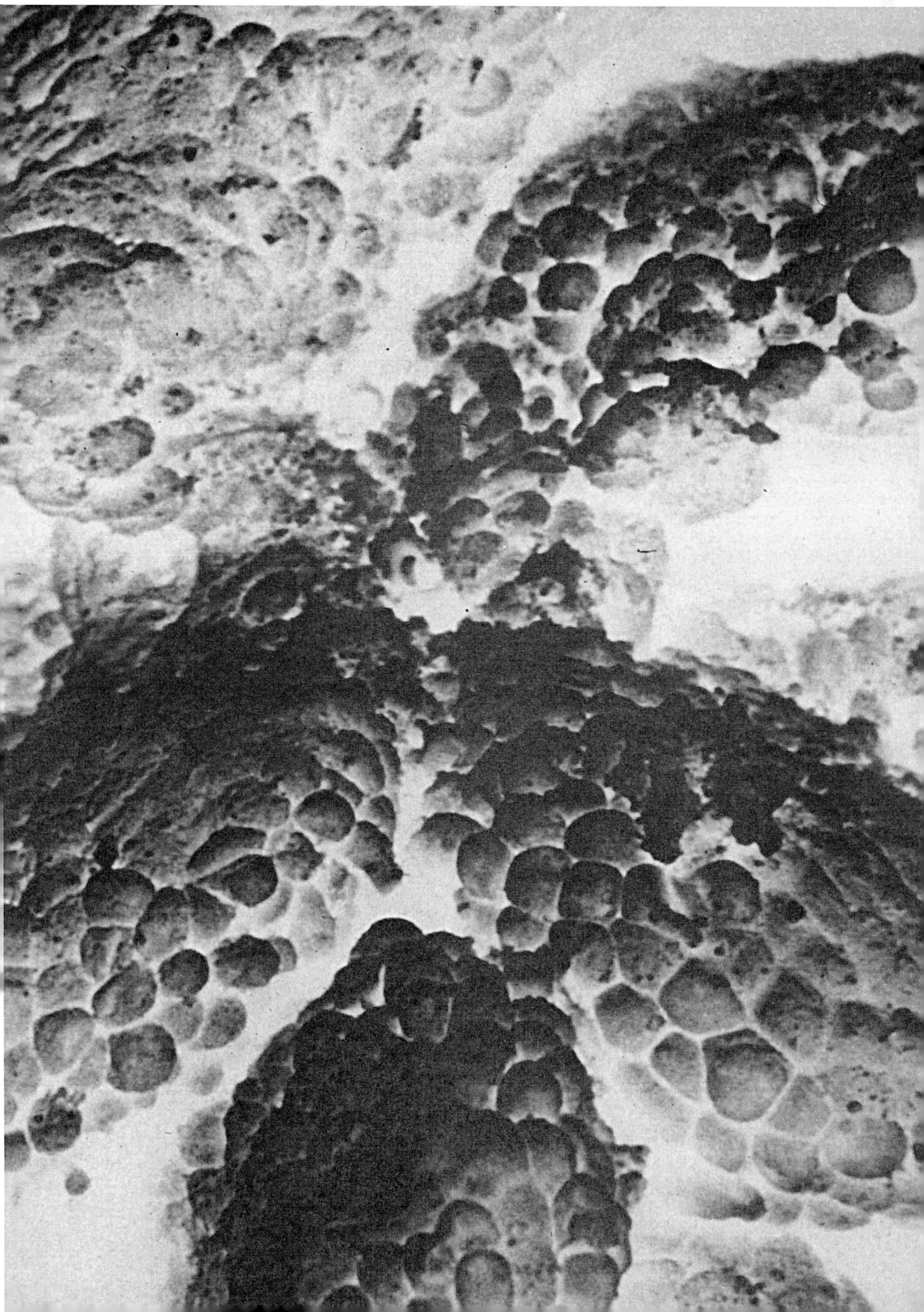

III. TESTICULAR PATHOLOGY

15. VARICOCELE: MECHANISMS OF ACTION AND DELETERIOUS EFFECTS ON THE HUMAN TESTIS

A.H. EL-BEHEIRY and E.S.E. HAFEZ

Since 1889, varicocele has been known to be one of the numerous possible causes of defective spermatogenesis (Bennett 1889). Several mechanisms have been postulated to explain the detrimental effect of varicocele on the testis but despite considerable investigations none has been proved (Donohue and Brown 1969; Zorgniotti and Mac-Leod 1973; Comhaire and Vermeulen 1975; Rodri-guez-Rigau et al. 1978). Testicular histology as determined by testicular biopsies has been evaluated in men with varicocele and several patterns have been described (Dubin and Hotchkiss 1969; Etribi et al. 1967; Ibrahim et al. 1977).

The purpose of this chapter is to give a short account concerning these mechanisms and the effect of varicocele on the testis (Figure 1).

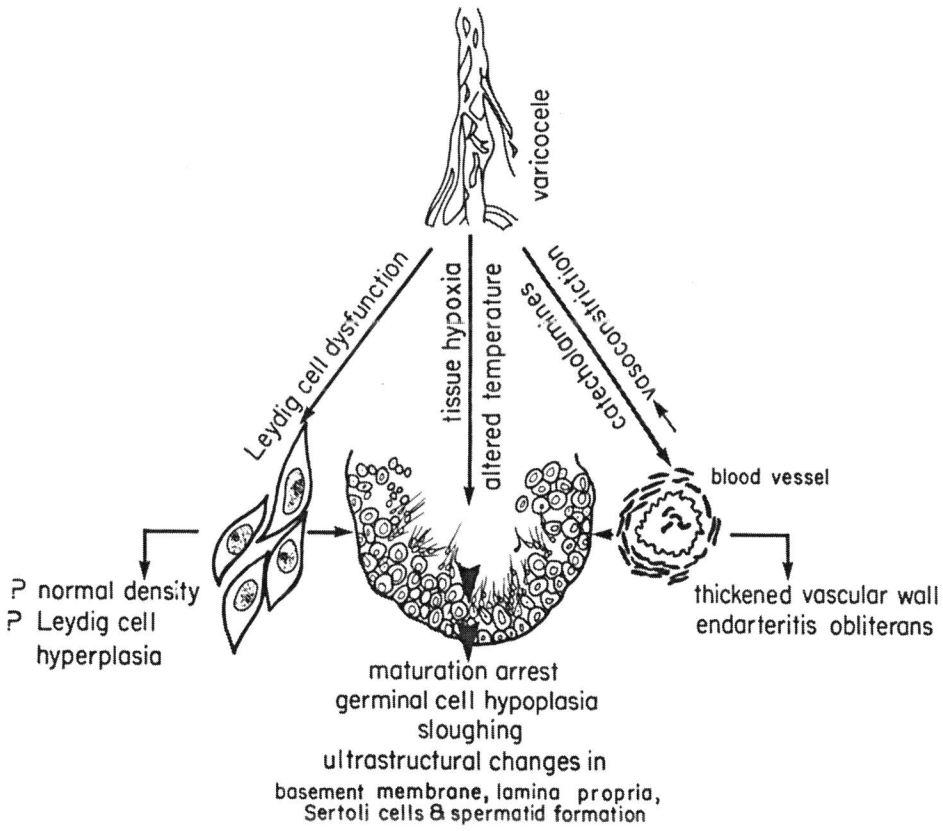

Figure 1. The possible mechanisms of action and deleterious effects of varicocele on the human testis.

1. PATHOPHYSIOLOGICAL MECHANISMS LEADING TO IMPAIRED SPERMATOGENESIS

1.1. Changes in the scrotal temperature

It is well documented that an elevated environmental temperature of the testis is associated with depressed spermatogenesis (Procope 1965; Robinson and Rock 1967; Robinson et al. 1968). The average difference between the intra-abdominal and scrotal temperature has been established to be 2.2 C° (Harrison and Weiner 1948). The question of whether varicocele produces a rise in testicular temperature has been met with conflicting reports. Studies done by Tessler and Krahn (1966); Stephenson and O'Shaughnessy (1968) failed to demonstrate a significant difference in intrascrotal or intratesticular temperature between the right and left testis or between the scrotal temperature of varicocele patients and controls. Recent information, both from direct measurements (Zorgniotti and MacLeod 1973) and from thermography (Gasser et al. 1973; Kormano et al. 1973) has shown a rise in scrotal temperature associated with varicocele. The supposition that scrotal temperature is indicative of the underlying testicular temperature has to be scrutinized carefully. In addition, the bilateral effect of varicocele on the testes due to temperature elevation has to be clarified owing to the fact that the raised scrotal temperature measured by thermography is confined to the same side of varicocele (Verstoppen and Steeno 1978).

1.2. Tissue hypoxia

The investigation into the role of varicocele in producing hypoxia of the germinal epithelium revealed an unexpected result. Blood pH, carbon dioxide, and oxygen pressure were measured in the testicular veins and peripheral blood of varicocele patients and controls. No substantial differences were noted in the pH and carbon dioxide pressure values. On the other hand the relatively higher values of oxygen tension in the testicular vein of varicocele patients tended to minimize the role of hypoxia in impairing spermatogenesis (Donohue 1969).

1.3. Toxic metabolic effects

1.3.1. Renin. Renin, a factor of renal origin has been

suggested to be responsible for testicular dysfunction in cases of varicocele, but a study of seven varicocele patients performed by Lindholmer et al. (1973) failed to demonstrate a significant difference in renin concentration between blood from the internal spermatic vein and peripheral circulation.

1.3.2. Cortisol. The situation regarding cortisol is unclear. Although the levels of cortisol have not been found to be elevated in the testicular vein compared to the peripheral circulation in varicocele patients, the cortisol concentration was found lower in the testicular vein of patients with varicocele when compared to controls (Agger 1971; Comhaire and Vermeulen 1974; Koumans et al. 1969; Lindholmer et al. 1973). A question to be raised is to what extent cortisone and subsequently cortisol are capable of adversely affecting spermatogenesis.

1.3.3. Catecholamines. Investigations done by Comhaire and Vermeulen (1974), and Cohen et al. (1975) demonstrated that the ratio of catecholamines concentrated in the testicular vein to that in the peripheral circulation was significantly higher in the case of varicocele than in controls. The authors suggested that this finding supports the hypothesis that chronic testicular vasoconstriction due to impregnation with catecholamine-rich blood could partly or totally explain the disturbance of testicular function.

1.4. Leydig cell dysfunction

Since the testicular meiotic division and the process of spermiogenesis are androgen-dependent (Weiss et al. 1978), the histologic disturbance found in men with varicocele could be explained by disturbed Leydig cell function resulting in decreased testicular androgen production (Rodriguez-Rigau et al. 1978). This possibility is supported by reports of decreased androgen levels in men with varicocele (Comhaire and Vermeulen 1975; Raboch and Starka 1971). The recent report by Dubin and Amelar (1975) of improvement in semen quality and pregnancy rate in oligospermic men with varicocele treated with human chorionic gonadotropins suggests a relation between Leydig cell dysfunction and disturbed spermatogenesis in patients with varicocele. It has been found that in patients with oligospermia and varicocele, the Leydig cell density, in vitro testosterone synthesis, and testosterone to luteinizing hormone ratio were also decreased in addition to impaired spermatogenesis (Rodriguez-Rigau et al. 1978). On the basis of these results, the authors concluded that the deleterious effect of varicocele on spermatogenesis is mediated by impaired Leydig cell function resulting in decreased androgen production and Sertoli cell dysfunction since the latter contain androgen receptors.

2. EFFECT OF VARICOCELE ON THE TESTIS

2.1. Histology

Histologic changes in the testis of varicocele patients are variable. They are usually reversible in varicocele with oligospermia (Figure 2), mostly irreversible in azoospermic individuals (Figure 3). Recent reports are summarized in Table 1.

2.1.1. Tubular compartment. A pattern of spermatogenic maturation arrest was observed in 23 varicocele patients studied by Charny (1962). The degree of histologic derangement was not uniform throughout each specimen, with no difference in the appearance of the biopsy from either testis in patients with unilateral varicocele. On the other hand, Etribi et al. (1967), in a study of 42 infertile men with unilateral varicocele, confirmed the finding of maturation arrest at primary spermatocyte or spermatid stage with pronounced changes on the side of varicocele. Germinal cell hypoplasia with premature sloughing of cells was the main pattern reported by Dubin and Hotchkiss (1969) in a study of 88 varicocele patients; both testes were similarly affected. More recently Ibrahim et al. (1977) have demonstrated the presence of disorganization and sloughing in 50% of their studied cases. This feature was more evident on the varicocele side. Bilateral testicular biopsies of 55 subfertile men with varicocele were studied by Rajan and Thomas (1978). Germinal cell hypoplasia and sloughing predominated. Testicular changes were of the same type on both sides though of more advanced degree on the side of varicocele. Peritubular fibrosis and/or Sertoli-cell-only syndrome are histologic features commonly met with in advanced cases of varicocele (Dubin and Hotchkiss 1969).

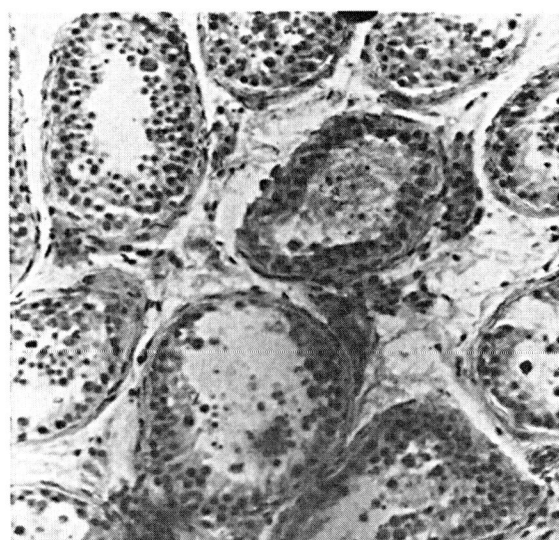

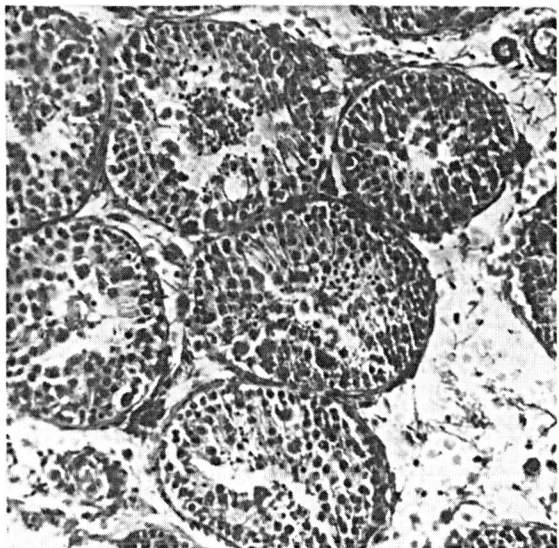

Figure 2. Testicular biopsy in varicocele with oligospermia. *Top:* Spermatogenic arrest at the stage of primary spermatocyte (×80). *Bottom:* Germinal cell hypoplasia with low density of all spermatogenic stages (×80).

2.1.2. Intertubular compartment. Despite the documented association between defective spermatogenesis and the presence of varicocele, no consistent relationship regarding Leydig cells has been demonstrated. While Leydig cell hyperplasia was observed in 50% of the cases studied by Dubin and Hotchkiss (1969) and in 34.8% of cases reported by Rafan and Thomas (1978), an association of varicocele with Leydig cell hyperplasia was not noticed by Ibrahim et al. (1977). Leydig cell density was evaluated quantitatively in bilateral testicular biopsies from 16 oligospermic men with varicocele.

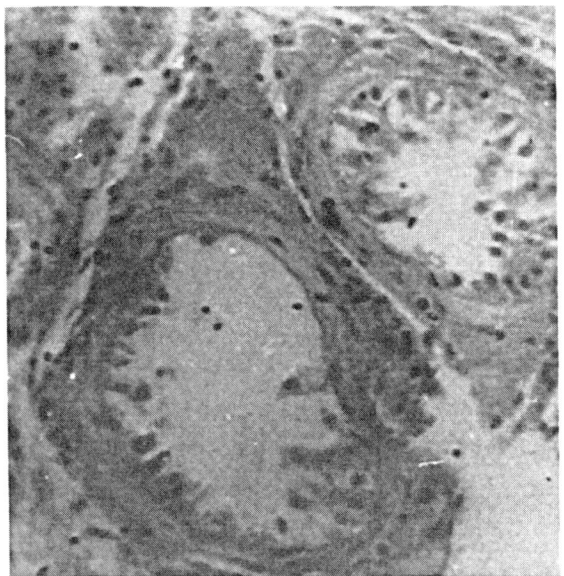

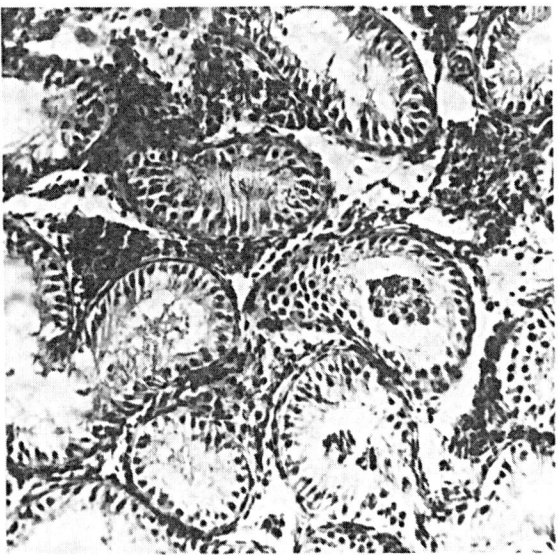

Figure 3. Testicular biopsy in varicocele with azoospermia. *Top:* Peritubular fibrosis (× 160). *Bottom:* Sertoli-cell-only syndrome: note the presence of some tubules with arrested germ cells denoting its acquired nature (× 80).

No significant differences in Leydig cell density between right and left testes were found and no correlation between Leydig cell density and site or degree of varicocele could be demonstrated (Weiss et al. 1978).

2.2. Ultrastructure

Ultrastructural features of the testis in cases of varicocele have been studied by Siew et al. (1977) and Cameron et al. (1979). Abnormalities were found in the basement membrane and lamina propria of the tubule, in the adluminal testicular compartment, and in blood vessels.

2.2.1. Tubular compartment. Changes in the basement membrane of the tubular wall consisted mostly in intratubular invagination with reduplication giving rise to the multilayered appearance.

Increase in the thickness of the lamina propria was a constant feature. It was usually due to an increase in collagen leading to wider separation of myoid cells.

Germ cell morphology and tissue architecture within the basal testicular compartment appeared normal. However, cellular morphology and intercellular association within the adluminal testicular compartment were altered. Nuclear and acrosomal profiles of some pre- and postspermiated spermatids were abnormal. Parenchymatous degenerative changes were observed and degenerated cells were found in Sertoli cells. Several investigators have suggested that the Sertoli cell may have a phagocytic activity acting like a reticulo-endothelial cell in removal of residual bodies and foreign material from their surroundings (Dietert 1966; Carr et al. 1968).

2.2.2. Intertubular compartment. The Leydig cells which have been reported as normal by histology were less prominent ultrastructurally as they were embedded in the increased fibrous tissue. They were identified mainly by their typical mitochondria and the predominant smooth endoplasmic reticulum. The intranuclear Reinke crystals described by De Kretser (1968) were seldom observed.

Thickened vascular wall with reduction in the size of lumen was a constant finding. In advanced cases, endarteritis obliterans with perivascular fibrosis was noticed. Both the intimal and medial cells were increased in size with aggregation of basement-membrane-like material in the intercellular spaces.

3. CONCLUDING REMARKS

It seems that impairment of testicular function in varicocele men is caused by a combination of factors. The mechanism responsible appears to be Leydig cell dysfunction resulting in decreased androgen production. This could be related either to disturbance of the scrotal temperature-regulating

Table 1. Main histological features in varicocele testis.

Author	No. of cases	Main histological features	
		tubular	intertubular
Charny (1962)	23	maturation arrest	no change
Etribi et al. (1967)	42	maturation arrest	no change
Dubin and Hotchkiss (1969)	88	germinal cell hypoplasia	Leydig cell hyperplasia
Ibrahim et al. (1977)	52	sloughing of germinal cells	no change
Weiss et al. (1978)	16		no change
Rajan and Thomas (1978)	55	germinal cell hypoplasia and sloughing	Leydig cell hyperplasia

system or to tissue hypoxia secondary to venous stasis or to impregnation of the testes with catecholamine-rich blood with consequent vasoconstriction and ischemia.

Varicocele effect is variably reflected in testicular histology. Spermatogenic maturation arrest, germinal cell hypoplasia and premature sloughing into tubular lumen could be demonstrated. Ultrastructural study of human testis biopsy proved to be a valuable adjuvant in varicocele investigations. It demonstrates findings such as abnormalities of the basement membrane, lamina propria, Sertoli cells and spermatid formation, which are not apparent by light microscopy.

REFERENCES

Agger P: Plasma cortisol in the left spermatic vein in patients with varicocele. Fertil Steril 22: 270, 1971.
Bennet WH: Varicocele, particularly with reference to its radical cure. Lancet 1: 261, 1889.
Cameron D, Snydle F, Drylie D, Ross M, Spellacy W: Ultrastructural alteration in the adluminal testicular compartment in men with varicocele: abstract. Arch Androl, suppl 11, 1979.
Carr I, Clegg EJ, Meek GA: Sertoli cells as phagocytes. J Anat 102: 501, 1968.
Charny CW: Effect of varicocele on fertility: results of varicocelectomy. Fertil Steril 13: 47, 1962.
Cohen MS, Plaine L, Brown JS: The role of internal spermatic vein plasma catecholamine determination in subfertile men with varicoceles. Fertil Steril 26: 1243, 1975.
Comhaire F, Vermeulen A: Varicocele sterility: cortisol and catecholamines. Fertil Steril 25: 88, 1974.
Comhaire F, Vermeulen A: Plasma testosterone in patients with varicocele and sexual inadequacy. J Clin Endocr Metab 40: 824, 1975.
De Kretser DM: Crystals of Reinke in the nuclei of human testicular interstitial cells. Experientia 24: 587, 1968.
Dietert SW: Fine structure of the formation and fate of the residual bodies of mouse spermatozoa with evidence of the participation of lysosomes. J Morphol 120: 317, 1966.
Donohue RE, Brown JS: Blood gases and pH determination in the internal spermatic vein of subfertile men with varicocele. Fertil Steril 20: 365, 1969.
Dubin L, Amelar RD: Varicocelectomy as therapy in male infertility: a study of 504 cases. Fertil Steril 26: 217, 1975.
Dubin L, Hotchkiss RS: Testis biopsy in subfertile men with varicocele. Fertil Steril 20: 50, 1969.
Etribi A, Girgis SM, Hefnaway H, Ibrahim AA: Testicular changes in subfertile male with varicocele. Fertil Steril 18: 660, 1967.
Gasser G, Strassl R, Pokieser H: Thermogramm des Hodens und Spermogramm. Andrologia 5: 127, 1973.

Harrison RG, Weiner JS: Abdomino-testicular temperature gradient. J Physiol 107: 48, 1948.
Ibrahim AA, Awad HA, Hagger SE, Mitawi BA: Bilateral testicular biopsy in men with varicocele. Fertil Steril 28: 663, 1977.
Kormano M, Kahanpaa K, Tahti E: Thermographic recording of the reaction of normal and varicocele scrotum to increased temperature. Andrologia 5: 201, 1973.
Koumans D, Steeno O, Heyns W, Michielsen JP: Dehydroepiandrosterone sulphate, androsterone sulphate and corticoids in spermatic vein blood of patients with left varicocele. Andrologia 1: 87, 1969.
Lindholmer C, Thulin L, Eliasson R: Concentration of cortisol and renin in the internal spermatic vein of men with varicocele. Andrologia 5: 21, 1973.
Procope BJ: Effect of repeated increase of body temperature on human sperm cells. Int J Fertil 10: 333, 1965.
Raboch J, Starka L: Hormonal testicular activity in men with varicocele. Fertil Steril 22: 152, 1971
Rajan R, Thomas M: Testis biopsy in varicocele as related to fertility. J Obst Gyn India 28(2): 291-295, 1978.
Robinson D, Rock J: Intrascrotal hyperthermia induced by scrotal insulation: effect on spermatogenesis. Obstet Gynecol 29: 217, 1967.
Robinson D, Rock J, Menkin MF: Control of human spermatogenesis by induced changes of intrascrotal temperature. JAMA 204: 290, 1968.
Rodriguez-Rigau LJ, Weiss DB, Zukerman Z, Grotjan HE, Smith KD, Steinberger E: A possible mechanism for the detrimental effect of varicocele on testicular function in man. Fertil Steril 30: 577, 1978.
Siew S, Troen P, Nankin HR: Ultrastructural study of human testicular biopsies in infertility. In: Male reproductive system, Yates RD, Gordon M (eds), New York, Masson, 1977, p 79-97.
Stephenson JD, O'Shaughnessy EJ: Hypospermia and its relationship to varicocele and intrascrotal temperature. Fertil Steril 19: 110, 1968.
Tessler AN, Krahn HP: Varicocele and testicular temperature. Fertil Steril 17: 201, 1966.

Verstoppen GR, Steeno OP: Varicocele and the pathogenesis of the associated subfertility III: theories concerning the deleterious effects of varicocele on fertility. Andrologia 10: 85, 1978.

Weiss DB, Rodriguez-Rigau L, Smith KD, Chowdhury A,

Steinberger E: Quantitation of Leydig cells in testicular biopsies of oligospermic men with varicocele. Fertil Steril 30: 305, 1978.

Zorgniotti AW, MacLeod J: Studies in temperature, human semen quality and varicocele. Fertil Steril 24: 854, 1973.

16. TESTICULAR TUMOURS IN CRYPTORCHID TESTIS

S. Omar and S. El-Badawi

The incidence of unilateral or bilateral undescended testis is estimated to be 14% amongst male children below the age of one year and less than 4% between one and five years. Cryptorchid testis is associated with a $20\text{-}40\%$ increased risk of development of malignant disease compared with scrotal testis (Smith 1974). Testicular tumours comprise $1\text{-}2\%$ of all malignant tumours in males and $5\text{-}10\%$ of these tumours develop in men with cryptorchid testicles.

Maldescent is not necessarily the direct cause of malignant transformation. Five factors may be responsible for the increased incidence of tumours: abnormal germ cells, elevated temperature, interference with blood supply, endocrine disturbances, and gonadal dysgenesis (Mostofi 1973).

The histologic pattern and progression of testicular tumours differ in the various age groups in which they are likely to occur: childhood, late adolescence, young adulthood (20-35 years) and above fifty years of age. Seminomas have never been reported in infants, whereas embryonal carcinoma and teratoma are the most common tumours of infants and children. Seminoma, embryonal carcinoma, teratoma and teratocarcinoma are common in young adults, but seminoma is more frequent in patients in the fourth decade.

Testicular tumours have been classified as follows (Dixon and Moore 1952):

    seminoma
    teratoma
    teratocarcinoma
    embryonal carcinoma
    choriocarcinoma
    teratoma with seminoma
    andro blastoma
        – tubular
        – mixed
    interstitial cell tumours

infantile adenocarcinoma of testis
malignant lymphoma

1. DIAGNOSIS

Tumours of the undescended testicle have special presenting features which depend upon whether the testicle is in the abdomen or the inguinal canal. An abdominal mass associated with the absence of a scrotal testicle should suggest the existence of a neoplasm of testicular origin. An inguinal hernia can be associated with an undescended testicle and a certain proportion of testicular tumours were found incidentally during herniotomy. Tumours developing in the inguinal canal may also simulate an inguinal hernia.

Associated inflammatory changes may increase the difficulty of distinguishing such tumours from a strangulated hernia.

Distant metastases may be the first clinical presentation of the disease.

1.1. Workup

1. Patients are subjected to routine x-ray chest examination for exclusion of intrathoracic metastases.

2. Excretory urography has a special role in this disease. It is required for radiotherapy planning. It is also a diagnostic aid to detect aortic nodal metastases which can produce displacement of kidney, distortion or compression of the ureters (Figure 1). Such changes were detected in 22% of patients with impalpable aortic nodes (Blandy 1966).

3. Lymphangiography is an essential diagnostic procedure. It is required for clinical staging upon which depends the overall treatment strategy

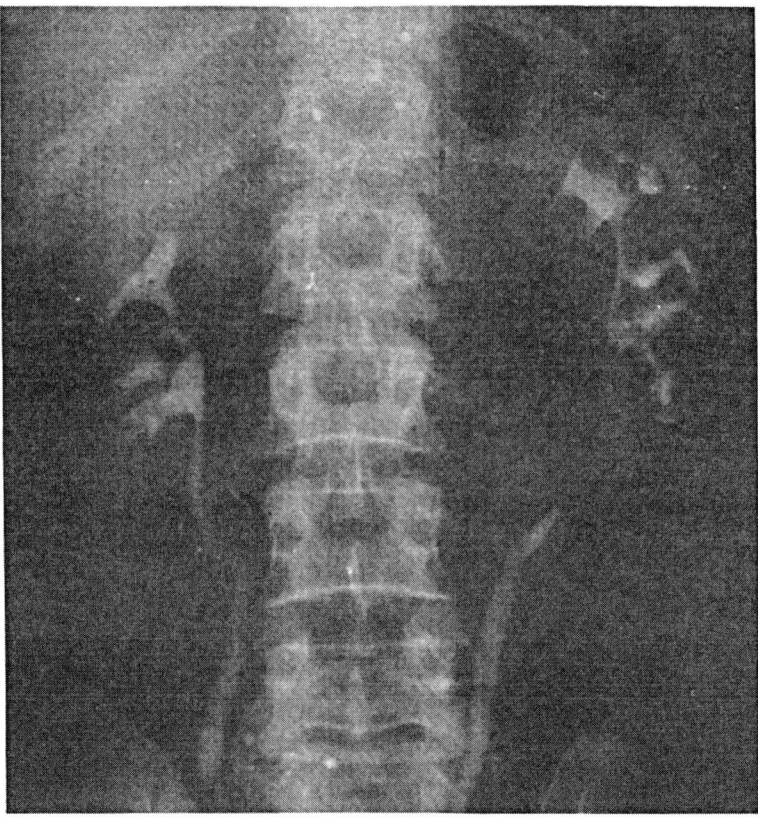

Figure 1. Intravenous pyelogram showing displacement of the left ureter by a mass of paraortic metastases.

(Figure 2). Lymphangiography findings often precede clinical detection of aortic nodal metastases. They are also useful in radiotherapy planning. The completeness of retroperitoneal lymphadenectomy can also be checked by plain radiography of the abdomen during and after surgery. It is also an aid to assess the response of aortic metastases to radiotherapy and chemotherapy.

4. Cavography has been abandoned as a routine diagnostic procedure since lymphangiography is safer and more informative.

5. Ultrasound is a newer diagnostic procedure. Its accuracy in detecting confirmed aortic nodal metastases was reported as 90% (Hendry et al. 1977).

The combination of lymphography and ultrasonography provides useful information on the presence, volume and position of paraortic lymph node metastases. It is likely that the precision of tumour localization will be enhanced by the use of computerized axial tomography.

1.2. Hormone studies

Gonadotropins may be detected in the urine of men with testicular teratoma and choriocarcinoma. This test has to be routinely performed during the initial workup and also to monitor responses to various therapies.

2. CLINICAL STAGING

Testicular tumours are classified according to the clinical, radiological, and pathological findings. The most frequently adopted classification is shown in Table 1.

3. MANAGEMENT

3.1. Prophylactic treatment

The ideal age for treatment is not established. It is

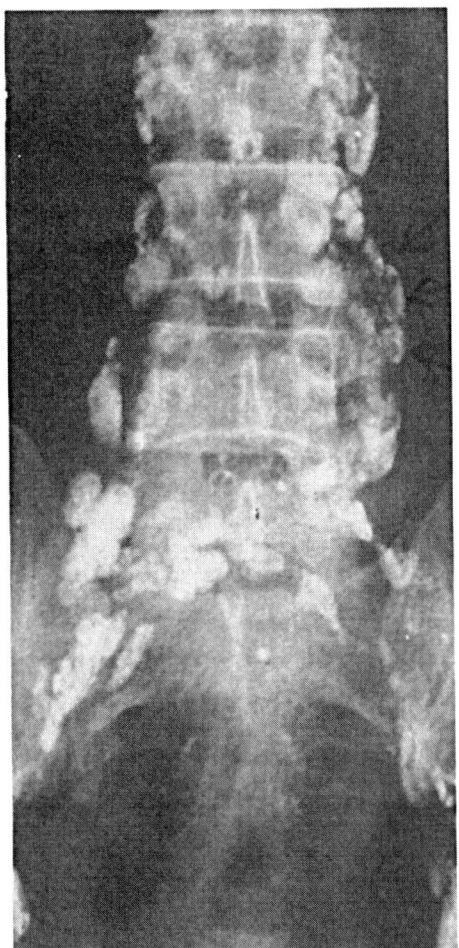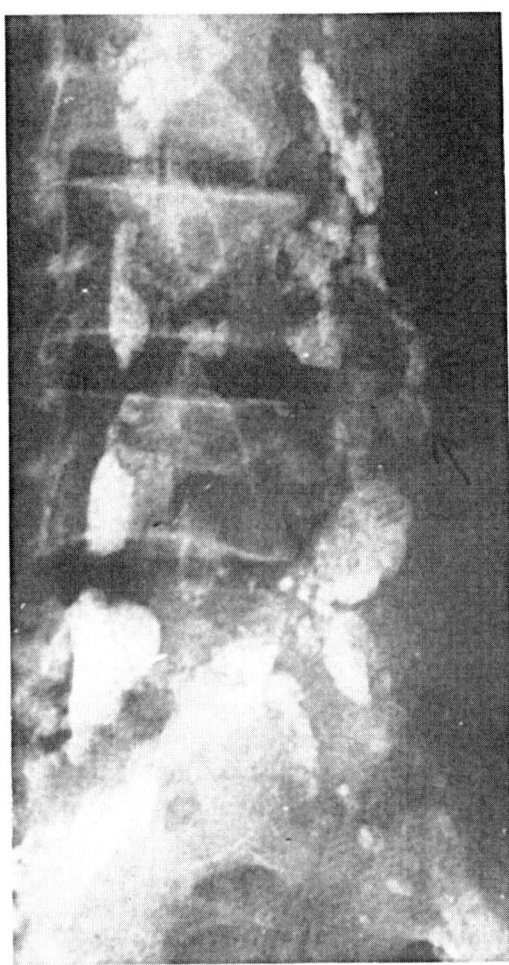

Figure 2. Lymphangiogram. a.p. and oblique views, showing enlarged left paraortic nodes with irregular filling defects.

Table 1. Walter Reed General Hospital staging system for testicular neoplasms.

Stage	Findings
IA	Tumour is confined to the testis with no clinical or radiographic evidence of spread.
IB	Tumour is confined to the testis with no clinical or radiographic evidence of spread. histologic evidence of metastasis to the iliac or paraortic nodes at time of retroperitoneal lymphadenectomy.
II	Clinical or radiographic evidence of metastasis to lymph nodes below the diaphragm but not to those above the diaphragm or to viscera.
III	Clinical or radiographic evidence of metastasis above the diaphragm or to viscera.

recommended not to delay the treatment of cryptorchidism beyond the age of five years. Spontaneous descent after this age is rare, with increasing risk of atrophic changes (Pinch et al. 1974). The incidence of the risk of testicular tumour development is not completely eliminated after orchidopexy. Careful follow-up and observation are thus necessary.

3.2. Treatment of germinal tumours in the cryptorchid testis

Surgical removal through an inguinal or abdominal approach is the initial step in management, the subsequent treatment plan depending on the histological type.

3.2.1. Subsequent treatment in seminoma. The risk of metastases in the paraortic and iliac nodes in stage I is estimated to be 10-19% (Maier et al. 1968). Elective irradiation of these territories is therefore indicated in both stages I and II. A tumour dose of 3000 rad in three weeks is generally recommended.

The inguinal nodes are included in patients previously subjected to orchidopexy or herniotomy (Blandy et al. 1970).

The presence of bulky nodal metastases requires whole abdominal irradiation. A total dose of 3000 rad in three weeks is recommended, but the kidneys must be shielded after a dose of 1500 rad (Castro 1973).

The risk of subclinical metastases in the supraclavicular area and mediastinum is significant in stage II. Elective irradiation of these regions is generally adopted.

The treatment of stage III is mainly by chemotherapy.

3.2.2. Subsequent treatment in teratoma. Teratomata have two specific features that influence the post-orchidectomy treatment plan:

1. Metastatic deposits are much less radiosensitive than seminoma. Thus retroperitoneal lymphadenectomy constitutes an important modality.

2. Vascular invasion is a relatively early feature. Prophylactic chemotherapy is often recommended. Retroperitoneal block dissection consists of removal of nodes en bloc with the cellulo-fatty tissue lying around the aorta, vena cava, common iliac and the proximal third of the internal iliac vessels. The dissection should extend upwards to the level of origin or termination of the renal vessels.

Irradiation following lymphadenectomy is recommended in patients with histologically confirmed ilioaortic nodal metastases. The recommended dose is higher than that used in the case of seminoma and amounts to 5000 rad in five weeks (Castro 1973). Removal may be incomplete, as reported by the surgeon or as indicated by a persistent radiological sign. Postoperative irradiation is mandatory in such cases and may require total abdominal irradiation.

4. CHEMOTHERAPY

Chemotherapy is administered to patients with stage-III testicular neoplasms and as an adjuvant in stage-II teratoma. The selection of agents is dependent on the histology.

Seminoma is extremely radiosensitive and is therefore expected to be chemosensitive. Radiomimetic alkylating agents, e.g. chlorambucil, have been used for this tumour.

Teratoma shows however a poor response to chemotherapy. Regressions were observed with a combination of Actinomycin D, Methotrexate and chlorambucil. Combinations of chemotherapy employing Vinblastine and Bleomycin have been used. Response rates ranged between 70 and 80% with partial responses, greater than 50% regression, amounting to 40% (Samuels 1975). Platinum compounds have been employed. As a single agent, this has not been rewarding, but in combination with Adriamycin striking regressions have occurred (Twito 1975).

ACKNOWLEDGEMENT

The authors would like to express their thanks to Professor H.K. Awwad, Chairman of Radiotherapy Department, Cancer Institute, Cairo University, for his help in preparing this chapter.

REFERENCES

Blandy JP: The surgical management of testicular tumors. Hosp Med 7: 133, 1966.
Blandy JP, Hope-Stone HF, Dayan AD: Tumors of the testicle, London, Heinemann, 1970.
Castro JR: Tumors of the Testis: textbook of radiotherapy, Fletcher GH (ed), Philadelphia, Lea and Febiger, 1973.
Dixon FJ, Moore RA: Tumors of the male sex organs. AFIP Atlas Tumor Path 8: 32, 1952.

Hendry WF, Tyrrell CJ, Macdonald JS, McElwain TJ, Peckham MJ: The detection and localisation of abdominal lymph node metastases from testicular teratomas. Brit J Urol 49: 739, 1977.
Maier JG, Sulak MH, Mittemeyer BT: Seminoma of the testis: analysis of treatment success and failure. Am J Roentgenol 102: 596, 1968.
Mostofi FK: Testicular tumors: epidemiologic, etiologic and pathologic features. Cancer 32: 1186, 1973.
Pinch L, Aceto T, Meyer-Bahlburg HFL: Cryptorchidism, a pediatric review. Urol Clin N Am 1: 573, 1974.
Samuels ML: Continuous intravenous bleomycin therapy with Vinblastine in testicular and extra-gonadal germinal tumors. Proc Am Ass Cancer Res 16: 112, 1975.
Smith JP: Management of testicular tumors in children. Urol Clin N Am 1: 593, 1974.
Twito DI, Kennedy BJ: Treatment of testicular cancer, Ann Rev Med 26: 235, 1975.

INDEX *

Acrosome   32, 33f, 35, 51f, 56, 58f
  Cap   54
  Formation   33, 44-61
  Granule   33, 51, 60f
  Malformations   38, 44-61
  Nucleus   54
  Phase   49f
  Vesicle   46f, 47f, 58
Allantoic diverticulum   5
Anaphase   26
Androgen   67, 80, 96, 98, 101
  Binding protein (ABP)   80, 99, 101
  Biogenesis   109
  Biosynthesis   109, 112
  Secretion   10
Andropause   114
Antehypophyseal cells   104
Aplasia   51
Aromatase complex   115
Aspermatogenesis   80
Atropic Leydig cells   144
Azoospermia   69, 89, 182f

B
Basal lumina   24f, 27f
Basement membrane   16t, 62, 64f, 66, 68f, 86, 182
Blastema   6, 7
Blood-testis barrier   62, 73-92, 95, 99, 100
  Mitochondria   82
  Postnatal development   80
  Testis   73

C
Capillary endothelium   73
Cauda epididymidis   142f
Centrioles   35, 44, 50, 52f
Chemotactic mechanism 6
Chemotherapy   188
Chromatin   35, 44
Coelomic epithelium   9
Collagen   65
  Deposition   67f
  Fibers   62
  Zone   63
Contractile cells   63, 65f, 68f, 69f
Corona cells   44
Corpus epididymis   173f

Cryptorchid   162
  Endocrine profile   162
  Leydig cells   159
  Morphology   158
  Sertoli cells   163
  Testis   148, 153f, 185
    hormone studies   186
Cryptorchidism   19, 90, 143, 144f
  Estrogen induces   166
  Prepuberty   19
Cytokinesis   44, 50
Cytoplasm   5, 15, 17, 21, 22, 44, 63, 69f, 86

D
Diakinesis   26
Descended gonad   172f
Descended Testis
  Function   15t
  Histological characteristics   15t
  Interstitial tissue   19
  Neonate   14t
  Prepuberty   14t, 15t
  Puberty   14t
  Sertoli cell   15
  Spermatogenic cells   16t
  Tubular wall   18
  Undescended testis   19
Diplotene   26

E
Efferent ductuli   90
Endocrine profile   162
Endoplasmic reticulum   63, 74, 76, 78, 101, 111, 162, 170f
Endothelium   73
Entoblast   5
Epitheloid cells   62
Epithelium   6, 64f
  Coelomic   9
Estrogens   109, 112
Exocytosis   49
Extra-hypothalamic CNS   105

F
Fetal spermatogonia   148
Fibroblasts   63, 68
Flagellum   39f
FSH   15, 68, 85, 86, 95, 97, 102

* f = figure
  t = table

G

Germ cells   7, 12, 17, 21-31, 79, 80, 85f-87, 100f
  Association   28, 30f
  Epithelium   6
  Lines   96, 148-157
  Morphology   182
Golgi apparatus   32, 33f, 44, 47f, 50, 52f, 56f, 58, 61, 162
Gonad   10
  Blastema   5
  Undifferentiated   5
Gonadotropin   73, 85, 86, 95-99, 106, 112
  Antehypophyseal   99
  Chorionic   111
  Hormones   89
  Hypophyseal   102
  Peptide   106
Gonocytes   7
Gubernaculum   10, 19, 125f, 143
  Morphology   128f
  Outgrowth   126
  Regression   128, 129f
  Testis   9

H

Hyalinization   18
Hypertonic solutions   91
Hypogonadism   66f, 112
Hypophysis   94, 103
Hypophysectomy   68, 69f, 89, 95, 97, 98
Hypoplasia   56, 59f
Hypospermatogenesis   64, 88
Hypothalamus   106

I

Impotence   112
Infertile males   51
Inhibin   80, 103-105
Interstitial cells   7, 14t, 97, 109; also, see Leydig cells

K

Karyokinesis   50
Karyoplasm   60
Karyosomes   83f

L

Lamina propria   64f, 94
Lanthanum   74, 75, 76f, 81f, 82f, 86, 89, 90f, 92
  Tracer   73
Laurence-Moon-Barden Bied syndrome   106
Leptotene   26
LH   19, 68, 85, 95, 97
Leydig cells   7, 8f-10, 18t, 19, 62, 99, 109, 111, 158, 168
  Androgenesis   113f
  Atropic   144
  Cytoplasm   170f
  Development   159f
  Dysfunction   180
  Tumors   116
Lymphangiography   185, 186, 187f
Lysosomal enzymes   58

M

Male gonad development   114
Meiosis   12
Membrana propria   95, 96, 99
Meromyosin   79f

Mesenchymal peritubular cells   65, 67, 68
Mesonephros   5, 6, 140
Microfilaments   76
Microtubules   17
Mitochondria   21, 24f, 25, 44, 46f, 47f, 54f, 59, 60, 63, 162
Mitosis   79f, 84
Morphogenesis   38, 40, 40f
Mullerian ducts   5, 12
Myoid cells   66, 66f, 68, 73-75, 95

N

Normal testis   150f

O

Oligospermia   89, 181f
Ovum fertilization   57

P

Pachytene   26
Peripheral hormones   98
Peritubular cells   9
  Connective tissue   14t
  Fibrosis   19
  Tissue   62-70
    endocrine factors   68
    hormonal effects   67
    lamina propria   62, 63, 66f
Phagocytic role   100
Phagocytosis   57
Pituitary
  Function   67
  Gonadotropins   15, 106
  Hormones   112
Pineal gland   105
Plasmalemma   44, 47
Plasma membrane   51f, 68, 95
Preleptotene spermatocyte   26
Prepubertal testis   80, 81f, 85
Primary sex cords   6
Primordial germ cells   5, 94
Prolactin   98, 99, 112
Pro-spermatogonia   94
Psammoma bodies   152, 155

S

Scrotum   12
Seminal epithelium   96-99, 104, 106
Seminal plasma functions   57
Seminiferous epithelium   21, 28, 30f, 57, 63, 68f, 74, 98, 100f
Seminiferous tubule   10-15, 32, 41, 62, 64, 73, 74, 79, 82f, 86-88, 89f, 94, 96, 109, 110f
Seminoma   187
Sertoli cells   7-18, 38, 56, 73, 79-85, 94-101, 116, 163
  Cryptorchid   163
  Crystalloids   83f
  Development   163f
  Estrogen   113, 118
  Junctions   74, 79
  Metabolism   96
  Proliferation   84
  Syndrome   65
  Tumors   116
Serum testosterone   133
Sexual differentiation of CNS   12
Short-tailed sperm   42
Somatic blastema   5, 6

Somatotropic hormone 98
Sperm head 35, 40
    Malformation 54
Spermatid 16, 32, 34f, 35, 37f, 40f, 50, 57, 58, 99
    Abnormal 54f
    Binucleate 52f
    Differentiation 38
Spermatocytes 26-28
    Primary 16t, 26, 29f
    Secondary 16t, 21, 26, 32, 44, 50
    Spermatogonia 10, 11f, 21-26, 27f, 28t, 94, 95, 148, 163t
Spermatogenesis 16-18, 21, 22f, 73, 79, 80, 86, 92, 96, 119
Spermatozoa 15, 21
Spermatozoon 44
Spermiation 38
Spermiogenesis 21, 44-51f
    Abnormal tail formation 41
    Acrosomic phase 45
    Axial filament 35
    Cap phase 45, 48f
    Defects 38
    Freeze-fracture aspect 36f
    Golgi phase 45
    Impaired 180
    Kinetics 15
    Metochondria 37
    Nervous factors 105
    Neuro-endocrine control 94
    Nucleus 36
    Vascular factors 105
Steinert's disease 105
Steroidogenesis 112
Steroidogenic activity 100
Subsurface cisternae 75, 78f, 80, 87

T
Teratoma 188
Testicular
    Capillary 73, 74f
    Cell types 109
    Cords 7
    Descent 125-136
        abnormal 129
        etiology 138-145
        fetal decapitation 135
        normal 125
        regulation 131
    Differentiation 5
    Estrogen biosynthesis 114
    Fluid 79, 80
    Histology 179
    Inhibin 102
    Neoplasms 188

Parenchyma 103f
Steroidogenesis 112
Tumors 185
Testis 62, 114
    Active migration 5
    Cryptorchid 17t
    Descended 17t
    Descent of 9
    Dorsal mesentery 6
    Embryo 5, 6, 8f
    Epithelium 6
    Evolution 10
    Fertilization 5
    Fetal 9, 10
    Functions 10
    Genetic control 12
    Genital ridge 6
    Genitalia 5
    Gonads 5, 12
    Gubernaculum 9
    Hormone causes 13
    Indifferent stage 5
    Mesonephros 9
    Migration 12
    Morphogenesis 7
    Normal 109
    Passive migration 5
    Prenatal stages 7
    Prepubertal 96
    Pubertal maturation 7, 10, 12
    Scrotum 7
    Tunica albuginea 7
Testosterone 10, 12, 41, 68, 85, 96, 102, 109
    Content of testis 171
Tissue hypoxia 180
Tunica propria 68
Two-cell hypothesis 116

U
Ultrastructure 32-42

V
Varicocele 179-183
Vasectomy 90
Vegetative nervous system 106
Visceral organs 10

W
Wolffian duct 5, 10, 173

Z
Zona pellucida 44
Zygotene 26